Pulling together

A snapshot of the first 70 years of the

NHS in Swansea Bay and Bridgend

Foreword *Michael Sheen*

Birth holds a special place within the NHS. And its own was very special indeed. The idea of it can be traced back to a number of beginnings but it was truly birthed out of the horrors and the triumphs of the Second World War. Everything we held dear, every value, every belief was being threatened by a hate-filled Hitler and his army of fascists. And we stood together. Every part of our nation, side by side, working for each other. Giving what we could when it was needed. Sacrificing for the greater good and bonded together in common purpose. And when the nightmare was over, inspired by the experience of that collective solidarity, something beautiful was born.

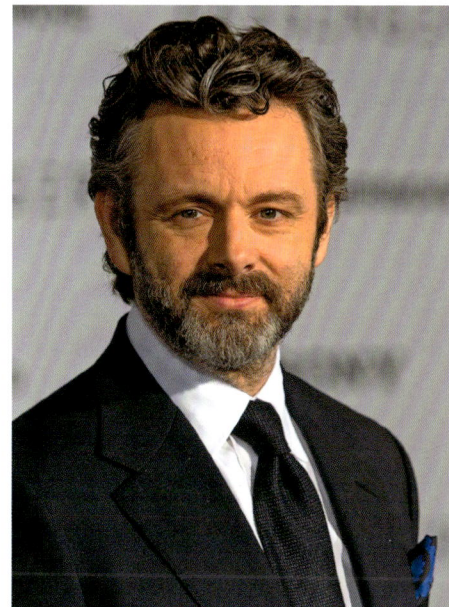

Something worth fighting for — our National Health Service.

And that's why those same values that sustained us through the dark days and all that they cost to champion lie deep in its DNA. The lessons we had learned from that terrible war would now be applied to our hard-won and most precious peace.

The vision of a new social compact that would reflect the power of a whole nation working together for the benefit of all. I would suggest though that that glorious vision was only able to become a living, breathing reality because of two things - firstly, because it already existed, on a smaller scale perhaps but with the same principles at its core, in the heart of South Wales in the form of the Tredegar Workman's Medical Aid Society and, secondly, because of Aneurin Bevan.

The principle of universal donation during fitness for universal provision during illness grew out of the realities of that Tredegar community that Bevan was formed by. And in turn, he gave form to what would eventually come to be known as "the most far-reaching piece of social legislation in British history."

And now it is 70.

It is the best of who we are. And of what we are. Born from the mother of all nightmares and a father from the Valleys.

And make no mistake - there's life in it yet.

3

Acknowledgements

We would like to acknowledge everyone who contributed to this book especially the patients, public and staff who have lived with and loved the NHS in the Swansea Bay area through the decades.

In addition thanks to

Kathy Thomas, Editor
The health board's Communications Team
Martin Thomas and Rebecca Kelly, the health board's Heritage Group
Douglas Neil and the Medical Illustration Department, Morriston Hospital
Richard Clayfield, Senior Procurement Business Manager
Lewys Rhys, Welsh language translator
All our volunteers
South Wales Evening Post
Jono Atkinson

Also Morriston Hospital: The Early Years by Dewi Glannant Williams and Diamond Days - 60 years of the NHS

Proceeds in aid of NHS charitable funds.

First Published 2018

Published by: Abertawe Bro Morgannwg University Health Board

Copyright Abertawe Bro Morgannwg University Health Board

ISBN 978-1-78926-317-6

Front cover picture:
July 1960 - Cefn Coed Hospital - staff tug of war

CONTENTS

Introduction

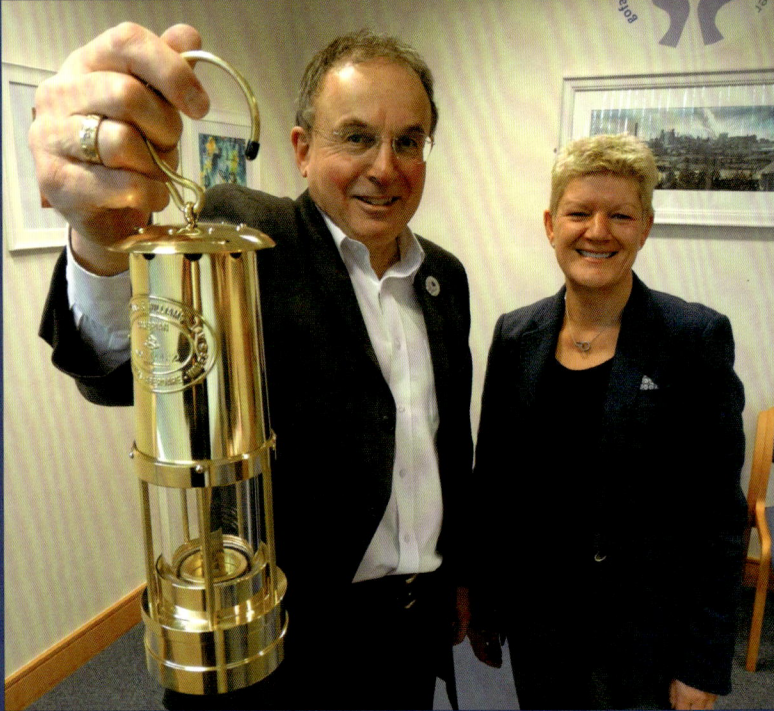

Introduction by Tracy Myhill, Chief Executive ABMU Health Board

Thursday 5th July 2018 is a very special date for each and every one of us; it marks 70 years of the NHS - when prevention, diagnosis and treatment were brought together to create one of the most comprehensive health services in the world.

The NHS transformed our society and we all owe the pioneers who helped establish such a remarkable service a huge debt of gratitude. It is very important that we not only mark their achievements since 1948 but also continue their legacy.

I am very proud to say I have spent all of my working life, since 1984 when I started my first job as a receptionist in the Dental Hospital in Cardiff, within the NHS in Wales.

That's nearly 34 years working in all parts of the Welsh NHS, across the whole country, and I look forward to being part of ABMU's celebrations when we take the opportunity to say thank you to our staff, look back at their contributions and look to the future and innovations that lie ahead.

These celebrations are also aimed at raising public awareness and understanding of local health services and encouraging members of our community to show their support for the NHS.

Pride of place at each of our health board events is a specially engraved miners' lamp as a symbol of ABMU's year of celebration. The lamp highlights the long-standing link between industry in South Wales and healthcare provision.

Aneurin Bevan, the politician heralded as the architect of the NHS, called on his own experiences as a miner in the South Wales valleys and his involvement with the medical aid society in his home town of Tredegar.

Both of my grandfathers were miners in the Rhondda Valley, where I was born and went to school. My Mam lost her father as a result of a mining accident when she was a toddler, leaving her mother a widow with six young children.

I spent many hours of my childhood talking to my father's father about his experiences as a miner so I feel I know a little about the difficult times that influenced Aneurin Bevan's actions and his passion.

During my career I spent 13 happy years in Aneurin Bevan's homeland serving the population of Gwent with a number at Blaenau Gwent Local Health Board so have some affinity there too.

Community-based organisations, like the medical aid society in Aneurin Bevan's home town, sprang up across the UK and saw industrial workers contributing a portion of their wages towards providing medical care and paying for doctors and the earliest hospitals. ABMU's own Maesteg Hospital opened in 1914, thanks to miners who contributed a penny a week towards the costs.

These hard-working pioneers helped inspire the NHS and the idea that good healthcare should be available to all, regardless of their wealth.

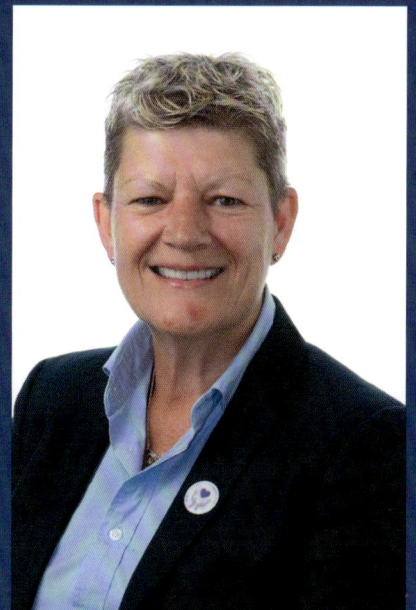

The NHS has shown the world the way to healthcare not as a privilege to be paid for but as a fundamental human right.

I am sure you will join me in not only celebrating its achievements over the past 70 years but also looking forward to its continued role at the very heart of our communities.

Tracy

Message from Professor Andrew Davies, Chairman ABMU Health Board

This is a remarkable year for those of us involved so closely with healthcare in the ABMU region.

We are the latest custodians of our National Health Service - the inspirational initiative founded by Aneurin Bevan 70 years ago in 1948, and which has been envied across the world ever since.

We take our responsibility for protecting and preserving the NHS as seriously as our predecessors, those pioneers who forged the services we have all benefited from.

Over those 70 years the hard work and skills of NHS staff, coupled with medical progress, has continually helped drive up standards and the quality of care for untold millions.

As the son of a nurse from Llandeilo in Carmarthenshire, I know that often it doesn't come easy and often it has involved staff making personal sacrifices to meet demands and provide quality services for the citizens and communities we serve.

I am very proud to be leading an organisation forward at a time of great change, especially for our region. The ARCH project (A Regional Collaboration for Health) sees us working with our partners in Hywel Dda University Health Board and Swansea University to shape a health and social care service fit for the 21st Century.

In addition, the medical advances, ground-breaking research and innovative techniques our teams are involved with across the health board demonstrate how dynamic today's NHS is.

It is a service that has constantly evolved to meet the changing needs of our patients and we know there are many more challenges to address in the future but we must never forget what it has achieved in those 70 years.

People now live on average at least 10 years longer than they did in 1948. The NHS has played a crucial role in that achievement. In

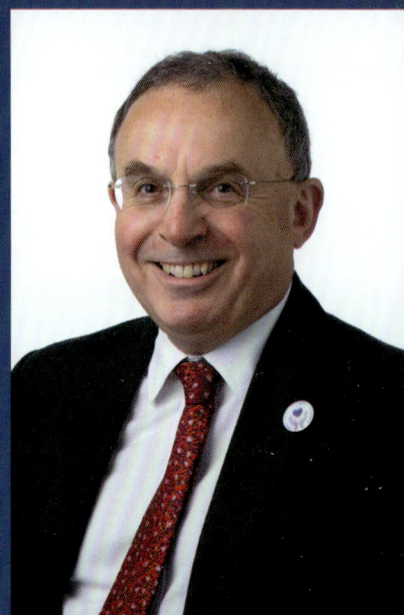

1948 infectious diseases such as TB and polio were a major cause of death and infant mortality was very high. In the last 70 years, survival rates from heart disease and most cancers have improved significantly and Britain is now one of the safest places in the world to give birth.

The principles on which the NHS was founded – namely, available to everyone who needs it, paid for out of general taxation and free at the point of use – remain as central today as they were when it was launched in 1948.

When I took over as Chairman in January 2013 I pledged to continue the work that had gone before me.

I know our staff remain dedicated and committed to providing excellent care and treatment for all our patients - so some things haven't changed, even after 70 years.

Andrew

Aneurin Bevan

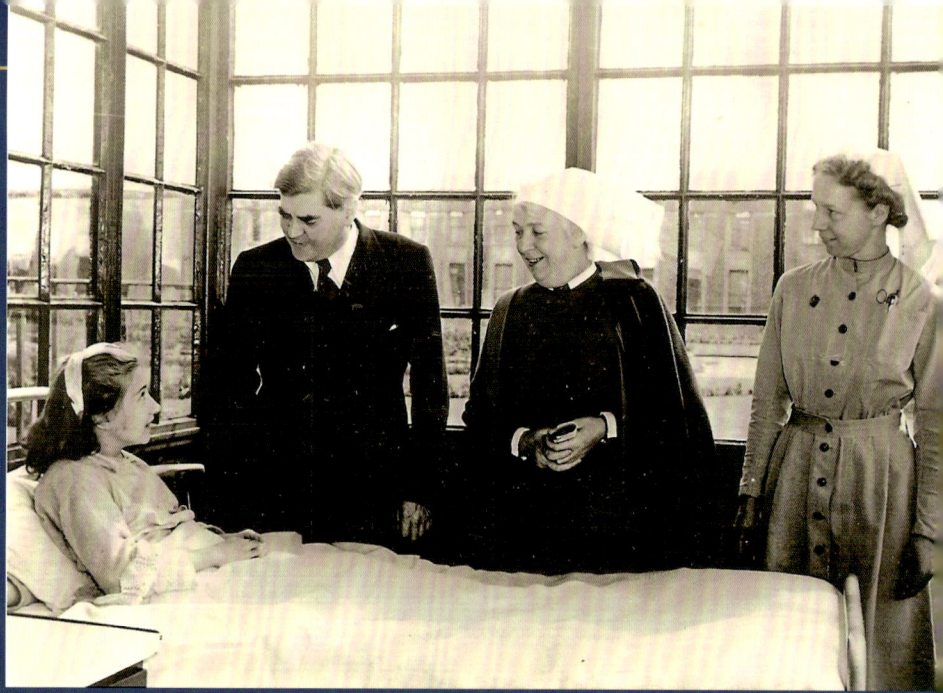

Welsh-born Aneurin Bevan was one of the most important ministers of the post-war Labour government and widely considered to be the chief architect of the National Health Service.

He was born on 15 November 1897 in Tredegar, the son of a miner, and grew up with first-hand experience of the problems of poverty and disease.

He left school at 13 to work in the local colliery and soon became a trades union activist. During the 1926 General Strike Bevan emerged as one of the leaders of the South Wales miners, and three years later was elected as Labour MP for Ebbw Vale.

He was appointed Minister of Health, following the 1945 election and made responsible for establishing the National Health Service. Just three years later, on the 5th July 1948, the Government became responsible for all medical services and the population of the UK enjoyed free diagnosis and treatment for all.

In 1959 Aneurin Bevan became leader of the Labour Party, although he was already terminally ill.

He died the next year, on 6th July, 12 years and a day after the NHS was established.

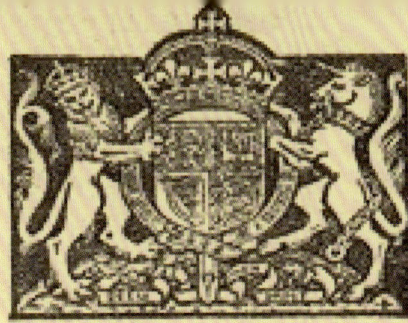

THE NEW
NATIONAL
HEALTH
SERVICE

The National Health Service Act, 1946

1 A totally free medical service provided for all. This included doctors' consultations, prescriptions, hospital treatment and all dental and ophthalmic services.

2 All hospitals were nationalised.

3 Twenty Regional Hospital Boards were formed to administer the hospitals.

4 Local authorities retained responsibility for the health services they already operated (e.g. ambulance services, maternity and child welfare, home nursing, school medical services).

5 Separate Executive Councils were set up to administer family doctor services, dental, ophthalmic and pharmaceutical services. There were 138 of these.

Aneira Thomas

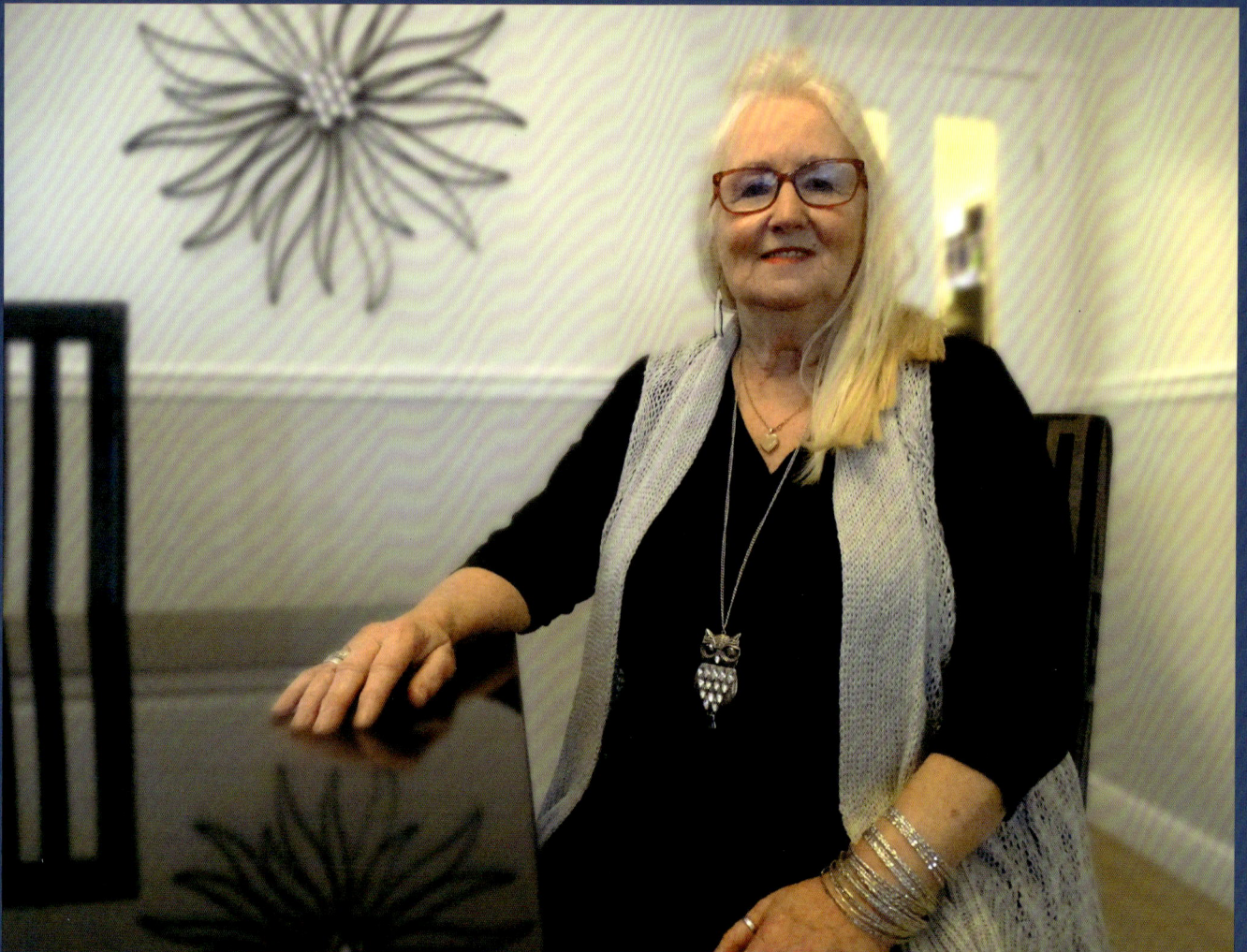

Being the very first baby delivered by the NHS means she celebrates her own 70th birthday on 5th July.

Aneira Thomas
has always known she was special.

Being the very first baby delivered by the NHS means she celebrates her own 70th birthday on 5th July and will definitely be raising a glass to the legacy of Aneurin Bevan, the minister of health who was the founding father of the service.

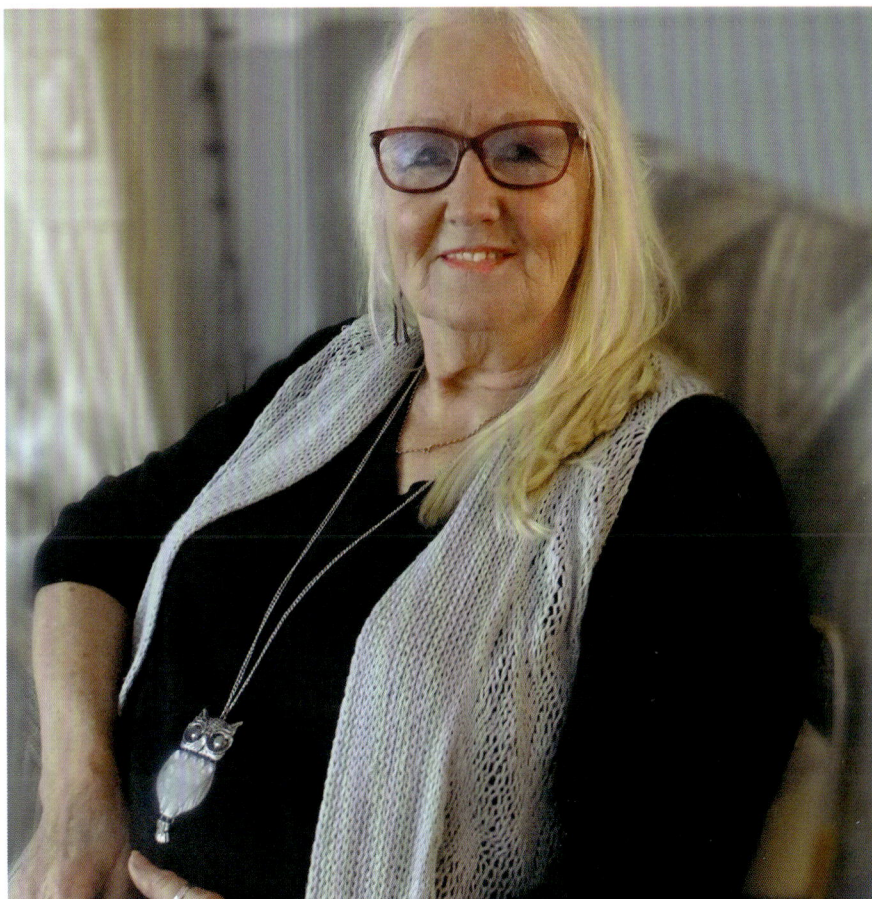

"My mother had been in labour for hours and it was coming up to midnight on Sunday, 4th July 1948. She wanted to push but the nurses and doctors said 'Hold on, Edna. Hold on.' They knew if they could make it to Monday they would make history.

"So I was eventually born one minute past midnight and became the first NHS baby.

"Because of that one of the team who delivered me, Nurse Richards, said to my mother that I should be named Aneira after Aneurin Bevan. It is a name I have been very proud of ever since – and I love telling the story of how I got it."

Now a great grandmother herself, Aneira was born in the Amman Valley Hospital in Glanamman, not far from her family home in Cefneithin.

Her dad Will and her mum Edna already had six children before Aneira's remarkable arrival.

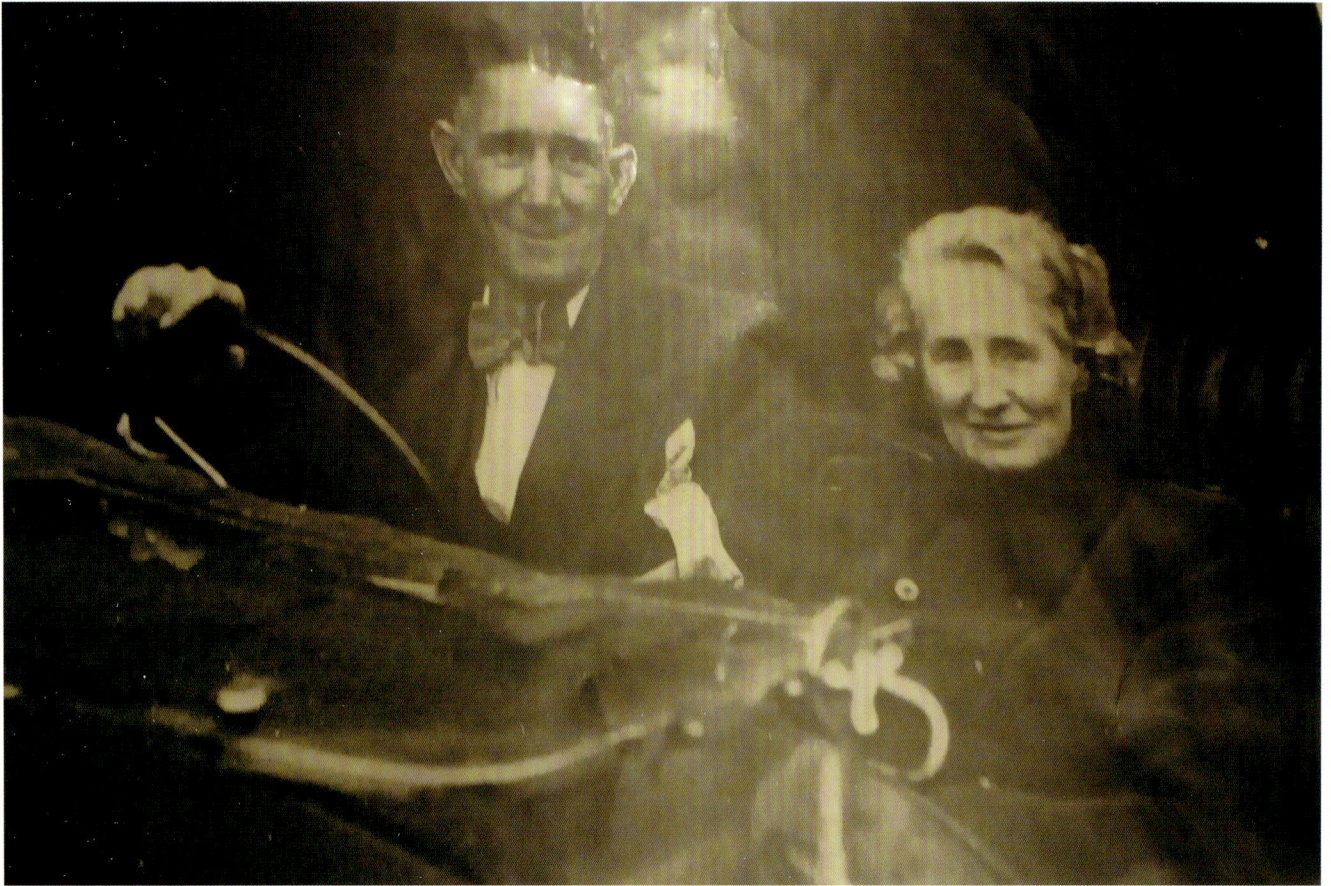

Aneira's parents Will and Edna Rees.

"Although my parents were both from Wales they actually met in Basingstoke while working as nurses."

She explained that they had left their respective valleys to find work in the more prosperous south east during the 1926 general strike.

"It was love at first sight apparently. My dad was a very imposing figure in his uniform, all 6ft 1ins of him, while my mum was just 4ft 10in."

After moving back to Wales and taking on a smallholding in Cefneithin, her father began working as a miner.

Aneira began to realise the proud legacy of her name when she was at school.

"When I was small I couldn't understand why I had my unusual name and I didn't really like it.

"I wanted to be called something like Sian, like my friends. But when I went to grammar school the teachers asked me about my name and I began to realise how proud I should be of it."

Healthcare has played a major part in her family's life. When Aneira – also affectionately called Nye by her family just like her famous namesake – passed her 11-plus exam her proud mum told her *"you can go and be a nurse like your sisters".*

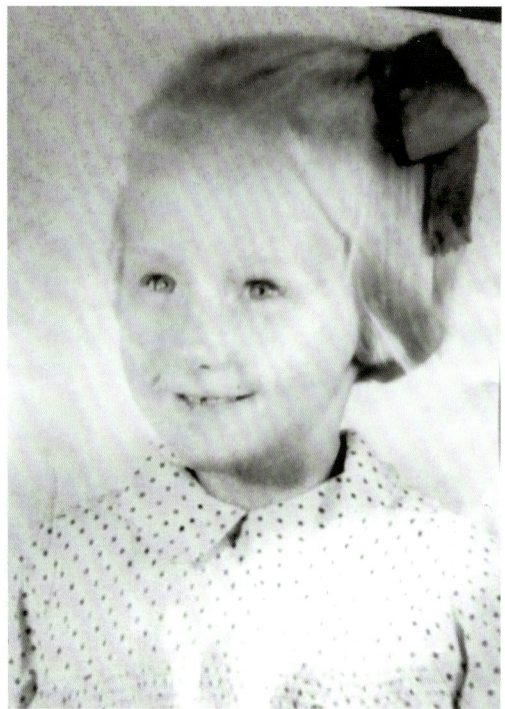

Aneira Thomas (then Rees) as a schoolgirl

"We were all brought up to have a caring nature, my three sisters and I all became nurses and my father's two sisters were matrons in Cardiff and Gloucester."

Although Aneira won a place to study to become an SRN at Morriston she put her training to one side when she and her late husband Dennis started their family.

But the lure of the wards was too much for her to ignore and she went on to work as an auxiliary nurse at Gorseinon Hospital before becoming a mental health worker in Swansea dealing with women suffering from a variety of conditions.

Now retired and living in Loughor, Aneira has two children, Kevin and paramedic Lindsey, six grandchildren and four great grandchildren.

Over the years they have all benefited from the NHS – particularly Aneira herself.

"It must have saved my life almost a dozen times. I have anaphylaxis - a severe allergic reaction to pain medication, pretty much anything that contains an opiate. I have even triggered an attack by taking Solpadeine.

"After my last incident my doctor said they may never know exactly how many things I am allergic to. But I have such an extreme reaction that I have to carry two EpiPens everywhere I go."

But, Aneira said she was grateful for the health treatment all her family members have had over the years.

She vividly recalls one of her most terrifying experiences when her then 10-month-old grandson Joe collapsed and had to be taken by ambulance to hospital.

"His blood sugar had dropped dangerously low and he had lapsed into a coma after suffering from a nasty bug.

"It was a terrifying time but he is now 21 and fighting fit – another example of what marvellous care we have had."

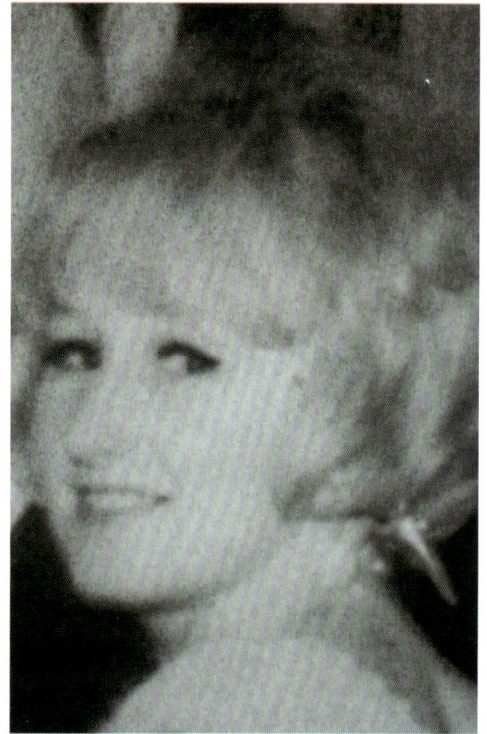

Aneira has always felt her unique position has brought with it a responsibility to represent the NHS.

Aneira Thomas (then Rees) as a teenager

"I am in a privileged position as the first baby born in the NHS and I feel I have a duty to speak up for the NHS and do whatever I can to protect it.

"What gets me is when the NHS was originally put forward the government came up against fierce opposition from political opponents and also from doctors and consultants who said it wouldn't work.

"But a plan was drawn up that meant doctors' and nurses' wages would go up as the service became established and became more successful.

"It was always obvious that the end result of a successful NHS was that people were going to live longer lives. This shouldn't now come as a surprise and certainly shouldn't be used as an excuse for why it is underfunded. Where has the planning been since then?

"It's no good just saying there's not enough money for it, the money has got to be found. This is people's lives we are talking about."

Aneira will also be seen as a judge during the latest season of BBC2's popular Great British Menu series which will see some of the country's best chefs competing to cook for a banquet being held in July to celebrate the NHS anniversary.

"I am indebted to the NHS, I owe it a huge debt of gratitude on my behalf and my family's behalf.

"I have made it to 70 because of the NHS, it has looked after me and I want to do what I can to return the compliment.

"The NHS is a national treasure and we have got to take care of it very carefully."

A more recent newspaper report looks back at how Aneira made history

So much to thank the NHS for

When we asked for your memories of healthcare in the area one phrase kept turning up – We have so much to thank the NHS for.

Whether it was saving a life, bringing a new one into the world or care and compassion shown when someone was at their lowest ebb, the words *"thank you"* were never far behind.

Here are some of your recollections about the NHS and how it has influenced your lives....

Ann Harrison

Ann Harrison is a familiar face to many visitors at Morriston Hospital. She is one of our long-serving volunteers who greets the public in the outpatients department. There is a very special reason why she is so eager to do something to help – it is her way of saying thank you for the care the NHS has given her.

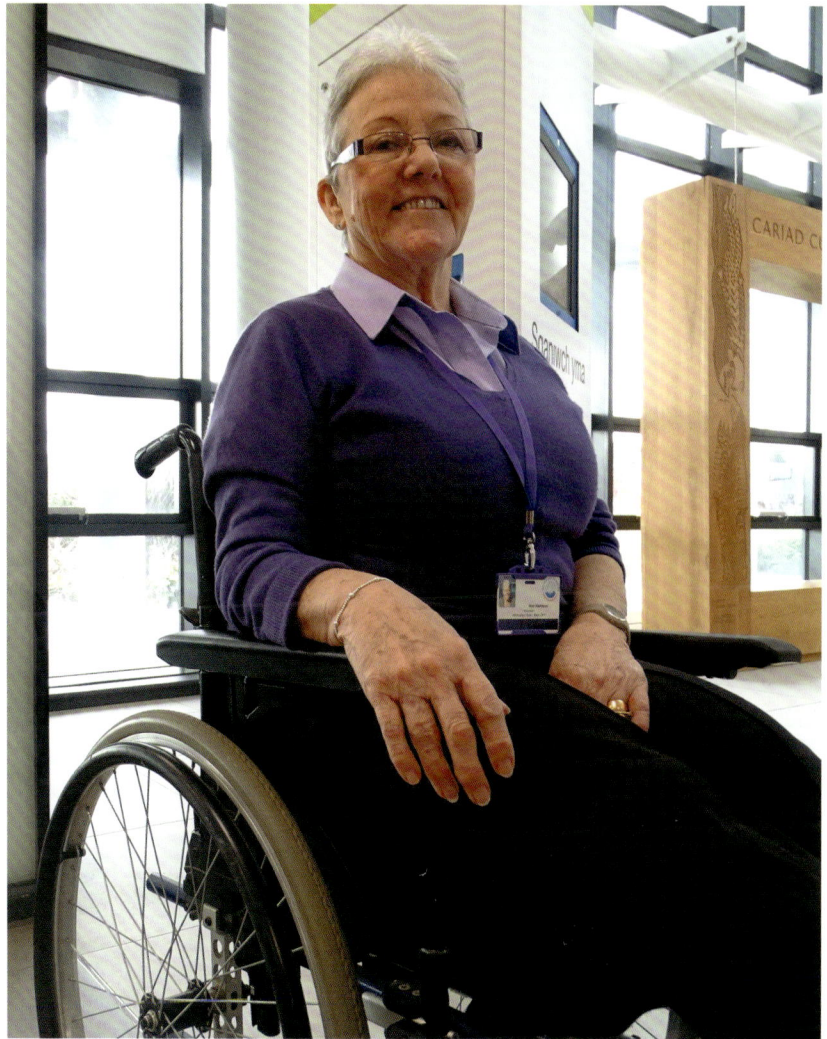

" I was born in December 1946 and my first visit to a hospital was when I was three months old in the spring of 1947. Our family doctor had said there was no more that could be done for me so mum took me to Morriston Hospital which was not yet part of the NHS but an American army hospital.

I was diagnosed with spina bifida and operated on by Mr Gordon Rowley.

He hoped that everything would turn out fine, and to a degree it did - I didn't have hydrocephalus but my right leg was paralysed, and I did have incontinence problems.

I had many operations at Morriston Hospital on Wards 7 and 11, and also Gorseinon and Swansea General which I didn't like at all.

I was very little and after been admitted to Swansea I remember that our parents were not allowed to visit us because it would upset us too much. Our beds were lined up at the top of the ward with a line of old fashioned screens at the bottom which our parents were allowed to peep through at us.

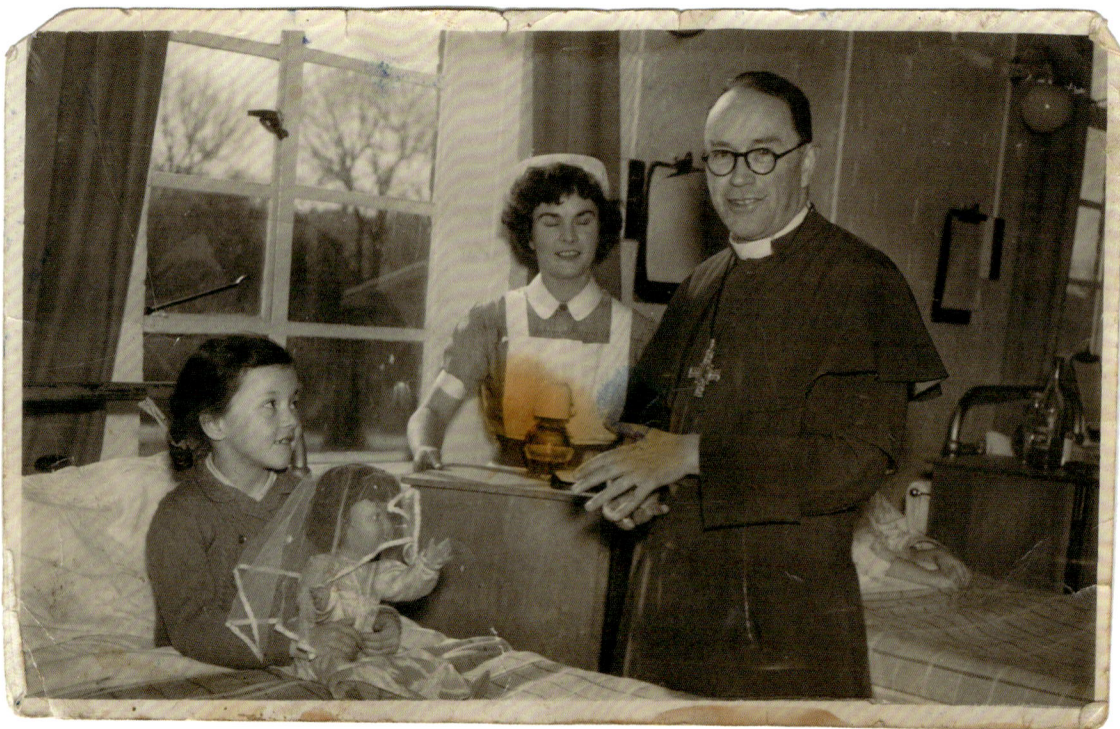

Ann as a child in hospital

I shouted: *"That's my mother, I want to see her."* They told me not to be silly, but I said: *"Yes it is, I recognise her shoes!"* Poor Mam must have been so embarrassed at people thinking she only had one pair of shoes!

I remember being very little in Ward 7, waiting for a porter to take me to theatre. When they arrived they laid me on a flat trolley and then sped down the big, long, steep corridor to theatre, with the lights flashing past above my head. Just as you reached the bottom there was a sharp turn onto the next corridor, you turn into it with such a force it was a wonder I never fell off!

My favourite ward was Ward 11 at Morriston where I spent many of my early teenage years under the watchful eye of Sister Morgan in her small bottle-like glasses, who ruled with a rod of iron.

I used to love to hear the peacock every day, which roamed the ground freely and used to come right up to the windows of the ward.

The ward was cleaned religiously every morning before Matron did her rounds with all the beds dragged into the centre and cleaned from back to front.

I often used to sit on the huge window sills and wave to the men on Ward 13. I was told off, they said it wasn't a very nice thing for a young girl to do in her pyjamas.

When visiting was over, and if you were lucky enough to have been brought fruit by your visitors, it would be taken away by the nurses to be cut up and served as delicious fruit salad for tea for all the patients equally.

Ward 11 was split into orthopaedic and neuro and for some reason I was put into the top third of the ward with the neuro patients. I could never understand why they had no hair and why their beds were suddenly empty, had they gone home? Later in life I realised they had died.

But it was far from a sad ward. I was a bit of a terror and got up to lots of tricks, anything to take away the boredom. One day I crawled under the cage that keeps the blankets off your legs and pretended I had had gone missing. They looked everywhere, very naughty.

I also threaded cotton through an empty strawberry punnet which I put on a table in the centre of the ward. When the nurse came in I asked her to pass me the punnet, which I then pulled and she screamed – this was not appreciated by Sister Morgan, may I say.

I used to whizz up and down the ward in my wheelchair, especially delivering the Evening Post which the paperboy gave to me for distribution in the evening. (I think his name was Dennis from Vicarage Road).

I had my left leg amputated in this ward in 1961 when I was 15. It wasn't a good time as I was a teenager and the hormones were going wild, but Staff Nurse Harris was wonderful with me, and talked me through the process. It was such a strange feeling after the operation, having phantom pains, and wanting to scratch toes which weren't there.

I had quite a few more operations after that. When I went into hospital to have my first child in 1969 Mount Pleasant Hospital – an old work house - was very depressing. It was a worrying time for me as there were no scans or amniocentesis so I was constantly worrying that he might have spina bifida.

I had to have a caesarean and was kept in that depressing hospital for 10 days after his birth. I had two more children at the same hospital who were both healthy and fine.

I started doing volunteering work around 1997, working on the reception desk in the old outpatients department which I had attended as a child all those years ago. Sadly it has now been pulled down and there is nothing recognisable of the old hospital anymore, which was a great part of my life.

But as always you adapt and the new outpatients department is a credit to the NHS which I am proud to say I am still a part of. Happily volunteering in the new outpatients department at Morriston 70 years after my first visit. **"**

Jan Cannon

"Like Ann Harrison, I was operated on by Mr Gordon Rowley and Mr Ambrose in Swansea General around about 1964. I had osteomyelitis in my hip. My parents were told I might have a limp but the operation was a complete success and to this day I have never had any more trouble with my hip.

"Our NHS is absolutely fantastic service and the people who work within it are amazing, they do a fantastic job."

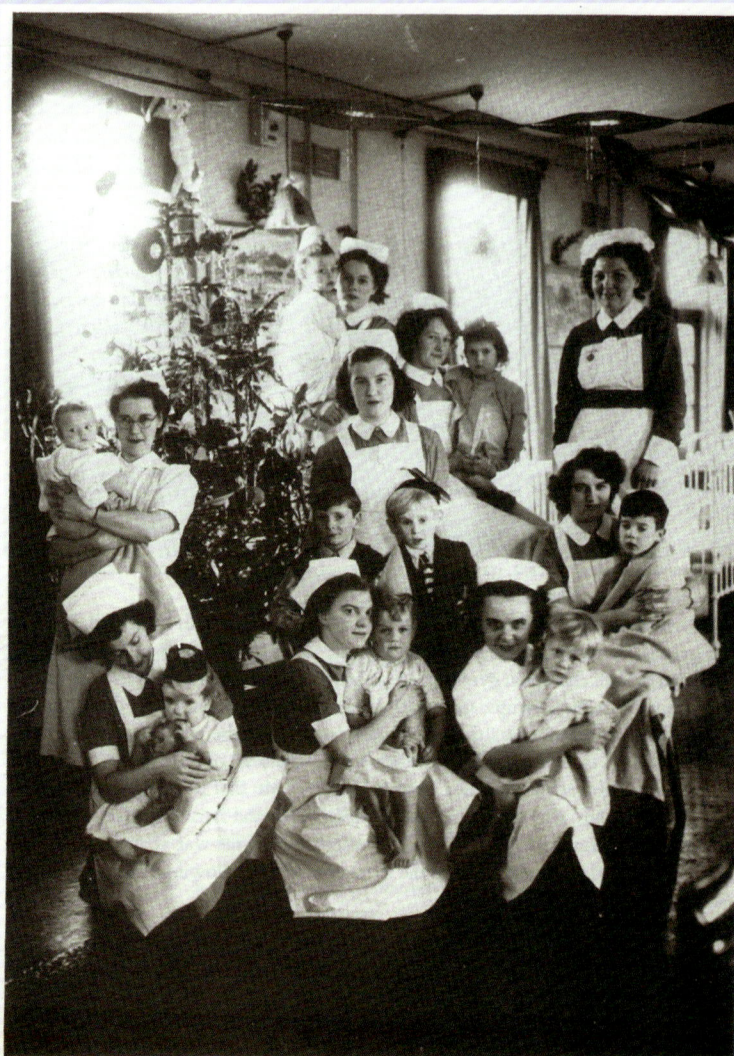

Children's Christmas Party, Ward 8, circa 1954
(Photograph courtesy of Mrs C. A. Bowen)

Lynda Shickell

Growing up in St Thomas, there was more than just four years separating sisters Ann and Lynda Davis.

Their father loved to remind them that because Lynda was born on 16th July 1948 – within days of the NHS being launched – her delivery had cost the family nothing.

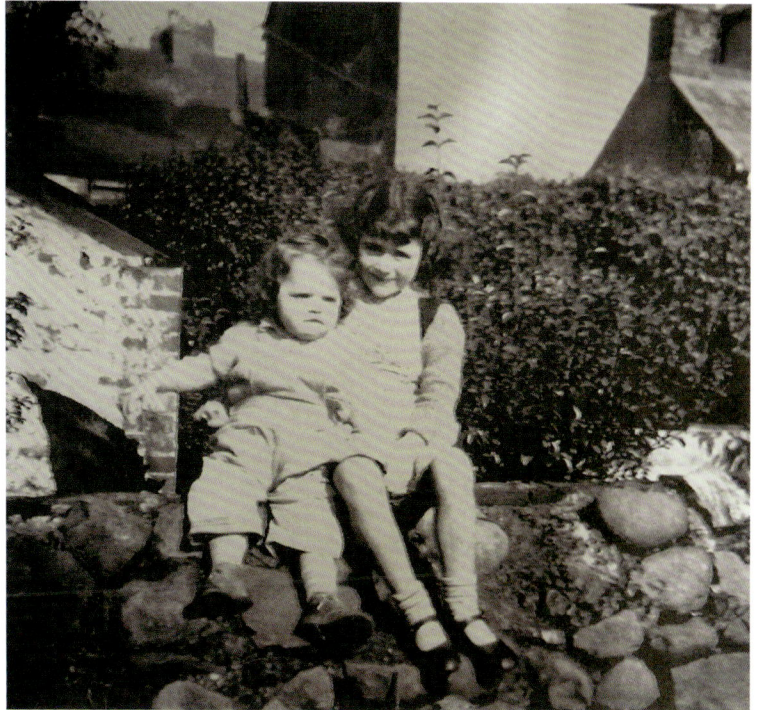

Lynda and her sister Ann

But big sister Ann, who made her entry into the world at Stouthall Maternity Hospital in Gower four years earlier, had to be paid for by the family – and her father Alan had the receipt to prove it!

"I always remember my father telling me he didn't have to pay for my birth - I was his bargain baby.

"He often showed us the receipt but unfortunately we can't remember how much it was they had to pay for her."

Mum-of-two Lynda said her father Alan was a railway worker and he and his wife Marjory were living in rented rooms near the docks when Ann was due.

"Back then babies were usually delivered at home but because of the war and the fact my parents were living in rooms, my mother went to Stouthall to have my sister.

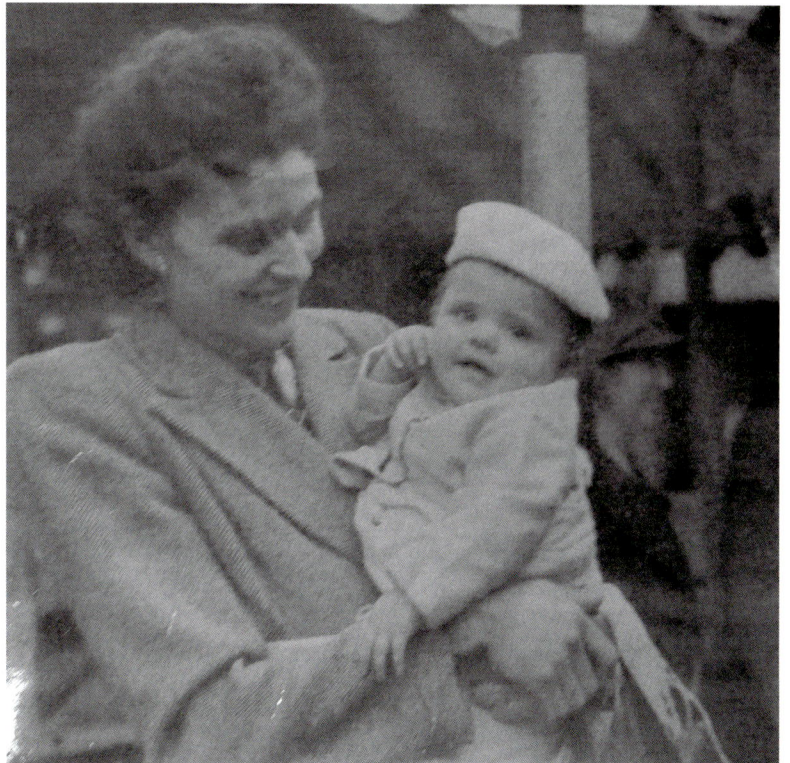

Lynda with Mum

"My father would tell us how he would go down to visit them on the bus along with the other fathers."

Alan still faced a bus trip when Lynda came along as she was born in Fairwood Hospital.

"When I was born they didn't have to pay for my birth and it seemed revolutionary. My father was a huge supporter of the NHS, and was very proud I was one of the first babies born under it."

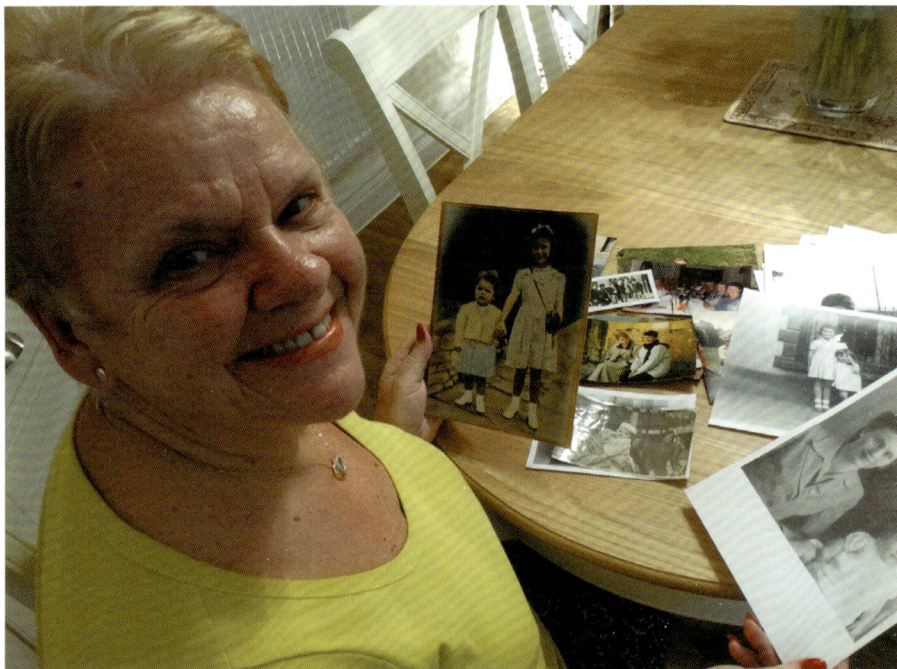
Lynda and her memories

Sadly Lynda and her sister have been unable to find the original receipt for Ann's birth among her late parents' papers but both have very fond memories of her dad sharing the story over the years.

Now Lynda Shickell and a mother-of-two, she is looking forward to her big birthday this year.

"I am delighted to be celebrating my 70th birthday at the same time as the NHS. I feel lucky to be one of the first recipients of its care. It is a fantastic service and we must always treasure it."

And she says her admiration for the NHS has grown over the years especially through her own experience.

"My grandson Cameron has the life-limiting condition Duchenne muscular dystrophy and without the care of the NHS I know he would not be with us now.

"A couple of years ago he was in intensive care at Great Ormond Street Hospital after an operation but now he is studying for A-levels, is about to turn 17 and is looking forward to learning to drive. We never thought we would see this.

"It is all down to the wonderful, wonderful NHS and I can't applaud it enough!"

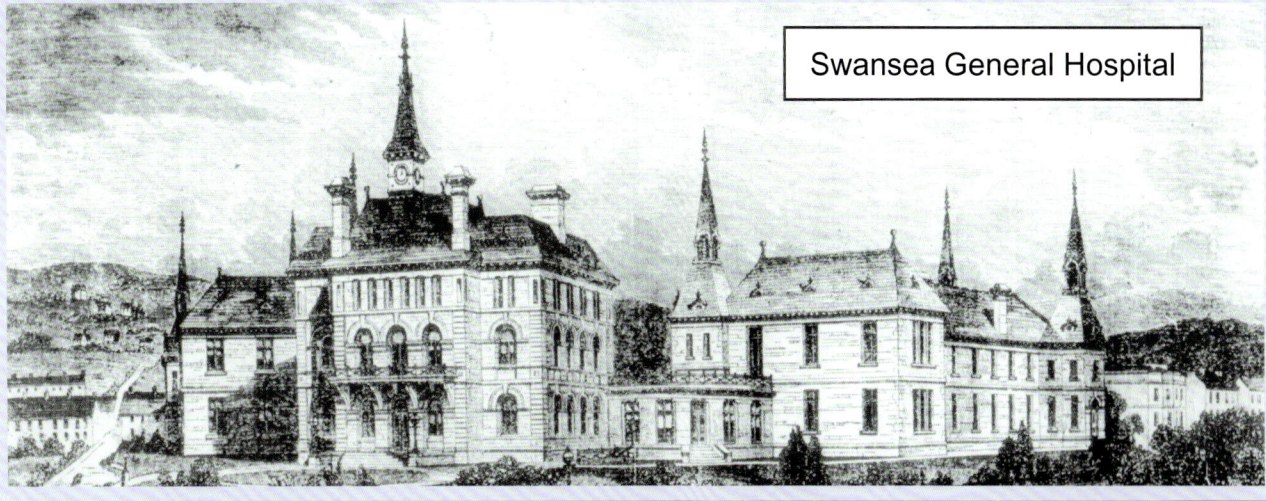

Swansea General Hospital

Charley Lemon:

"I wouldn't be here without the NHS! I got rushed into Morriston Hospital after having a seizure, was diagnosed with a brain tumour and operated on by an amazing neurosurgeon named George Eralil and his team in Cardiff. I had radiotherapy followed by chemotherapy at Singleton Hospital under Professor Roger Taylor, as well as being able to freeze my eggs for the future, free of charge, in Neath Port Talbot Hospital. The medical and emotional support I've received throughout is something I don't think you'd get anywhere in the world, especially without having to worry about costs. Eternally grateful."

Glenys Hall:

"So much to thank the NHS for - from saving of my life when I fell on a broken bottle and cut an artery at the age of two and a half in 1950 (grateful thanks to Mr Tanner at Swansea General, we were fortunate we lived seconds away from the Casualty Department in Phillips Parade) to my recent surgery at Singleton Hospital and the on-going care I have been receiving from the NHS."

Josephine Williams:

"We have so, so much to thank the NHS for - saving my brother's life, all their care and hard work fighting for my mother's life, the staff and doctors who work endlessly and the nurses doing far and above their duty. We are so lucky in this country."

Beth Carlisle:

My first memorable experience was having the sleeve of my favourite "fishy jumper" cut so my greenstick fracture could be bound in sticky plaster. Worse was to come. Pulling it off a few weeks later, with hairs of my arm pulled with each tug, at four years of age was no joy!"

Alice Harris

When Alice Harris was diagnosed with a cancerous lump on her knee nearly 60 years ago, the treatment at Morriston Hospital was drastic. Nearly a quarter of her body was amputated, leading to her needing a prosthetic tin limb with buttons and gears to restore her mobility.

She faced a challenge which would have overwhelmed many. But the determined and plucky farmer's wife, then just 41, refused to let her disability hold her back. She carried on working on her farm, went dancing with her husband, Frank, and even passed her driving test when she was 72!

Sadly, Alice passed away in 2007, aged 92. But her family have paid a warm tribute to her, and the care she received in the early years of the NHS

Speaking in our publication Diamond Days, released to celebrate the 60th anniversary of the NHS her daughter Ann, said: *"Nothing ever slowed my mother down. She lived on a farm in Cwmgors and didn't let her disability stop her from carrying on doing all the jobs she had before as a farmer's wife."*

Mrs Harris had a special prosthetic limb made for her fashioned from metal and attached to her body with a leather corset which laced up tightly around her. It was very heavy and she had to push a button to release her knee joint if she wanted to sit down. But she refused to let it get in her way, and she was even able to scale the steep wood staircase in the farmhouse by negotiating them sideways.

She stood for house doing the family laundry (no washing machine then) and would even confidently balance on a chair when she was re-decorating.

Her family believe the limb was designed by the same specialist who helped the Second World War legend Douglas Bader walk again after he lost both his legs.

Her grand-daughter Joanna Miles added: "I didn't see my grandmother as disabled, it was just the way she was. We used to call her Nana Knock-Knock because her leg was made of tin. She was very open about it and didn't try to hide anything from us. She had tremendous gumption."

Over the years her prosthetic limb was replaced, and eventually Mrs Harris began to rely on a wheelchair to get around.

But the courageous great-grandmother of 17 had proved to all who knew and loved her that determination can overcome the greatest odds.

One patient still remembers his time spent in Swansea General Hospital as small boy.

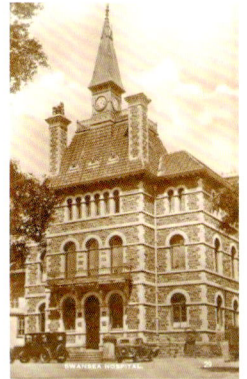

"It was 1952. I was a 10 years old and it was Easter when I had a bad stomach, and it turned out it was my appendix. I went into Griffith Thomas ward at the old Swansea General Hospital – it was a men's ward, I don't know if they had a children's ward as such.

"I remember vividly the large bowl and jug which was passed around at 6.30 am every morning for us to have a wash, and the huge kettle and mugs of tea we were given.

"I remember being taken up for my operation and told I was going to theatre. I asked what I was going to see … and I was told I would see some very bright lights and to count backwards. The next thing I knew I was waking up in bed.

"I was in hospital for 10 days, and in the bed next to me was an old man named Mr Bidder. He used to let me borrow his wheelchair so I could go for a ride.

"Only one visitor at a time was allowed in to see us, and after they had gone, at 7.30 or 8pm, matron came around and put the lights out.

"I remember seeing the nurses in their camel-coloured cloaks looking very smart.

"It was the only time I've every been in hospital in my life."

Three-and-a-half days is along time in hospital when you're just seven years old, but another patient remembers spending three-and-a-half years in hospital.

He was a patient in both Fairwood and Hill House hospitals between 1945 and 1948 – at the dawn of the NHS being treated for a hip displacement.

In those days the treatment involved tying his legs to a bed, raising the bed on bricks, and letting gravity take its course.

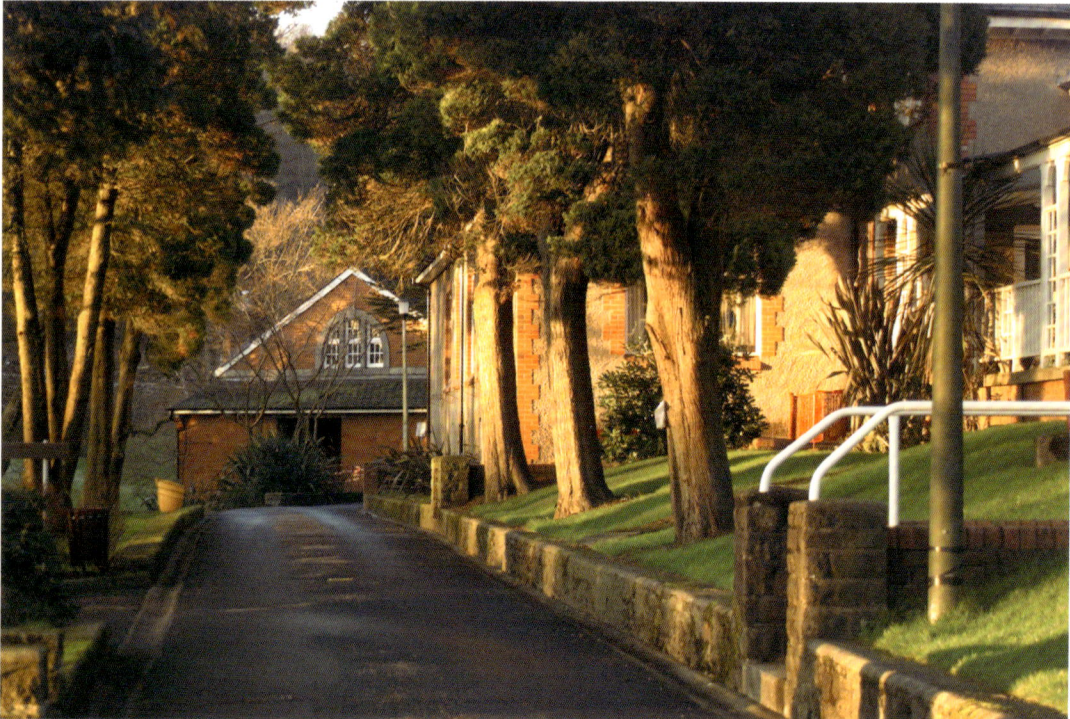

Hill House Hospital

He recalled:

"My mother took me to the doctors because I was lame on my left side, and he decided I needed to go to hospital as an orthopaedic patient. I remember being taken in an ambulance which was all-blue. It belonged to Hill House, the hospital I was taken to, and it was used to collect their patients.

"I was put in a single room and in the room next to me was an iron lung. It was a big box which looked like a coffin and as it worked the lungs on the patient inside it, it made a terrible noise.

"I was in a bed which was up on blocks and my ankles tied to the foot of the bed. It was an early form of traction."

He was later transferred to Fairwood Hospital, where he spent most of his three-and-a-half years on a general ward with patients of all ages.

He was put into a special frame, made up of iron bars across his chest to stop him falling out, and leather straps which also held him securely.

"I was like that for 12 months. I was in plaster from my ankles to my thighs with a broom stick holding my legs apart."

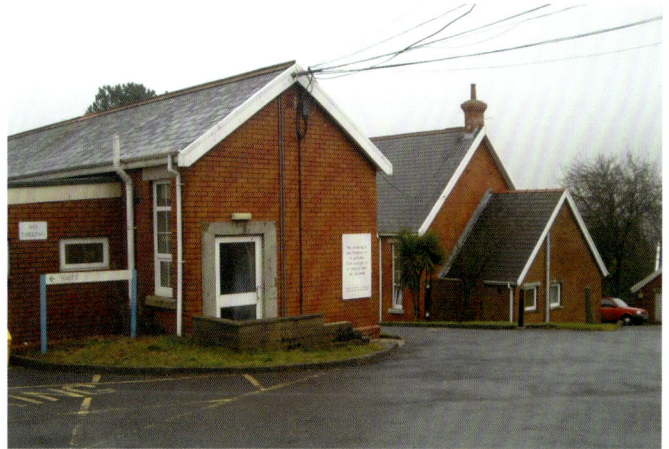
Fairwood Hospital

On sunny days the patients were wheeled outside in their beds, where they would watch RAF pilots stationed at nearby Fairwood aerodrome swoop overhead in Spitfires.

But days were long when they were on the ward, and the youngsters among the patients made their own entertainment. Knotted bandages served as cricket balls and newspapers were fashioned into bats, and the "balls" hit from one bed to another.

Perhaps the hardest part for the youngster was the separation from his family. Fairwood was an isolation hospital and there were patients there suffering from infectious diseases like diphtheria and scarlet fever.

"Every visitor had to stand outside the window, they weren't allowed inside.

"We couldn't have any physical contact with each other. I had to talk to my family through the window - not even my parents could come in and see me."

But despite the years of forced inactivity, he had nothing but affectionate memories for his time in hospital.

"They were lovely cottage hospitals and I made some good friends during my time there."

When matron ruled the roost

Nursing as a career has seen so many developments, adaptations, innovations and changes since 1948.

From the uniform and training to facilities, equipment and the influence of the ever-present Matron - so many things are different.

But, as one of our long-serving former nurses says, over all those decades there has been one constant –

> *"the role of the nurse has not changed from that of curing sometimes, relieving often but caring always."*

Here some of our nursing staff – past and present – share their experiences....

Alison Kingdom

When Alison retired from her role as Singleton Hospital site manager she completed a career that began and ended there. She was so determined to be a nurse she spent every Saturday and school holiday for two years helping on the wards at Neath General Hospital before beginning her training with the Glantawe Group School of Nursing in 1972.

66 When I started my training there were 44 female and one male student in my set. I completed ward placements at Singleton, Morriston, Mount Pleasant and Cefn Coed hospitals where I was part of the ward team and learned how to care for patients under the watchful eye of the ward sister.

In those days ward sister was someone to behold! She would say jump and I would say 'how high?' During my first year I felt I would never get out of the sluice!

As well as learning to physically care for patients, I learned to keep a clean and tidy ward, always ensuring that the opening of the pillowcases faced away from the door. I always stood up when a senior nurse came into the office and would only go in the office if invited - I used to hover outside.

Nurses' uniform consisted of a striped dress with a starched white apron, collar and hat. I used to pin up the corners of my apron so it would not get creased on the journey from Park Beck to the hospital – appearance was everything! After qualifying, my nurses' hat had to be sewn so that it had a ruffle in the back and the sister's hat was very lacy.

In my student days, nurses were responsible for laying up the breakfast trolley, buttering the bread and then cooking the patients' boiled eggs for their breakfast.

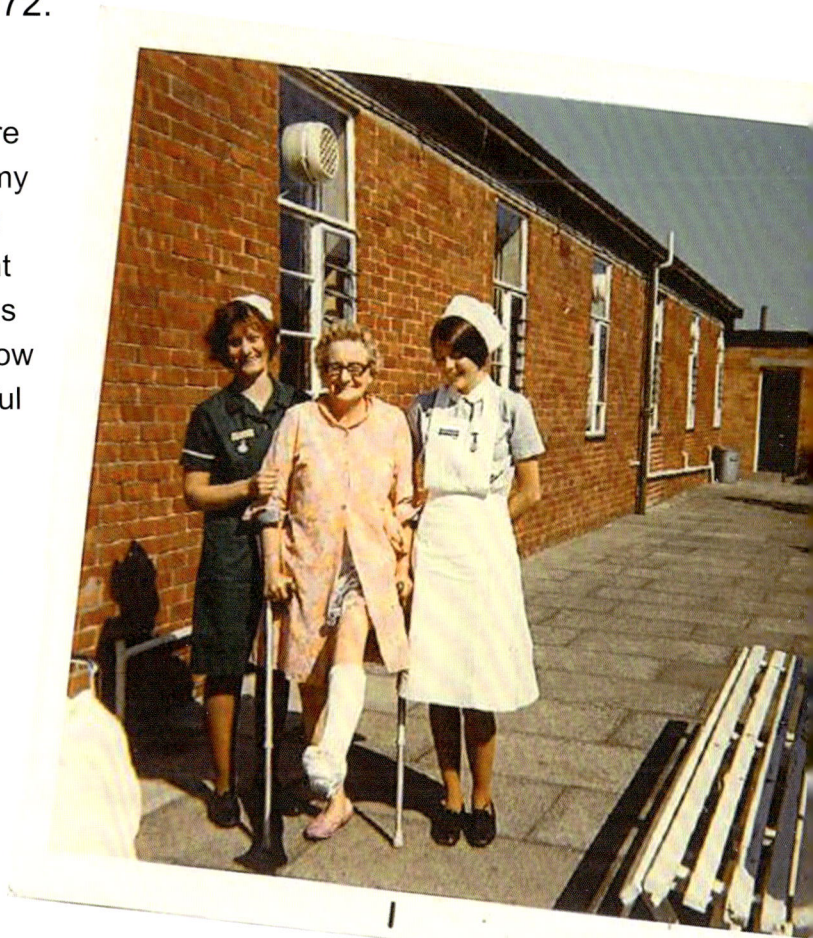

Patient meals came up in bulk, not plated. Sister and the senior staff nurse would serve the meal with more junior staff delivering it to the patient and assisting them as necessary. It was quite a ritual and there was always ice cream, jelly and cake served at afternoon tea.

I lived in Park Beck Nurses Home in Sketty where we were allowed two late keys a week, otherwise we had to be signed in and in our rooms by 11pm.

Every morning at about 6am whether you were working or not, you would be knocked up. They were very happy days. As a student I earned £30 a month after accommodation was deducted. I wasn't that bothered about wages because I was so pleased to be training to be a nurse.

After qualifying in 1975 I received a letter of congratulations from Matron Miss Daniel, who informed me that she was placing me on Ward 4 which was a 40-bedded trauma ward - A&E was based in Singleton in those days.

It was a very busy ward with many elderly patients being nursed on traction, not like today where operation and early mobilisation is advocated.

Matron knew everyone by name, the nursing staff were her girls. She used to periodically move staff around. Every six months or so the change list would go up and nurses were moved to work on a different ward.

Over the years I worked in many different roles.

In many respects the science of nursing has changed as new treatments have informed practice. However, the role of the nurse has not changed from that of curing sometimes, relieving often but caring always.

It is very pleasing to me that I am ending my career where I started 44 years ago. If asked whether I would do it all again, my answer would most definitely be YES!! **"**

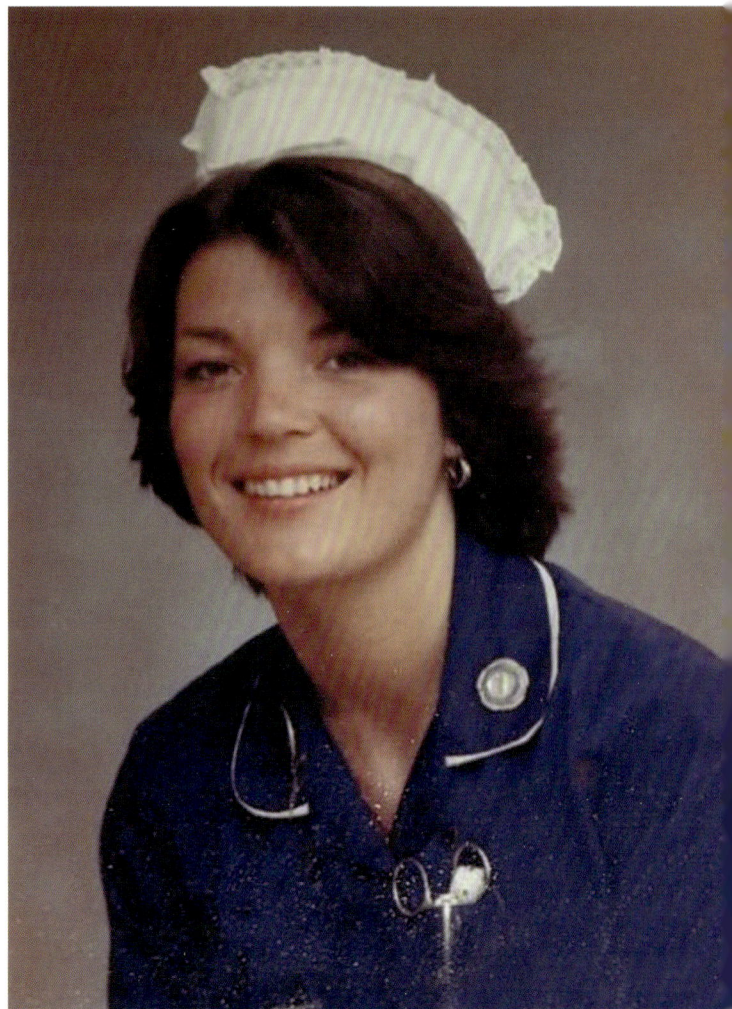

Eira Rees

Approaching the nurses' home at Morriston Hospital after coming off duty something caught the eye of student nurse Eira Pugh.

Fluttering from the flag pole above the building wasn't quite what you'd expect to see – it was a selection of bras and briefs flapping in the wind.

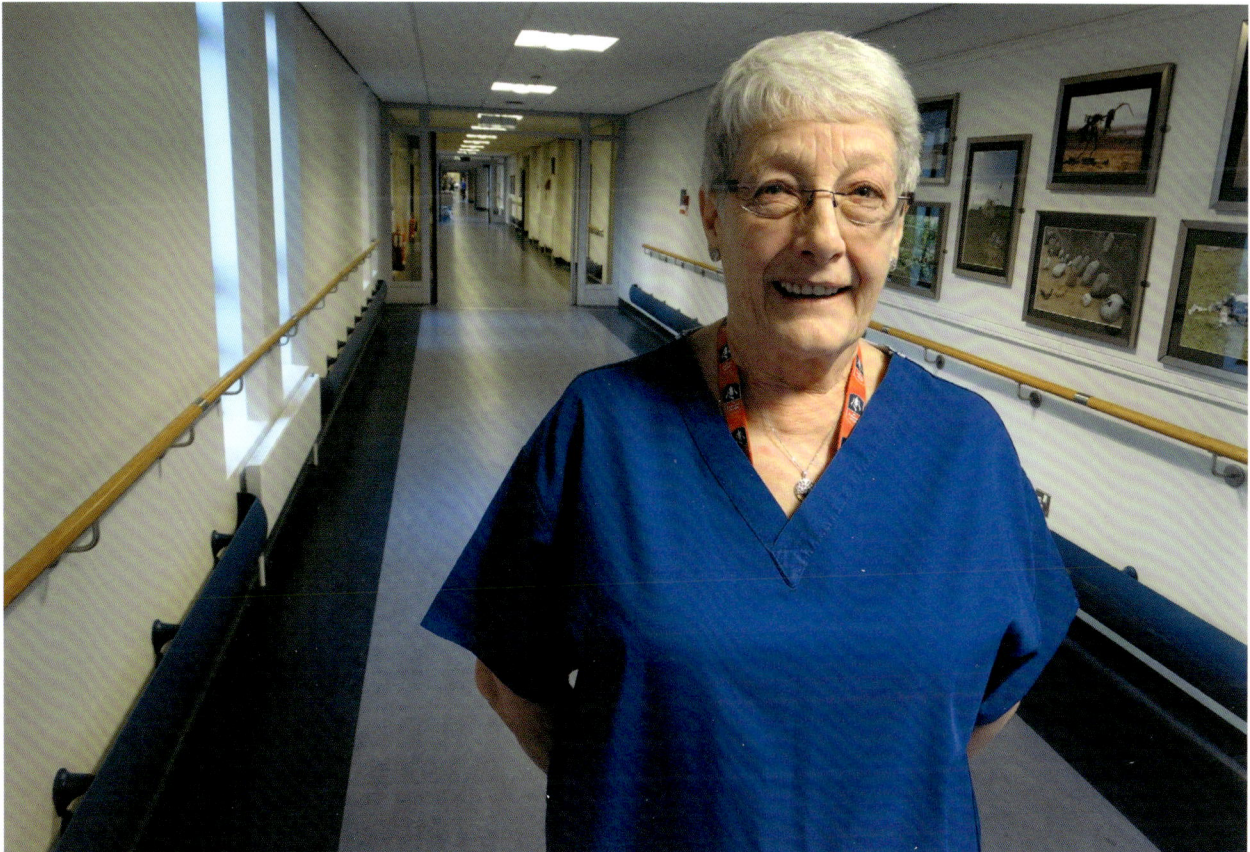

Eira – now staff nurse Eira Rees – explained:

"The junior doctors had raided the laundry room, grabbed our underwear and run it up the flagpole."

It was the kind of prank that wasn't so unusual when she was training in the 1960s - the doctors were also to blame for hiding towels and removing fuses from lamps - but she says those days were among the happiest of her long career.

"We were naughty, more mischievous really, but it was all harmless fun.

"The home sisters in charge were tough but then we wouldn't have had the fun we had if they weren't."

She remembers the strict rule that every nurse had to be signed in and tucked up in their room by 10.30pm.

"But you would still go out for the evening and just get someone else to sign in for you and to let you back in later."

And the rules were just as rigid during the day.

"When you would get back after doing night shifts you would have a bath, go to your room and get into bed but leave the door open.

"Home Sister would come round with a mug of Ovaltine or Horlicks – if I'd had a sink in my room I would have chucked it away – and when you finished your drink you left your mug by the door.

"When she came back round to collect the mug she would shut your door and you were supposed to go to sleep – but once she shut the door I would go out shopping!"

It wasn't so easy to escape the strict regime.

"When you wanted to move out you had to have your Matron's permission along with your parents'*"*

She explained that Matron noticed everything – especially the length of nurses' uniforms back in the days when mini-skirts were the rage.

"She would pass nurses in the corridor and ask them to kneel down. If your skirt didn't touch the floor when you were kneeling you would be handed a scissors and told to unpick the hem and stitch it to the correct length immediately!"

A young Eira at work

Eira is now 72 and one of ABMU's longest serving members of staff, clocking up 51 years with the NHS. She works three days a week as a theatre nurse at Morriston Hospital and still loves her job as much as ever.

Eira initially hoped to become an enrolled nurse but once she started training she caught the eye of the matron in charge.

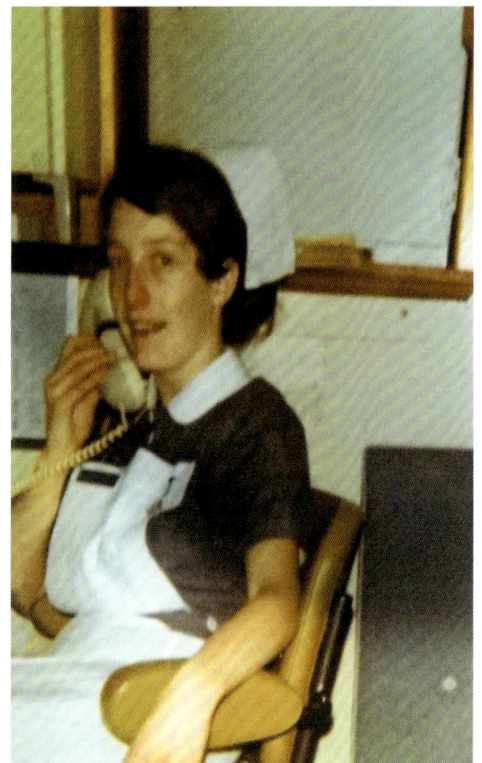

"She spotted something in me and she said she didn't think the course offered me what I needed. She encouraged me to train as a State Registered Nurse instead.".

Eira was 19 when she started training at Morriston with the initial aim of becoming a health visitor which required her to train as a midwife, a role she undertook at Mount Pleasant Hospital in Swansea for five years.

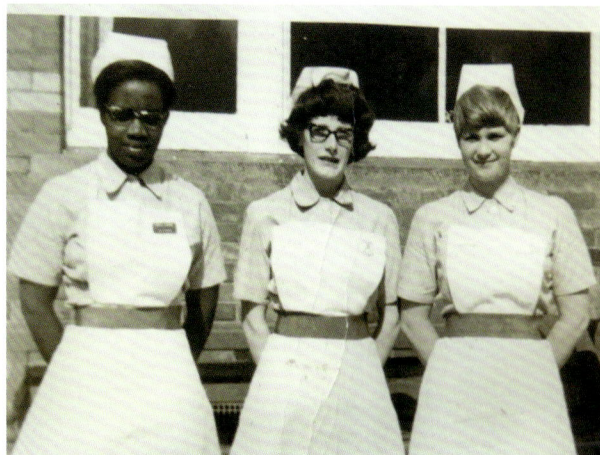

Eira and two colleagues

"When I worked as a midwife I was always amazed by every single delivery. I still have a record book of every single baby I delivered."

She went on to swap the labour ward for the operating theatre before working at BP Llandarcy and as a school nurse, gaining teaching qualifications and lecturing in health and social care at Swansea College.

However eventually Eira returned to her role within surgery at Morriston.

Eira says she has seen many changes in her days working in theatres.

"When I started nurses on night shift would have to scrub the theatre from top to bottom and clean it with a hose. We'd also be responsible for preparing the instrument trays and preparing piles of swabs ready for the next day's surgery. It was a really good way of getting to know your instruments.

"We'd often get two sets ready then one would be in use while the other was in the autoclave being cleaned after use.

"Back then the operating theatres had doors and windows and if it got too hot we would just open a window.

"Over the years we have seen the expansion of our knowledge and that has helped improve outcomes and what we can do to help people.

"Some of the drugs we use have been around a very long time but we have now found uses for drugs that we didn't know before and techniques have certainly improved."

Helen Goldring

ABMU research nurse Helen Goldring devotes her time to ensuring the smooth running of vital clinical trials. The studies she is involved with take her all over the health board as she helps to find new treatments to improve patient care for the future.

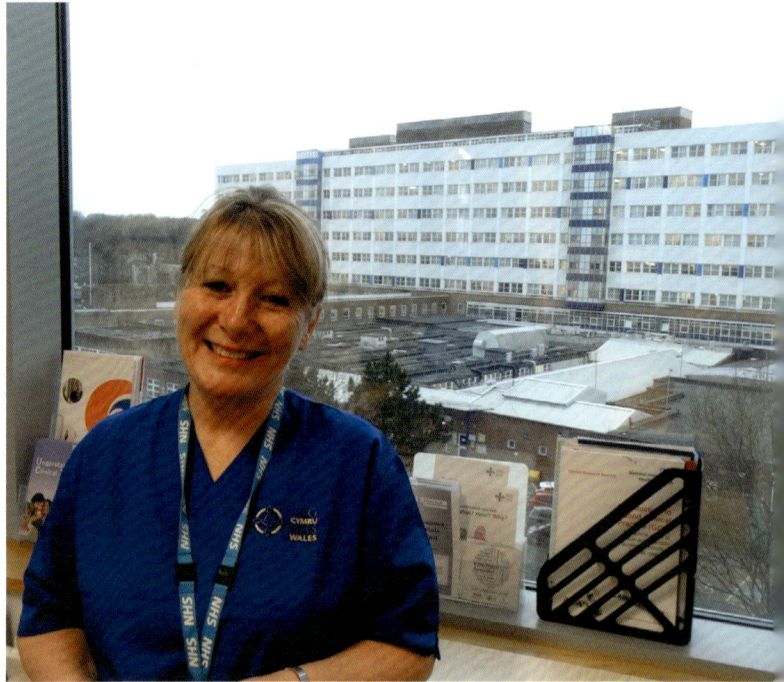

Helen in her office overlooking Singleton Hospital

" This is now my 42nd year of nursing and as I was walking through the corridors of Morriston Hospital, it struck me that I was born at this hospital and only survived because of the NHS.

I grew up in a post-war council house in Cathan Crescent, Portmead, Swansea. My mum and dad, Dolly and Bert, were both born in 1912.

My mother had lost four boys due to pre-eclampsia before the NHS was created - with no health care and no one except relatives to care for my mother as my parents had no money to pay.

They eventually adopted a boy before I was born but I was an accident, as she was told not to have any more babies.

Mum was 42 when I was born at Morriston Hospital. She had full blown eclampsia of pregnancy and I was an emergency caesarean section and weighed in as 4lbs 3.ozs.

It's a miracle we both survived and I only lived because of the NHS.

Not only am I grateful for my life, but also of the life of my father. When I was 13 back in 1967 he collapsed at home with a perforated appendix and sometime after surgery he had what they called a twisted bowel and bowel obstruction as a complication of initial surgery.

I remember the police arriving at our house and taking my mother and me to hospital to see him. We didn't have a car then and nobody had phones so it was the only way we found out about it.

I can recall sitting in one of the alcove waiting areas in the old corridor leading to outpatients at Morriston, just hoping to be able to see my dad after his operation.

By this time he only weighed about 5 stone and he survived thanks to a brilliant surgeon from Africa - I think his name was Mr Okeke - who took a chance on performing further surgery on a dying man who had nothing to lose.

After three months convalescence in Stouthall, my father survived and lived to be 89. I was always very grateful for the hospital for saving my father who I adored.

I always had a caring instinct - my husband calls it a compulsive need to care. My earliest photo is of me aged two in a nurse's uniform holding a baby.

I met my future husband Colin and moved to Essex. I trained as a nurse there.

When Colin retired about 12 years ago we came back to Swansea and have lived in Gorseinon ever since.

Initially I spent four years as a continence specialist nurse in the valleys before taking up my post as research nurse in Swansea where I have been involved in managing clinical trials and seeing them through to completion.

We generally have six or seven running at a time and I hope the work that we are doing will help to shape healthcare for the future.

Good quality research is one way that patient care can be improved and that is always our long-term aim.

It is very satisfying but I have to say I have been very lucky, I have had a varied and rewarding career in nursing and have enjoyed every minute of it.

I love the NHS and feel so proud to have been able to give something back over the years. 🙶

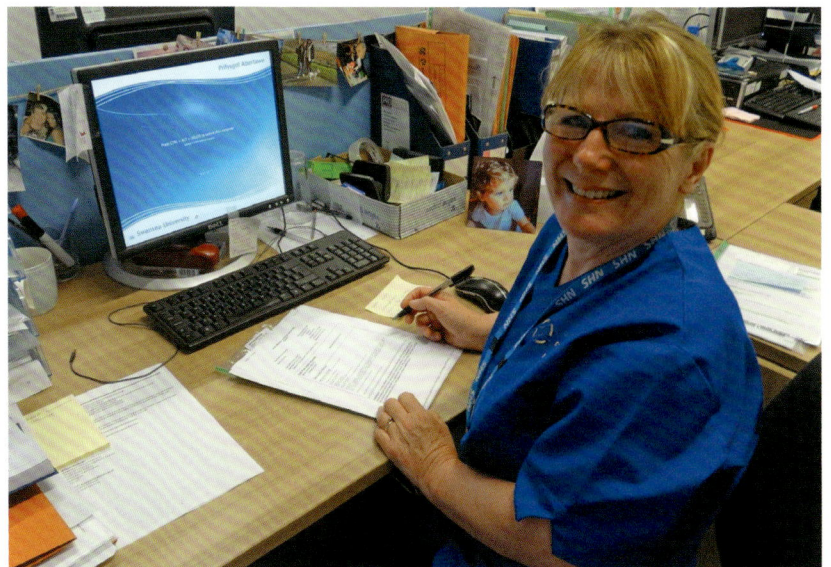

Julia Thomas

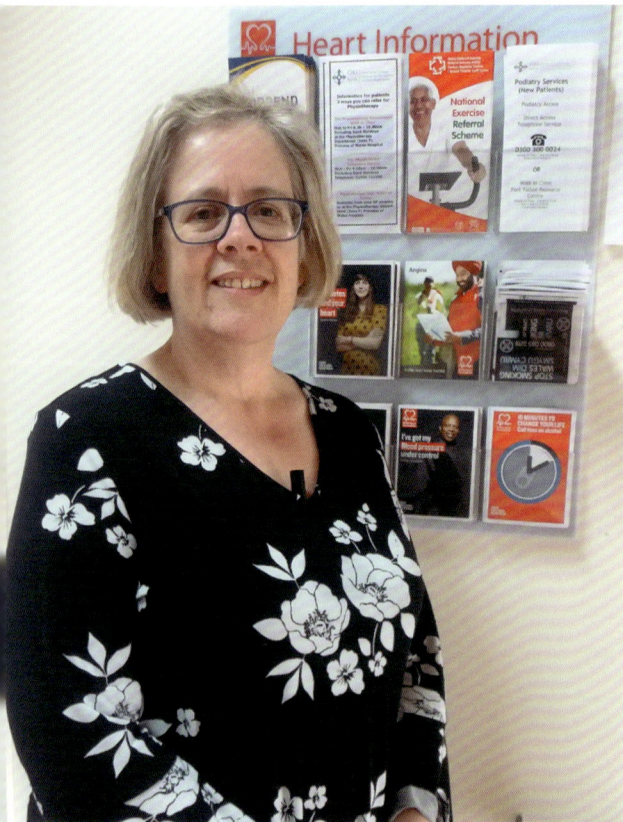

After clocking up almost 40 years of nursing Julia Thomas has seen many changes – particularly in her chosen field of cardiac care.

Now a cardiac rehabilitation nurse specialist at the Princess of Wales Hospital, she looks forward to time spent talking to her patients.

"We are so fortunate that our role involves talking with people. I can walk onto the cardiology ward and sit down to talk with anxious patients.

"When I started working in Bridgend in the 1980s nursing and medical care were very different. We were never allowed to sit and talk to patients."

After training at Bridgend School of Nursing Julia qualified as a staff nurse in 1983 and began working at the old Bridgend General.

"There were so many nursing traditions, as a first year student it was a huge learning curve. I was mystified why 'Mrs Brown might want to talk to me in the kitchen' – that meant having a cup of tea. I can remember sister telling me to clean the sluice twice because there was nothing left to do on the morning shift."

And heaven forbid if anything didn't come up to Matron's standards.

"She would hold her arm out straight to ensure the beds were aligned and even check that the wheels weren't sticking out. She would also check the water in the flower vases and what patients were keeping on their lockers and bed tables.

"As an idealistic first year student nurse I must have looked a bit scornful because she smiled very sweetly and asked me how I would ensure rigorous standards were met in all aspects of patient care. 'It starts with the basics' she said and I've always remembered that.

"I was also once asked by a nursing officer to climb down off a bed whilst doing CPR to put my cap back on after it had been accidentally knocked off by a doctor."

In 1985 Julia was able to pursue her real love – nursing cardiac patients when she took up a role as staff nurse in the coronary care unit.

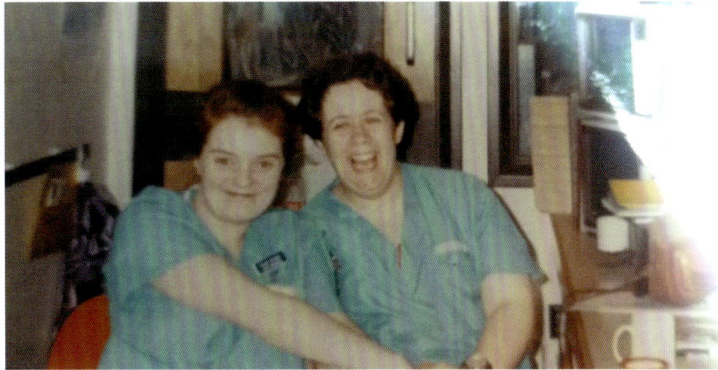

Staff nurses Ann Harvey and Julia Thomas (left) on a night shift in CCU in the early 1990s. Both are now nurse specialists in cardiac rehabilitation.

She said diagnosing a heart attack or myocardial infarction (MI) was not as sophisticated then and only those that had had full blown MI would be diagnosed.

"In the 1980s the initial nursing treatment for an MI would be at least seven days bed rest. Patients would be bed bathed, some would have their teeth brushed for them and they would only be allowed out of bed to use a commode.

"They would not even be allowed to swing their legs to sit at the side of the bed. Patients would also have bed cradles to take the weight of blankets off their feet.

"After a week, if the consultant agreed, they would sit out of bed for five minute increments increasing until they were mobile."

Julia explained that the intensive care/coronary care unit in Bridgend General was on the ground floor with five beds, some next to large sash windows.

"Some enterprising patients would occasionally work out that their monitor leads were long and maybe the nurse wouldn't be checking them for a few minutes and so would climb out of the window for a cigarette!

"It was an old hospital and there were cockroaches, ants and sometimes even rats but I loved it. We all knew each other and it had a lovely local feel to it."

However, life changed dramatically when Julia was among the first staff to move into the new Princess of Wales Hospital in 1985.

"We couldn't believe the new coronary care unit (CCU), it seemed huge, lots of bed space and plenty of electric sockets and oxygen piped through the wall, no more cylinders.

"Apparently there was no sluice in the original plans because there was a thought that critically ill patients would not be using bed pans!"

In 1986 the first cardiac rehabilitation programme in Wales was set up by Dr Linda Speck with Dr Guy Chappell and Sister Angela Smith. Shortly after that, the CCU nurses began inpatient counselling for people who had had heart attacks.

"The treatment of MIs was changing fast. We started getting patients out of bed within 24 hours and new drugs were becoming available. The most amazing thing was the advent of clot-busting drugs thrombolysis

"As nurses, we were well used to palliative care for many of our patients because there was no way to stop the damage done by a heart attack, and so many of our patients died in the first few days.

"Now with thrombolysis we were seeing patients who not only survived but were feeling well within hours. It was a miracle to us."

More recently angiography and echocardiography have revolutionised the care of heart attack patients, said Julia, a former ward sister on the unit.

Now Julia is delighted to be part of an expanding cardiac rehabilitation programme offering an eight-week programme to patients who have had MI, stents, coronary artery bypass grafts, valve surgery and patients and partners diagnosed with heart failure.

"I love feeling that I can make a difference to my patients and that all my years of experience can help to support newly qualified staff - after all, they may well be looking after me one day and I want the standards to be high."

Byron Morgan

Byron Morgan was the first male nurse to be trained as a pupil nurse at Singleton Hospital.

Swansea-born Byron initially signed up as a ward orderly because he was too young to start his SEN training.

He had experience of the NHS because his dad had spent time as a night porter at Singleton and he had cousins who were nurses.

Byron, who later progressed to become a registered nurse, started training at Singleton was part of the first group to be trained jointly between Morriston and Singleton.

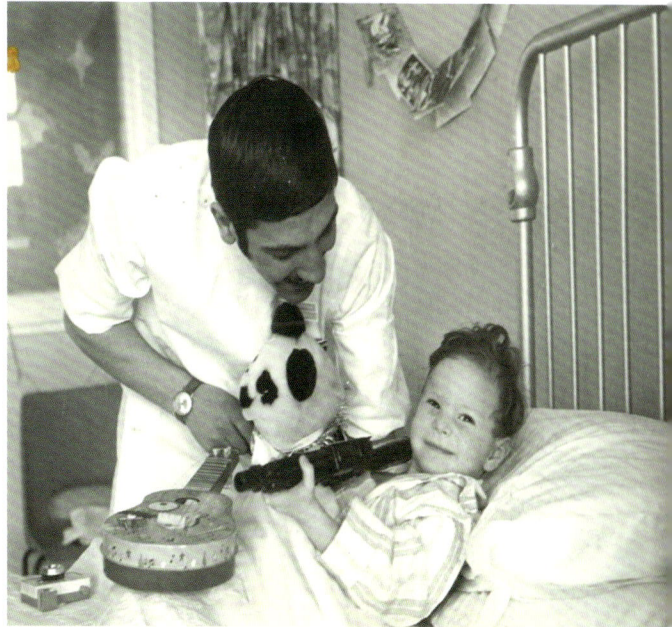

This picture of Bryon with a young patient was taken in 1969, the first Christmas he worked on the children's ward in Singleton. It was Ward 3, with Sister Annie Jenkins.

"We spent three months at training school in Parc Beck, our first year was in Morriston and second year was Singleton and also geriatric training in Mount Pleasant Hospital."

He explained that the student nurses had to follow very strict rules.

"You didn't get many parties in those days because the nurses had to stay in Parc Beck nurses home and because I was the only male nurse there was no accommodation for me so I went home.

"I was only allowed to be on Parc Beck grounds when I was on my training block. If I was caught on the grounds I would have been disciplined.

"It was very strict, they kept the males and the females apart so if you valued your job you didn't go there!

"There were only two children in and on Christmas Eve I had put this child to bed, tucked him up, left him with the night nurses and then the following morning I came on duty and helped him open up the presents Father Christmas had brought him.

"I remember he was a very happy child. Parents would bring in some gifts

but everybody who was in on Christmas Day would get a gift from the hospital's League of Friends.

"Back then half the ward was paediatric and the other half was general surgery/urology – so you had adults on one side and children the other – it was very different to today."

After qualifying in 1972 Byron's first job was as an outpatients plaster technician and minor ops nurse in Singleton.

He took a break from the NHS, working in industry and studying at theological college, before returning as a theatre nurse in Kent. He came back to Swansea in 2004 to work in manual handling training, his current role

Byron has now spent about 30 years in the NHS and over that time has also been a patient.

"It can be difficult because of my position now people know who I am. When I go to a ward as a patient staff are very conscious of watching what they do correctly with regards manual handling.

"So much so that on one occasion when I was in hospital I was in a room of four other people when I noticed a healthcare support worker bending down to put the brakes of a hoist on with her hands. I eventually spoke to the nurse in charge and said 'That's dangerous, she could trap her fingers. I don't want to interfere but I can't let that go'. Within an hour I was put into a single room with the door shut!"

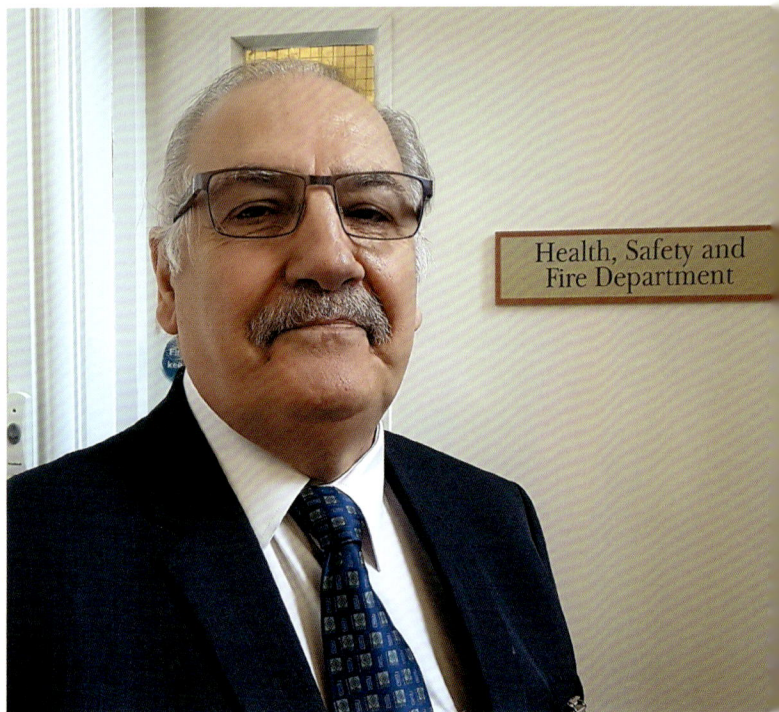

Byron today

Caroline Kirk

When Caroline Kirk began her career at Maesgwyn Hospital back in 1976 nurses wore paper hats with plastic studs that had to be made up every day.

"Those were the days when you had an elastic belt with a buckle which you could only wear once you were qualified and long black capes with red lining,"

"When a young colleague died the family requested that all the nurses attended the funeral wearing full uniform with capes and walked behind the hearse – it was a dramatic sight and something I will never forget."

Caroline has fond memories of her days as a nursing auxiliary at the hospital which provided valuable basic nursing care on its four wards and day hospital.

"In 1978 we were snowed in and some nurses where stuck there for three days, sleeping in the day hospital on hard examination beds for a few hours at a time, as nurses could not get in to work."

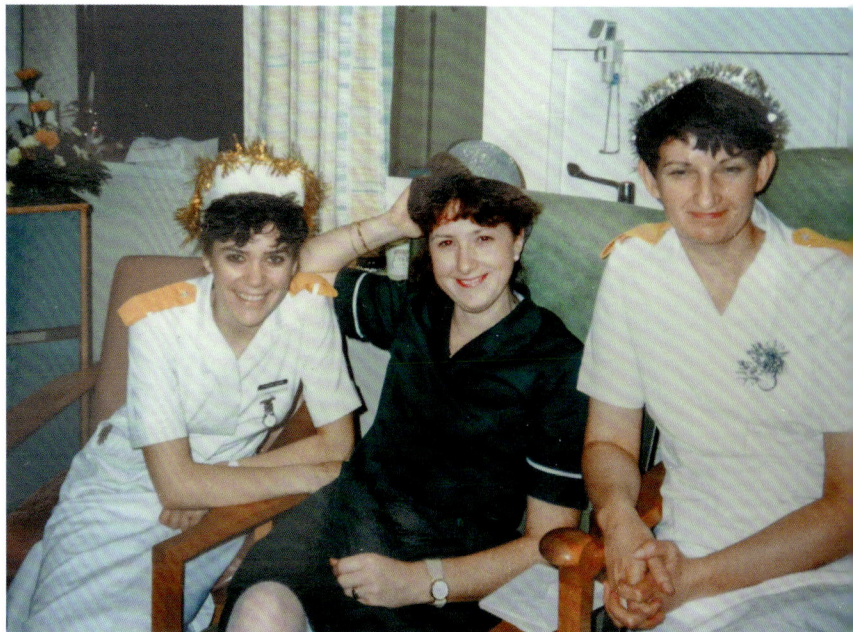
Caroline Kirk (centre) with colleagues

In 1985 she was transferred to the Princess of Wales Hospital in Bridgend.

Caroline Kirk (centre) at the newly opened Princess of Wales Hospital.

"It was a brand new hospital and I can remember getting the wards ready for the first patient which was quite exciting.

"Every Christmas most wards would have a cubicle which the nurses would decorate and patients used to bring in chocolates and the odd bottle of sherry."

After training as an enrolled nurse Caroline's first job was on the new paediatric cardiac ward (Heulwen). She went on to undertake a conversion course to RGN and then trained as a RSCN (Registered Sick Children's Nurse).

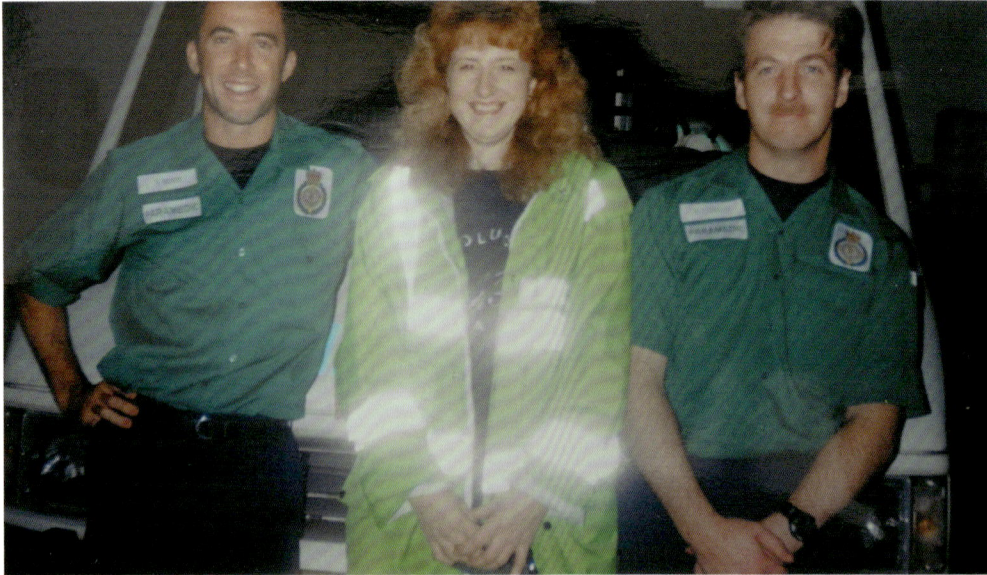

Caroline Kirk with some paramedic friends

"I worked there for many years supporting parents and families with children with heart conditions.

"One on occasion the family of a very sick baby wanted to attend their church before the baby died. The child was on continuous oxygen and so I accompanied them – something I felt privileged to be able to do."

The family of one of Caroline's young patients showed their appreciation in a very memorable way.

"I was looking after a very sick child with a heart defect. His recovery was slow and problematic but after several stressful weeks for the family he made a full recovery.

"His grateful parents owned a hotel in Pembrokeshire and his father invited 10 nurses to stay to thank them for the care his son received on the paediatric cardiac ward.

"We had a lovely time - they had arranged a hovercraft trip to Ireland as well as a chance to go out on the lifeboat which was very exciting. It was a weekend I will never forget."

Caroline went on to swap hospital wards for community nursing, as a paediatric sister managing a team of nurses caring for children with complex health needs.

After time with the Community Resource Team, Caroline now works for the Acute Clinical Team.

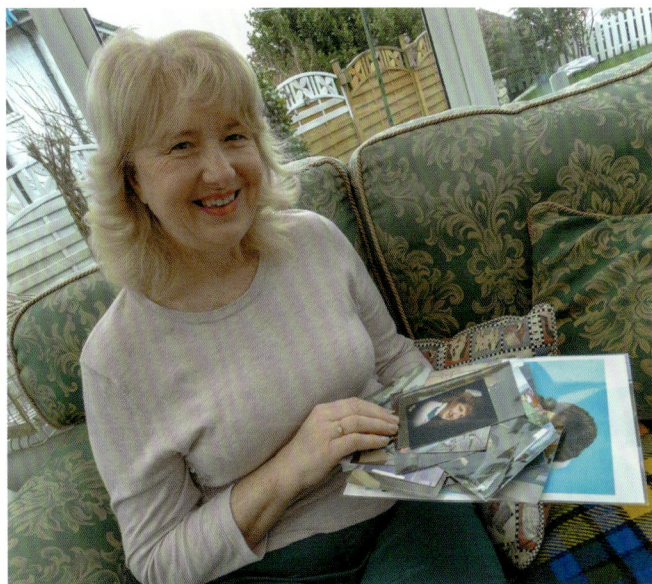

Caroline Kirk looking back at some of the photographs that record her nursing career.

"In the last 42 years I have seen many changes. I could not have seen myself doing anything else. It's been a great privilege to be a nurse and, although it has had its challenges there have been many rewards.

"Recently I retired and then returned which gives me the best of both worlds - more time with my family but still keeping up my registration by working two days a week."

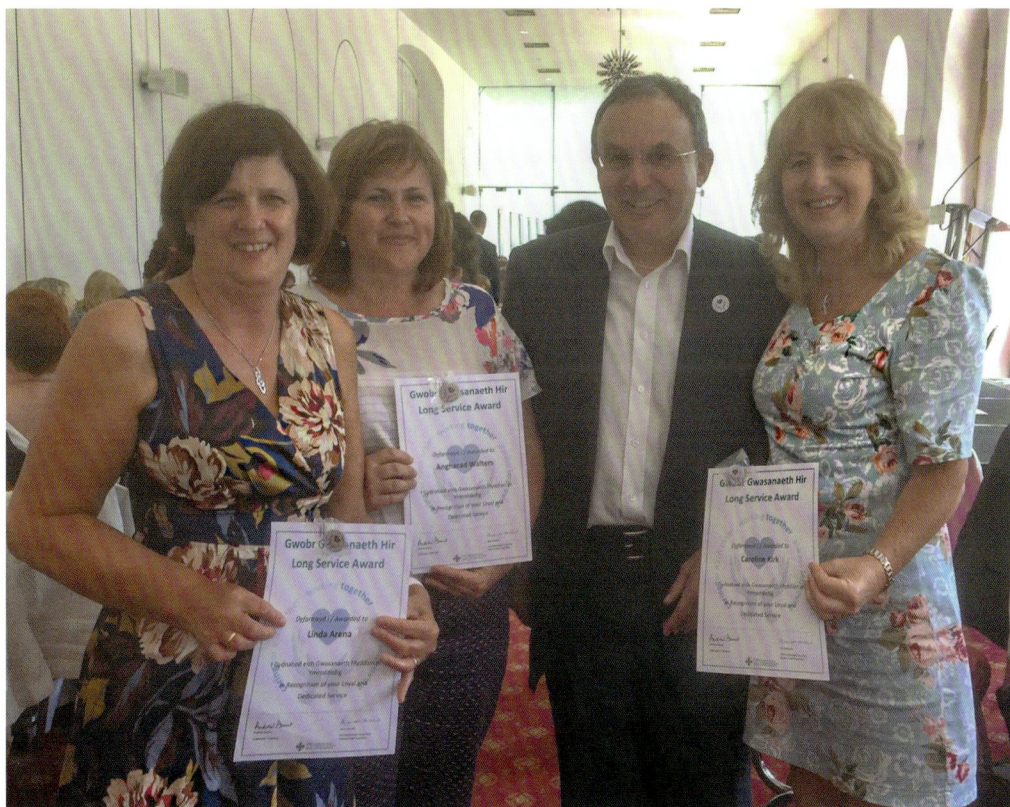

Caroline Kirk *(far right)* with colleagues and ABMU Chairman Andrew Davies at a special long service awards ceremony in 2017.

Mount Pleasant midwives

It may be 32 years since it closed but the memory of Mount Pleasant Hospital's maternity unit lives on – thanks to the group of midwives who still meet up regularly.

They have held annual reunions, organised by Carol Evans, every year since the Swansea hospital closed.

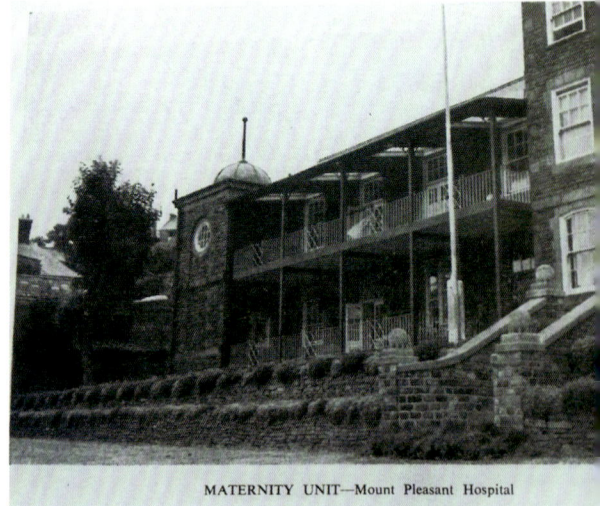

MATERNITY UNIT—Mount Pleasant Hospital

"There were 21 of us at our last reunion. At our first reunion there were about 60 of us but numbers have declined over the years.

"It's nice to keep the reunions going because it's all about friendship. It was a very nice family centred hospital and we all say if it was still open we would still be working there."

Carol, who lives in Morriston and is now a grandmother of four, worked at the unit from 1977 until it closed. She looks back with fondness on her long career.

"We enjoyed going to work. With every child you had a wonderful experience of being able to deliver new life and see the smiles on the faces of parents.

"I spent part of my childhood in a children's home and after I left Mount Pleasant I went on to support an orphanage in Zambia with my husband Graham. I love being able to help children."

When Carol was at Mount Pleasant the hours were long – midwives were expected to work 48-hour weeks – and the rules were strict.

"You never addressed senior members of staff by their Christian names and uniforms were never worn outside unless you were on district duty."

During her time as a midwife Carol worked in all areas – the delivery suite, post and ante natal, special care baby unit and domiciliary *"where we cycled to the home to deliver at all times of day and night".*

Having a baby was very different experience for the mums back then.

"At one time only the partner was allowed in the delivery room, now any immediate family member is allowed and they can take photos or even video.

"All the baby's needs used to be met by the health service when it came to providing nappies gowns and so on. Now the mother brings everything in with her."

Carol also explained that while security of newborns had always been important, during her career new measures had been introduced to ensure babies' safety.

"Back then there was one label for the arm and the foot. Now every new baby is tagged and an alarm system will go off if any cot is moved without mother's permission. There are alarms on all entry doors along with cameras to see who is coming in."

Other differences in maternity care include how babies were looked after.

"At one time the baby would be nursed in a nursery at night and the midwife would feed the baby to enable the mother to rest, unless she was breastfeeding. Now every baby stays with their mother."

Carol is looking forward to many more happy reunions with her colleagues.

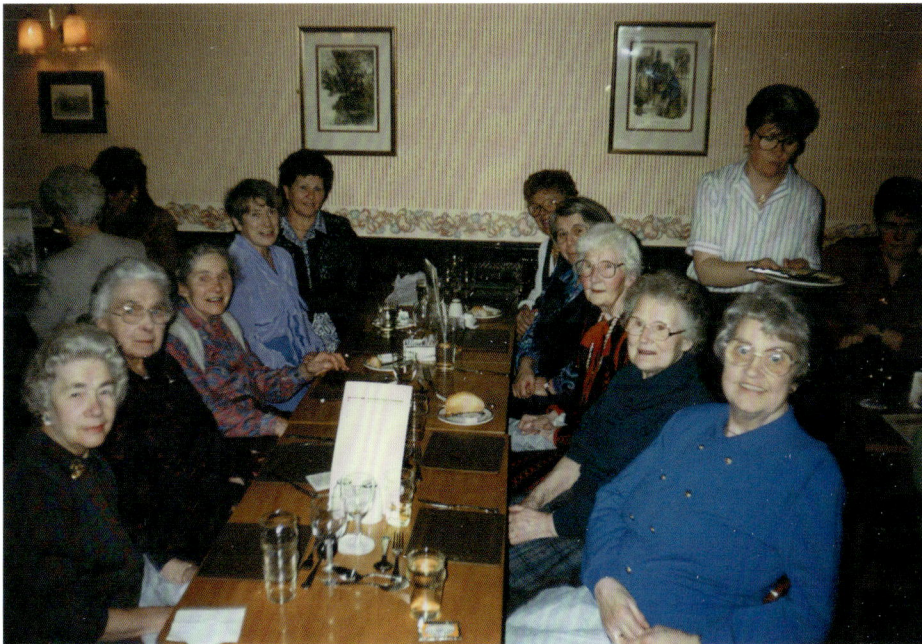

"We were all very much involved with each other. I think midwives are like that, you develop a comradeship because your job is about dealing with people.

"With every child you had a wonderful experience of being able to deliver new life and see the smiles on the faces of the parents."

One regular figure at the reunions is former director of midwifery services at Singleton hospital **Gwyneth Stewart.**

"We do still enjoy getting together, it was a very close-knit community at Mount Pleasant."

When Gwyneth started her nursing career at 16 as a care assistant at the Tumble Isolation Hospital in 1948 she was pursuing her childhood ambition – she had wanted to be a nurse since she was 10 years old.

She started her nurse training at Swansea General Hospital when she was 17. She remembers well the annual ball held at the Brangwyn Hall in Swansea when all the nurses living at Parc Beck nurses home had to ask Matron to approve their partner for the evening.

Gwyneth then went on to join the first cohort of staff to be trained at the Mount Pleasant School of Midwifery in 1954.

"It was very enjoyable training and working there."

Back then, she says it was very like *Call The Midwife* – you could walk home at 3am from a delivery quite safely, as everybody had such respect for midwives.

She remembers well how the geriatric patients at the hospital, a former work house, would be treated to special entertainment by the midwives who would perform Christmas concerts for them every year.

Later after studying for her Advanced Diploma in Midwifery, Gwyneth went on to become Chief Nursing Hospital Officer advising and supervising the closure of the Morriston maternity unit and the opening of the Singleton unit and the Special Care Baby Unit

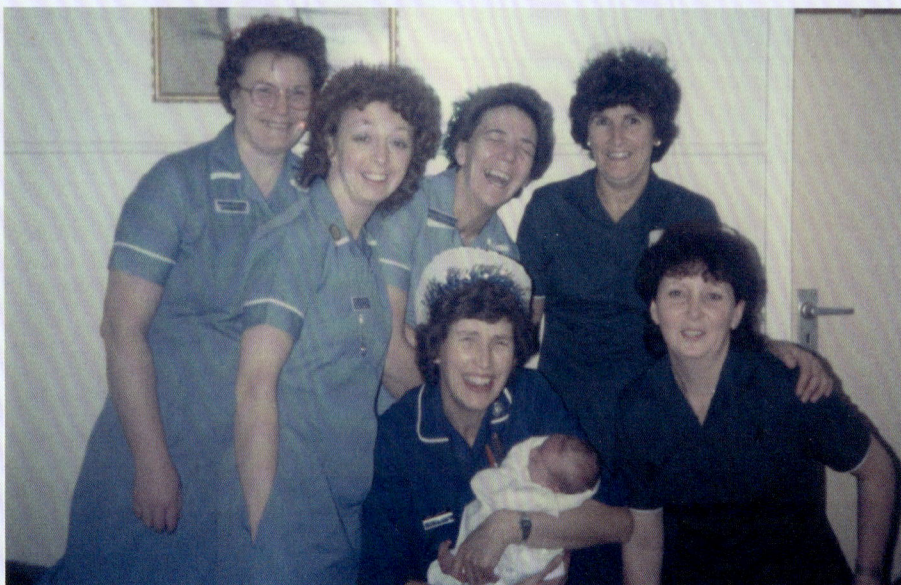

Madge Williams

When a neighbour told Madge Williams she had found her the perfect job she never dreamt she would end up doing it for 45 years.

Neonatal nurse Madge eventually retired from her role at Singleton Hospital last year after caring for newborns and their families since 1972.

But Madge, from the Swansea Valley, actually started her nursing career in 1966, training at Mount Pleasant Hospital before taking up a post on the wards at Morriston Hospital.

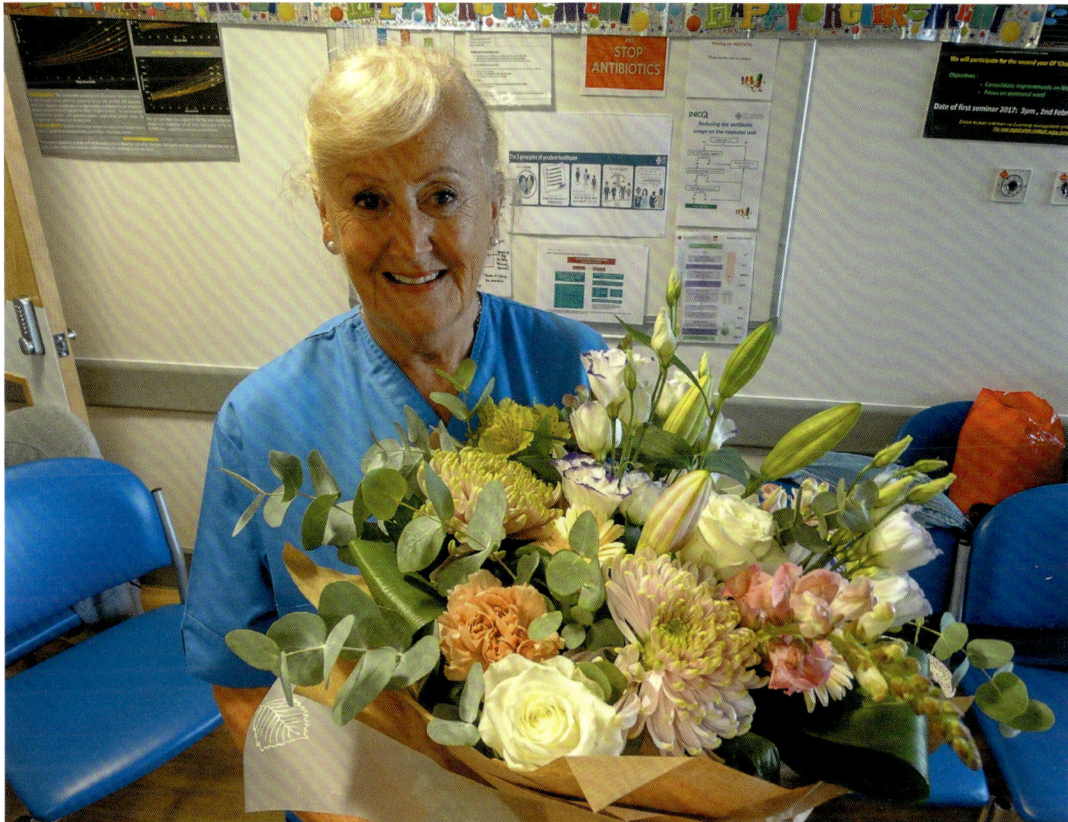

Madge retires after 45 years dedicated to neonatal care at Singleton

"I had given up work to have my first baby and a neighbour, who was a midwife, came round one day and said 'Madge, I've got you a job'.

"My son was only four months old so I just laughed but she said she was serious and that I couldn't turn it down. 'Madge, you can work any day you want, any hours you want, they are absolutely desperate for staff.'

"I had never done neonates before but she said not to worry and to take the job and that's how it started here at Singleton."

When Madge began her job the neonatal ward saw fewer premature newborns.

"It was totally different then, it wasn't such a specialised role.

"The main difference is babies born earlier now have a better chance of surviving. Technology and modern equipment have changed the job entirely."

"When I first started there were no ventilators at all, then we progressed to what was called a Gregory box which was put around the baby's head and provided oxygen. The service has really developed over the years."

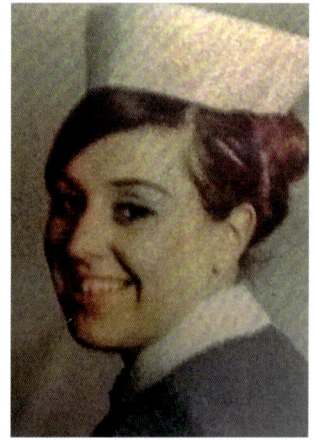

Neonatal nurse Madge Williams at the start of her career.

However despite the advances some things never change she says, including the anxiety felt by her tiny patients' families.

"I always told parents to take things second to second, minute to minute, and to remember every hour is precious.

"This ward is unique in every way – we touched families' lives and I always felt privileged to work there," she added.

"My colleagues made my career and what a wonderful career I had."

Ursula Arnold

Ursula Arnold was a student nurse when she caught the eye of a fellow trainee in the corridor of Parc Beck nurses home in Sketty who plucked up the courage to say hello to her.

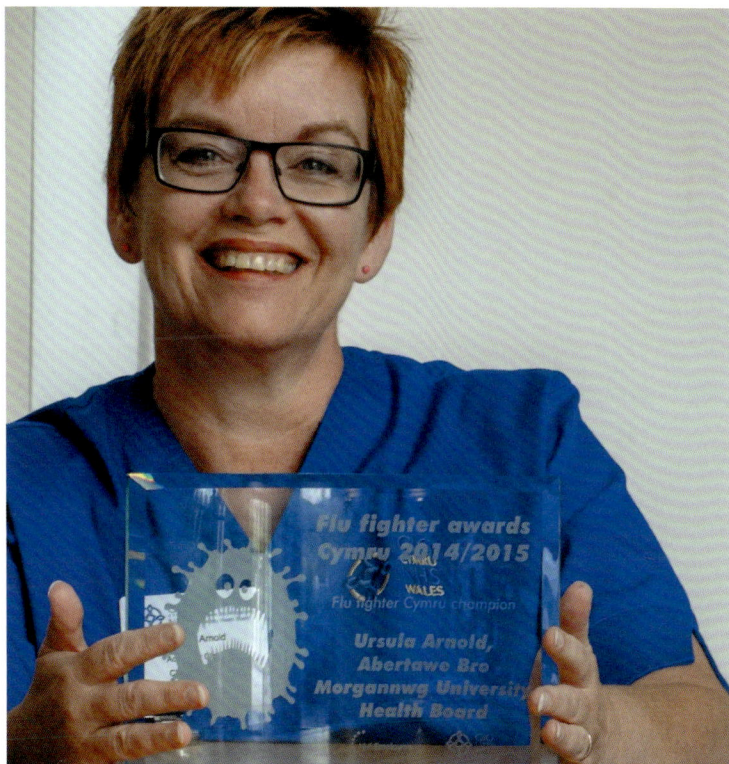

"He says I ignored him but I'm hard of hearing - that's my excuse - and Mark and I have just celebrated 30 years of marriage!"

The couple married in 1987 when they were still working at Singleton.

Ursula has fond memories of her training days at Singleton Hospital where she says she had a fantastic time and made life-long friends even though things didn't always run smoothly.

"I got sent to theatre as a student nurse on orthopaedics for a long weight but I got a long wait instead!"

Mark trained from 1984 to 1986 as an SEN and was also in the Territorial Army, going to the first Gulf war in 1991 as a medic.

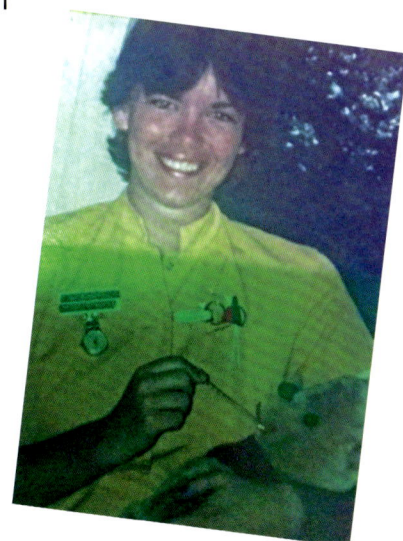

"He was on ITU in Morriston then and we had our son Tom exactly nine months after his return from the war!"

Ursula in her early years as a nurse

Ursula moved to Morriston Hospital's Emergency Department in 1993 and has been there ever since – working as a staff nurse, then a sister, then an emergency nurse practitioner (ENP).

In 2015 Ursula, was named Flu Fighter Cymru Champion of the Year for increasing the number of staff in the emergency department who have their flu vaccination every year.

She swapped the bays of ED for the bays of the Caribbean and South East Asia with a four-month stint as a ship's nurse on cruise liners in 2016-2017 but is now back working full-time as an ENP in the Emergency Department .

"I am loving being part of such a strong and dedicated team that has to work in some amazingly stressful and challenging situations, all the while attempting to support each other and give excellent care to the hundreds of patients who attend every day."

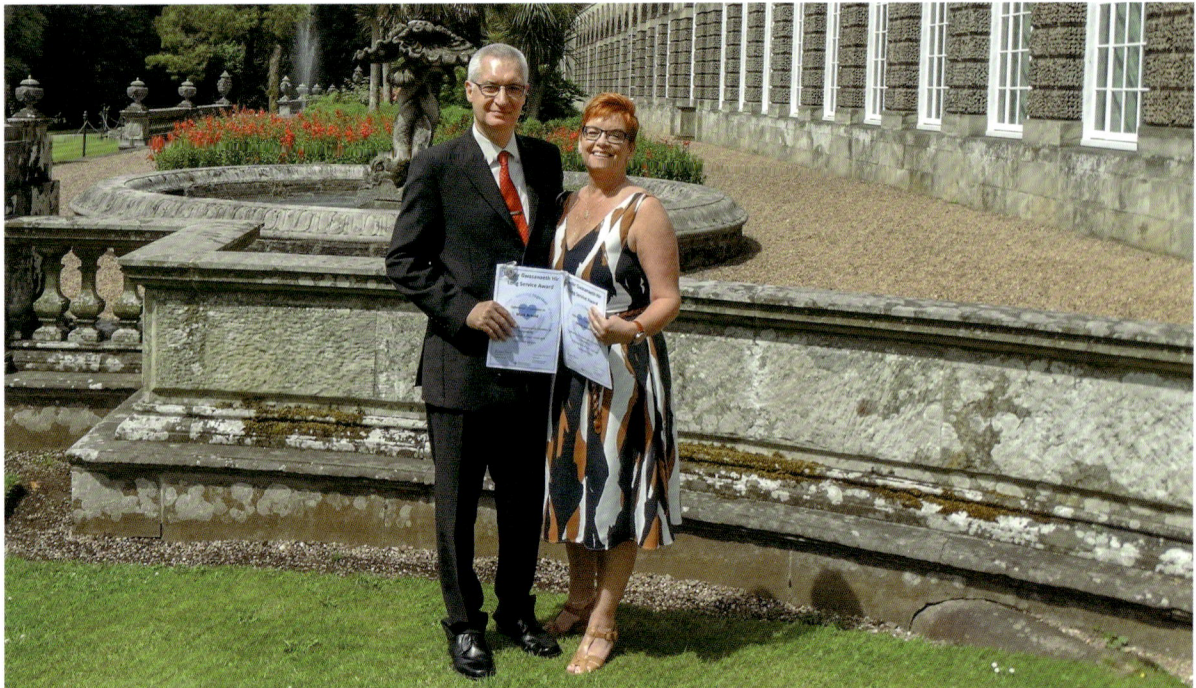

Ursula and Mark

Mark spent 16 years at NHS Direct before returning to his first love, intensive care, three years ago but was set to retire in April after 34 years with the NHS.

But he will have a while to wait before Ursula joins him by hanging up her scrubs.

"I can retire next year but am not decided yet, we shall see!"

Lynette Jenkins

A diagnosis with type 1 diabetes in 1982 was life changing for Lynette Jenkins in so many ways.

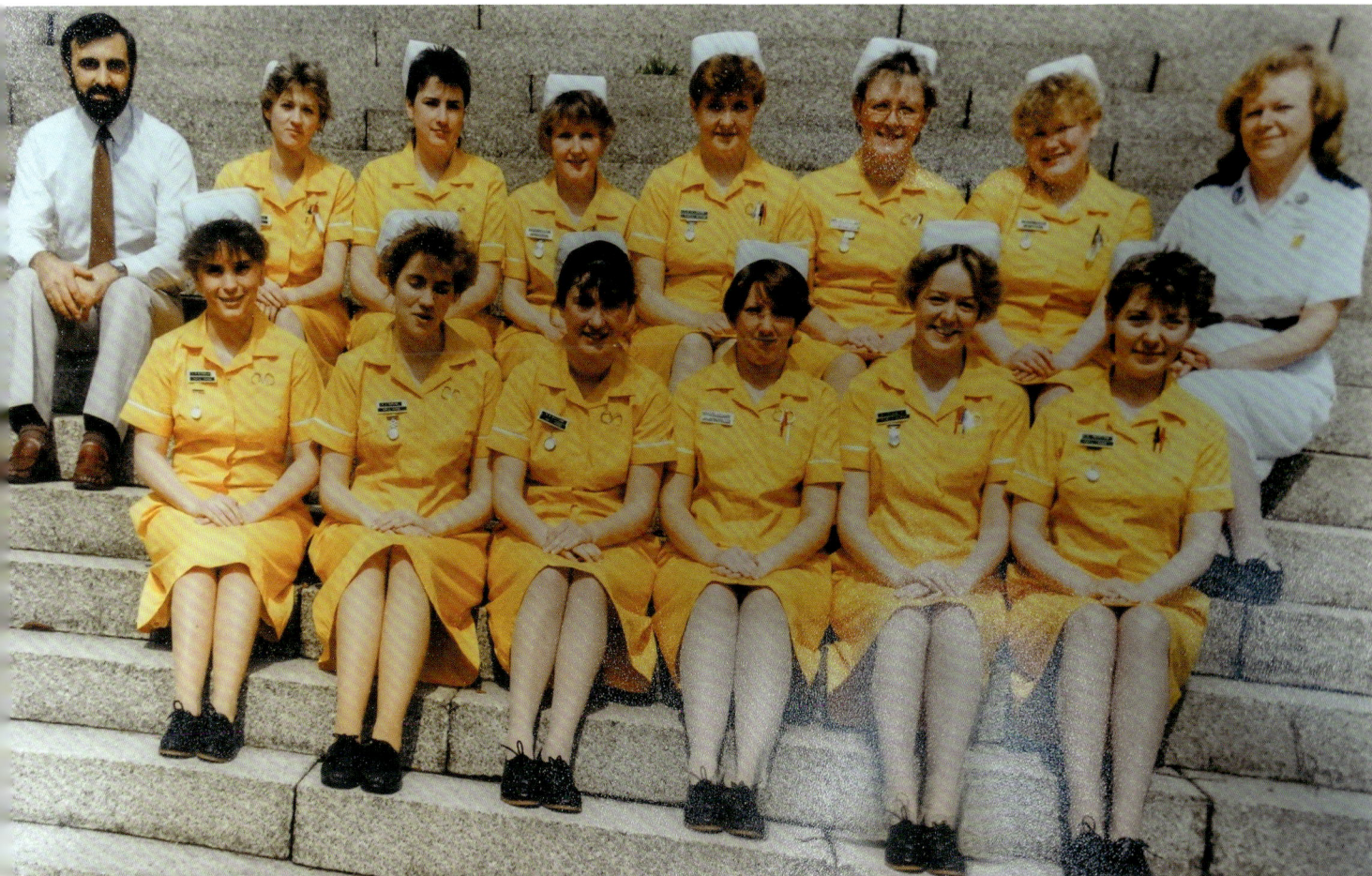

Lynette (back row, third from right) as a student nurse.

Twenty two, newlywed and working for the civil service, Lynette did not want to spend time in hospital and certainly had no interest in nursing.

But all that changed after she met nurse Nancy Kent.

It was Nancy who explained to Lynette how her condition could be managed with daily insulin injections and arranged for Lynette to become the first patient in Swansea to be treated with insulin injections at home.

"Diabetes care as we know it now was just evolving back then. For many people having diabetes meant going into hospital to be treated but I was lucky, she showed me how I could do it myself at home.

"It was this experience that gave me an interest in diabetes nursing. It was life-changing and it made me realise the other opportunities that nursing presented."

She decided it was time for a career change and started her training at Morriston Hospital, living at Parc Beck in 1986.

"I really enjoyed my time in general nursing but diabetes nursing was always my long-term goal."

At the time Nancy Kent was working at Singleton Hospital, helping to create the diabetes service that we know today.

"This was the start of it all for me. Patients were more included and there was a youth group for younger patients. The aim was to keep people from being hospitalised."

Now Lynette is senior specialist nurse who manages the diabetes service based at Morriston Hospital and she and her team are kept busy with the challenges presented by rising levels of type 2 diabetes.

The mum-of-one who has nursed in Swansea throughout her 32-year career said: *"Our ultimate goal is to keep people healthy and out of hospital and, if they do have to come into hospital, to get them home as soon as possible. It is a very important role and my journey towards it started back when I was first diagnosed."*

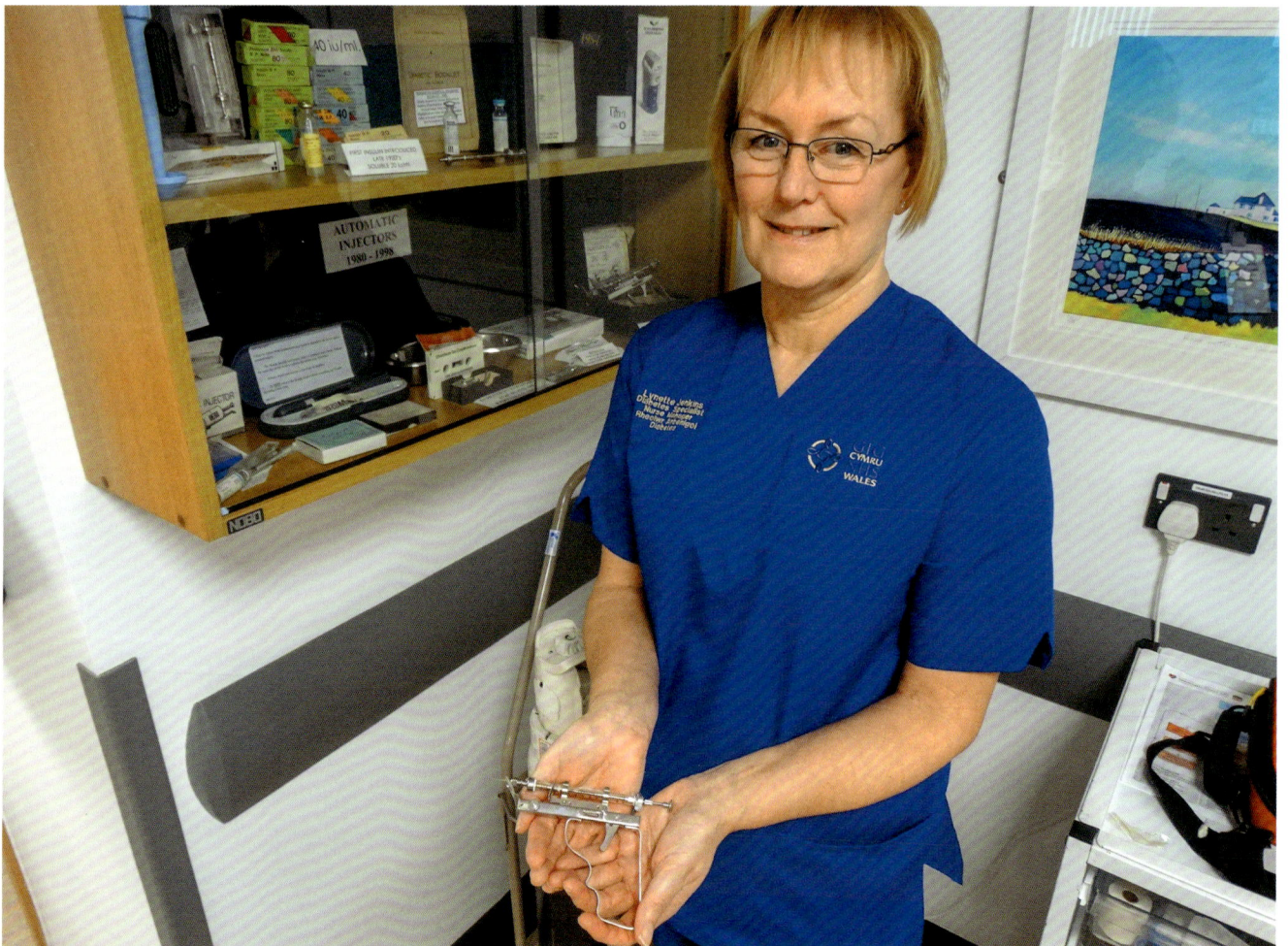

Fiona Dix

Fiona Dix's life is inextricably linked to the NHS.

A nurse since 1991, after spending time as a chronic conditions nurse in the community she is now part of the acute clinical team working out of Bonymaen Clinic in Swansea.

And while Fiona has nursing to thank for a long and satisfying career, it is also the reason her parents got together.

Her mum Enfys was a third year nurse at Morriston Hospital when she met a young Neath RFC player called Alan Dix who had been admitted after breaking his jaw in a match.

Fiona says he must have been impressed by her bedside manner during his time on the ward:

"Mum always says they had their first date in what is now the garden at Ty Olwen. They married in 1968 and are now looking forward to celebrating their golden wedding."

Enfys went on to qualify as a midwife and enjoyed a 43-year- career in the community and at Gorseinon Hospital.

But Fiona, from Clydach, says her own decision to become a nurse was not inspired by her mum's choice of profession.

"My mum was very surprised when I decided to become a nurse because I didn't like blood. She always told me not to become a nurse because you will be working when your friends are going out!"

Despite those words of warning Fiona started her training at Morriston in 1991 and went on to spend 14 years working in the hospital's ITU before swapping for life in the community.

Debbie Evans

Debbie Evans is now a diabetes specialist nurse at Morriston Hospital but she has clear memories of her days as a student nurse. She still has her first ever contract from 1980 which sees her employed at the princely sum of £2,542 a year.

"I trained as a pupil nurse and became a state enrolled nurse before converting to becoming a staff nurse. We trained in the West Glamorgan School of Nursing.

"The first six weeks were spent in the classroom being taught things like how to make beds, bedbathing and how to wash someone's hair while they were in bed! We were then let loose on the wards and from day one you were hands on.

"As new recruits to the nurses' home you had to stay on the top corridor. There were no plugs in the room and you shared a kitchen and bathroom.

"The girls used to laugh at my orange and white battery operated record player (the lid came off and was the speaker).

"I soon had the last laugh as I listened to Queen, Michael Jackson , The Police and the Bee Gees.

"We used to go to the café which was next to the red telephone box at the bottom of the hospital and have pie and beans!

Debbie's training contract dated 1980.

Debbie is pictured with friends during her training placement at Mount Pleasant in 1980.

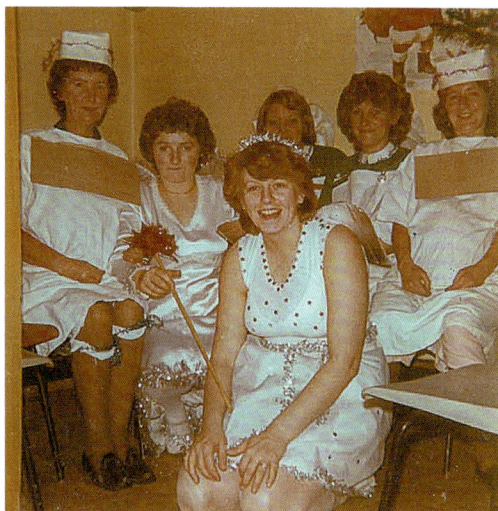

"I spent 16 years working in Singleton before becoming a nurse in the Diabetes Centre in Morriston. I was employed by Jackie Dent who pushed and encouraged me to do the conversion to staff nurse. She then encouraged me to take on the role of diabetes specialist nurse.

"If it wasn't for her I wouldn't be where I am today. Coincidentally my grandfather was a diabetic patient of Jackie's and she also nursed my gran when she died and was a patient on Jackie's ward.

"Unfortunately she passed away in 2016 but I have always been grateful to her."

Debbie pictured at the Brangwyn Hall for presentation of certificates.

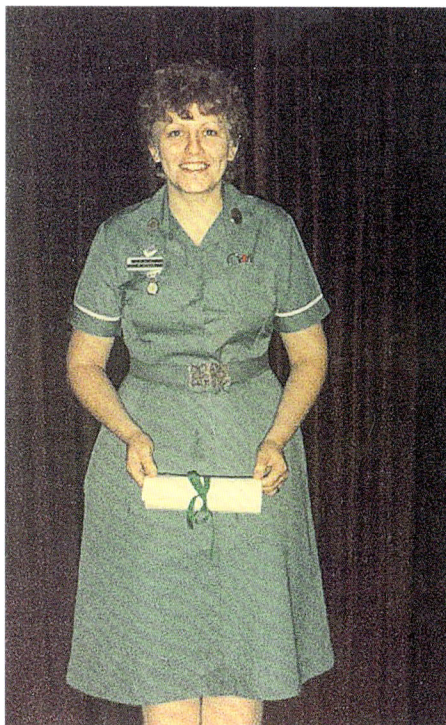

Jennifer Torkington

A long-serving member of Princess of Wales Hospital's cardiology team has seen quite a few changes since she started her career in the early 1980s.

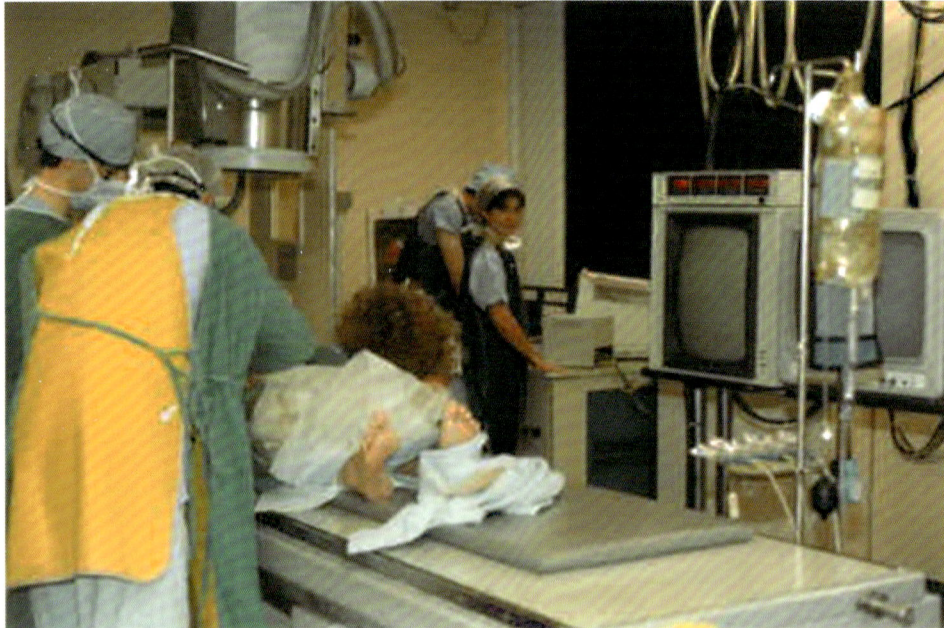

Jennifer, at machine on right, pictured at work in the early stages of her physiology career

Jennifer Torkington has worked as a cardiac physiologist for 34 years – most of them in the Bridgend hospital.

Cardiac physiology involves the diagnosis and assessment of heart disease, although Jennifer's role extends beyond that.

She began her career in 1983 in the University Hospital of Wales, moving to Princess of Wales Hospital in 1990.

When she first arrived in Bridgend there were four cardiology members of staff and no echocardiogram machines, pacemaker service or cardiac catheterization investigations.

"I am delighted to say we now have 20 members of staff and six echocardiogram machines and other services – so we have come a long way in my 34 years of service."

Cardiac physiology involves the diagnosis and assessment of heart disease – though Jennifer's role now extends beyond that.

In 2012, Jennifer and colleague Hugh Pascoe set up a physiologist-led valve clinic so patients did not have to be seen in a general cardiology clinic.

More recently they also set up a solely physiology-led stress echocardiography service – the only one of its kind in South Wales.

Both initiatives improved patient care and reduced waiting times.

Jennifer has received an NHS long service award, while last year she was presented with the Lynda McGurk Award for Welsh Cardiac Physiologist of the Year *(pictured below)*.

> *"I didn't even know I'd been nominated. I was shocked but I was also extremely honoured that my colleagues felt I was worth nominating."*

Jennifer said the award had only been possible thanks to the support she had received from all her colleagues.

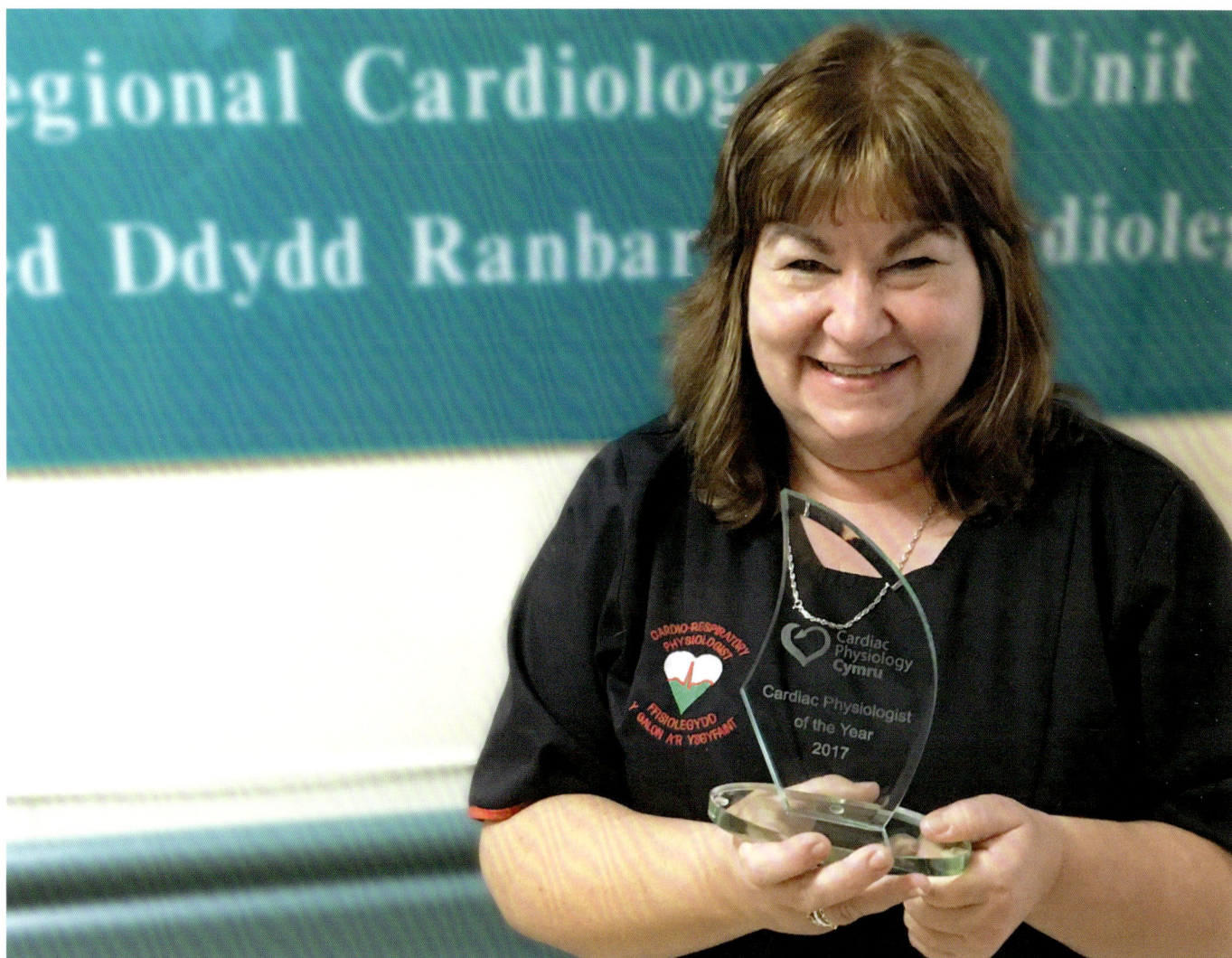

Amanda Hopkins

A serious accident led Swansea mum Amanda Hopkins down a very different career path.

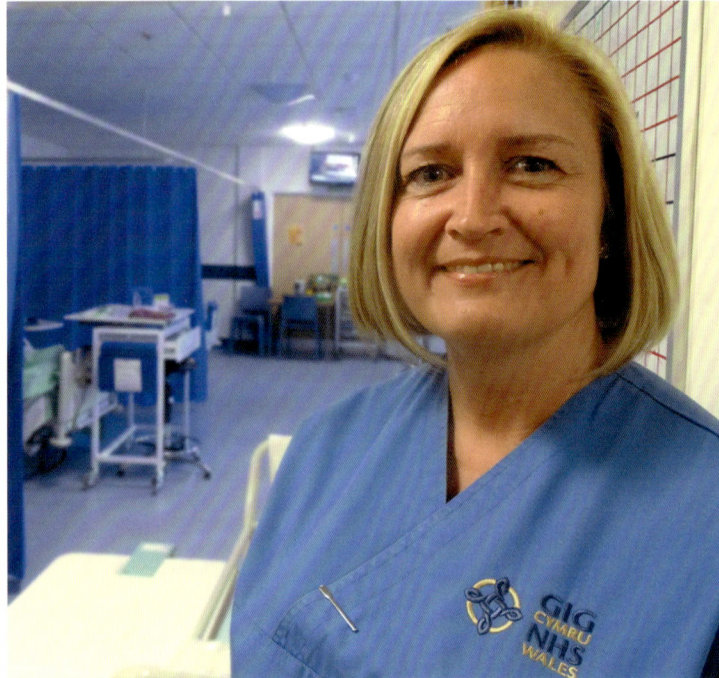

Amanda suffered multiple injuries including a fractured skull, a broken leg and two broken arms.

It happened while she was crossing the road in her home town of Pontarddulais in 2006.

She was resuscitated twice, once on the roadside after paramedics arrived, and again in Morriston Hospital's Emergency Department.

"I'm really lucky to be here today. It was touch and go for a while.

"After surgery I was in ITU for a couple of days, then transferred to Ward J where I spent about another six weeks. Then I went home in a wheelchair with a collar on for three months.

"I had lots of physio after that and more operations – I think I've had 11 operations in total.

Mother-of-two Amanda had worked in a bank for 16 years. But she was so impressed with the care she received in Morriston Hospital that she decided to retrain as a nurse.

This despite the fact that, following her accident, she'd been told she would be unable to work full-time in any job that kept her on her feet, while her head injury meant she was unlikely to be able to study for a degree.

Amanda said:

"I finished with my job and applied to do an access course in Gorseinon College.

"After that I applied for university, got my nursing degree in 2014 and here I am today, doing 12-hour shifts on the ward."

Amanda, who works in Ward T, one of Morriston's surgical wards, said she had no regrets about her career switch.

"You get a lot of gratitude from people in their time of need, not just from patients but their families too.

"After the accident I was out of it for about a fortnight but my family couldn't praise the staff enough for the support they had.

"My children were aged five and eight at the time, and it was very difficult for them.

"So I think that when people come in for surgery it's the support you give the families as much as the patients.

"I experienced it and my family experienced it, and it's nice to be able to give it back."

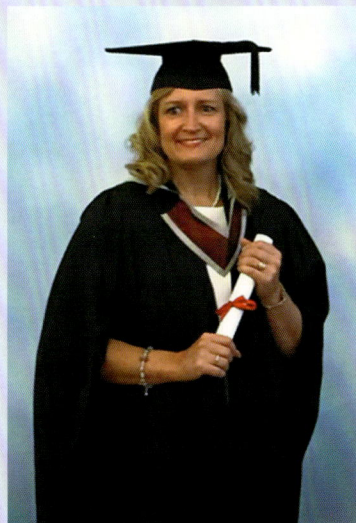

A proud day as Amanda gains her degree

Parties, pantos and ghosts

From consultants to carpenters, receptionists to radiographers – the workforce keeping the NHS running has been many and varied.

Here some of our staff – past and present – share their memories of their times, from ghostly goings on in the dead of night to new techniques that helped transform patient care .

Jayne Caparros

Lower the lights, cue the music and raise the curtain – it's panto time!

A regular highlight in the calendar for staff at Singleton Hospital was the annual panto, staged by the enthusiastic members of its Amateur Dramatic Society.

Drawn from departments across the site, the members would take to the stage in the old Outpatients' Department Waiting Hall and perform to packed houses.

The society put on its first production in 1968 – Cinderella – and it continued until the early 1990s performing not only an annual panto but also variety shows and plays.

Staff nurse Jayne Ellis was an enthusiastic member during the society's final years.

Now Jayne Caparros, she still works at Singleton as research delivery manager in the Cancer Institute and has very fond memories of her days treading the boards.

"The stage area was where Costa Coffee is now and we had fantastic facilities. They were wonderful productions with great lighting and sets - all very professionally done.

"We would use the rooms in the outpatients' corridor as changing rooms and for make-up."

She explained that the society was a long-standing part of Singleton history.

"When I joined I was a student nurse and the leading light was Pat Francombe and before that it had been Fran Purchase. I was a student working in coronary care at the time and my friend and I thought we'd have a go at it."

Jayne, who went on to co-direct Peter Pan in 1990, said: *"I remember when we did Cinderella in 1988,*

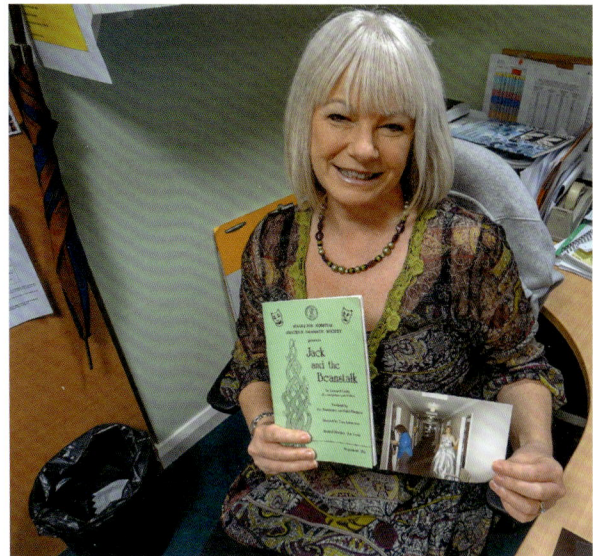

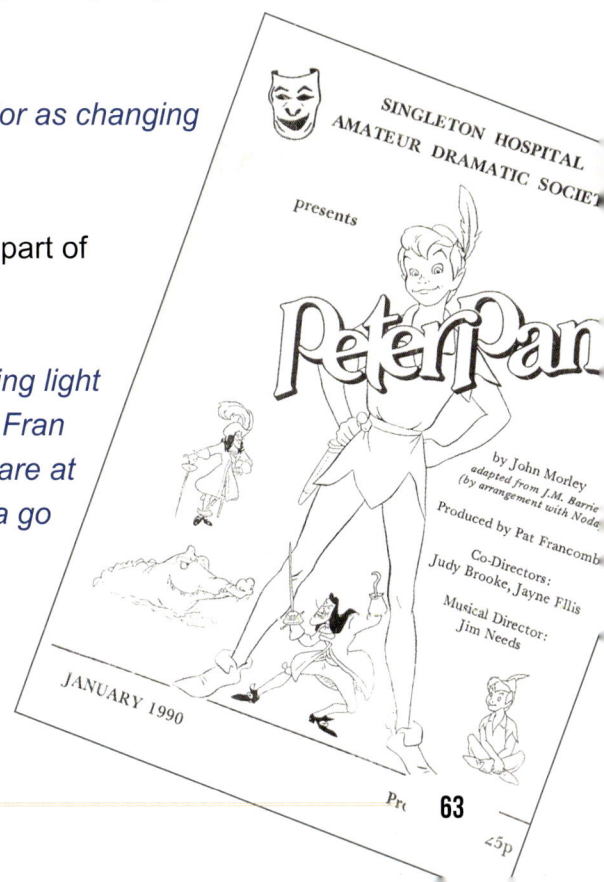

SINGLETON HOSPITAL
AMATEUR DRAMATIC SOCIETY

presents

Peter Pan

by John Morley
adapted from J.M. Barrie
(by arrangement with Noda)

Produced by Pat Francombe

Co-Directors:
Judy Brooke, Jayne Ellis

Musical Director:
Jim Needs

JANUARY 1990

25p

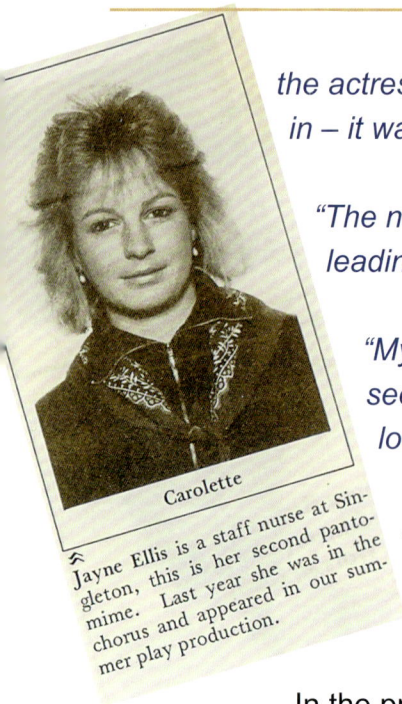

the actress who was going to play Dandini was off sick so I had to step in – it was amazing.

"The next year I was Princess Carolette in Jack and the Beanstalk, the leading female role.

"My husband Elliot, who is a radiographer at Singleton, remembers seeing me on stage before we had met - you could say he fell in love with me from afar!"

Carolette

Jayne Ellis is a staff nurse at Singleton, this is her second pantomime. Last year she was in the chorus and appeared in our summer play production.

Jayne, who has kept pictures and programmes from the shows, explained that the society folded when the stage space was no longer available for its shows.

In the programme for the production of Peter Pan in 1990 the society's honorary life president Frank Tromans wrote: "The Health Authority's decision to utilise the stage space for a fundraising development or, to use the current jargon 'income generation' has been received with dismay by the Society whose members have already felt that their activities formed a serious contribution to the corporate life of the hospital.

"I refuse to believe that the Singleton Hospital Dramatic Society with a 23-year-history of enthusiasm and achievement will allow itself to be defeated by the set-back."

Sadly it was but it will always be remembered fondly by Jayne Caparros and many others.

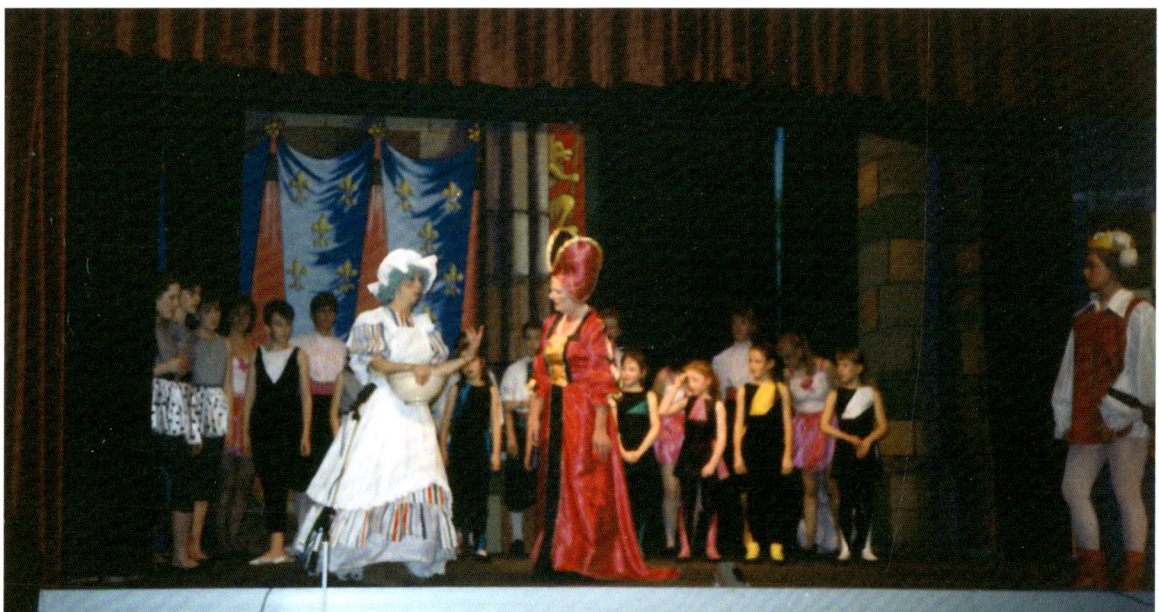

"I loved being involved – it was one big family, a real team spirit!"

Julie Nedin

Julie Nedin, who retired from her role in ABMU's Nutrition and Dietetic Service in 2016, saw many changes during her 34-year career.

"Over 30 years ago when I trained and started working in the NHS, the numbers in my profession were tiny.

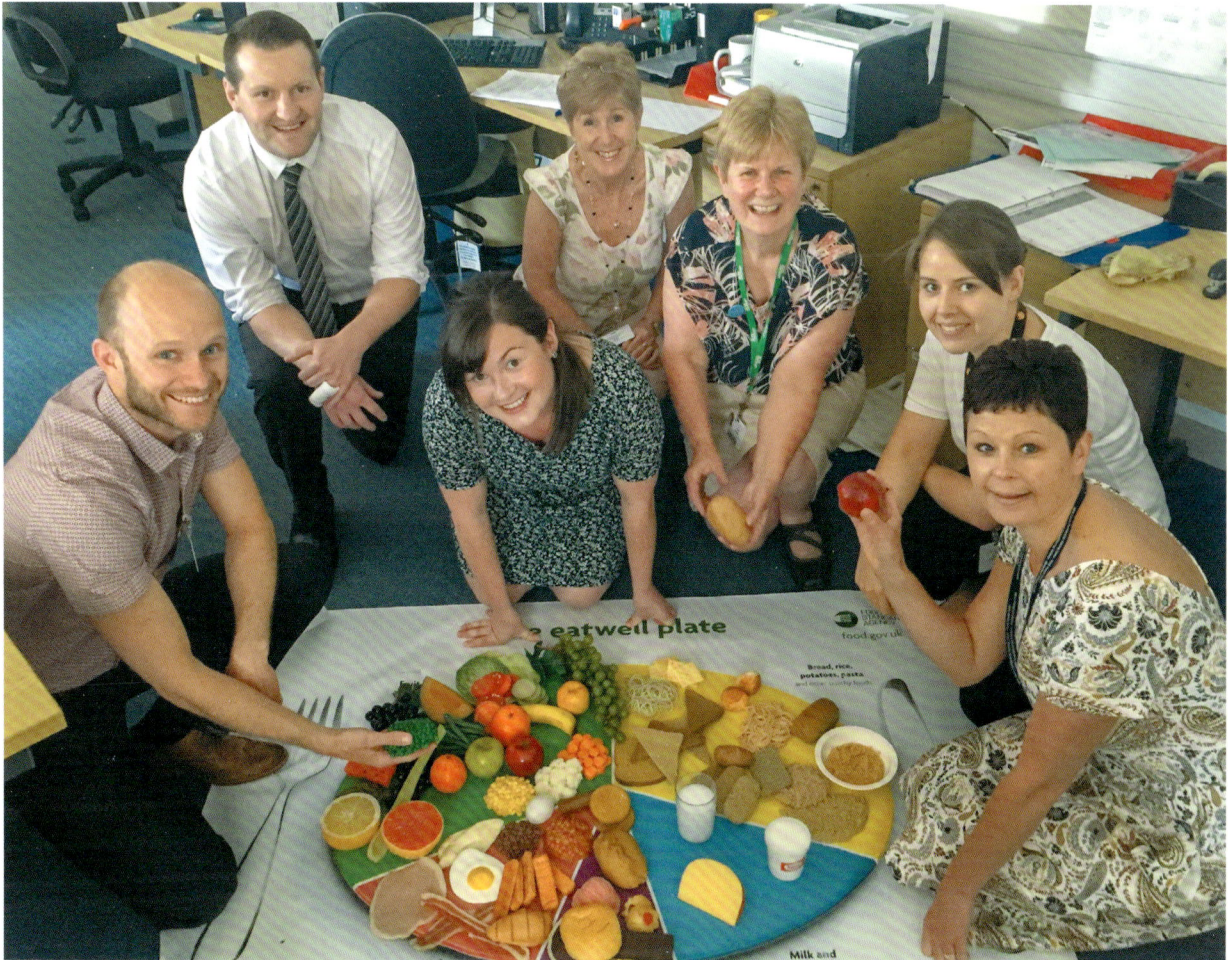

Julie Nedin (third from right) and colleagues demonstrate how to eat well

"It's still quite small compared to the numbers of doctors, nursing and some therapy staff, but I feel privileged to have worked through a time of growth and development.

"It's amazing to look back at what we achieved both in numbers and specialities.

"Medical staff understood the value of support from dietetics but it was, and still is, hard work proving our worth to gain funding. I'm thinking of fields like renal, paediatrics, public health, gastroenterology and critical care, but even our 'bread and butter' work (excuse the pun!) of diabetes, nutritional support and weight management badly needed improvement.

"But there have been marvellous initiatives and better techniques have been developed to help individuals find solutions to the challenges they face living with a chronic condition.

"I'm pleased there has been a big increase in cross-professional team work in the past 20 years. By working with all parties-medically trained or not -we have the only chance of finding solutions to the challenges that face our patients and staff.

"Areas of food and nutrition touch everyone and have to be everyone's responsibility.

"The dramatic change in technology over the years has helped and hindered working life. We don't have to travel to have a conversation with a number of people at once anymore but misuse of emails has resulted in more time spent at desks and less talking when that's what is really needed. They are not as efficient as we've been led to believe!

"What has caused me the most amusement when looking back has been two documents dating back to 1980s which illustrate the monumental change in our thoughts over the decades."

The first was a discussion paper, *Can Computers Be Used in Dietetics?*, the second a booklet called *Computer Guide for Dietitians.*

"At the point when I was retiring I showed staff these documents and found the reactions quite telling. The older set of staff thought it was really funny but younger staff looked really confused. So much a part of their life has that technology been that they could not be expected to know that there was a time before computers!"

Yvonne Watkins

Yvonne Watkins is now ABMU's laundry linen manager but she began her career a fresh-faced teenager back in July 1977 in the laundry at Mount Pleasant Hospital.

" When I walked in that first day I was given a very large, dark green wraparound overall. It was like something worn by ladies in a munitions factory in a wartime film, not very appealing to a fashion-conscious 16-year-old.

My abiding memory of that day was all the ladies had their hair in rollers with a scarf tied around their head and everyone looked like Hilda Ogden from Coronation Street.

In those days the work was extremely hard. On a Friday morning I remember having to starch and press thousands of nurses' caps as every nurse had to have a pristine white cap.

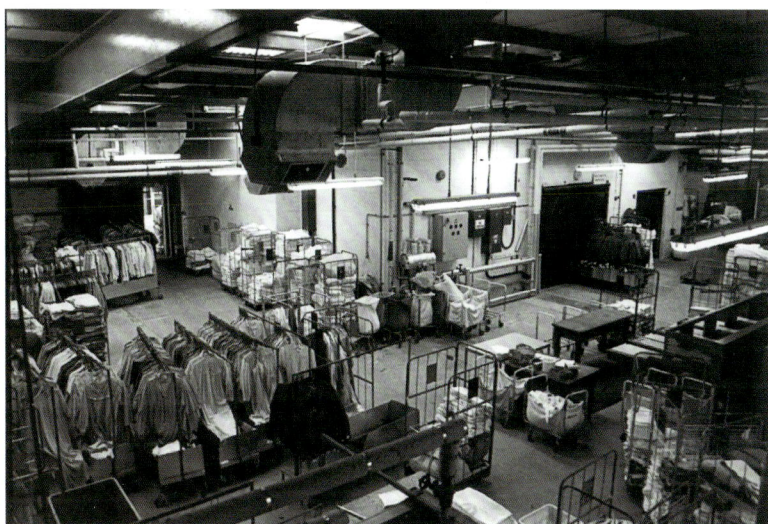

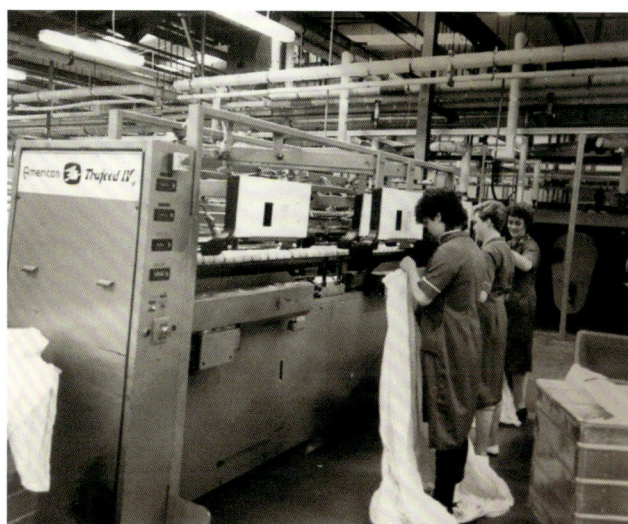

During the 1970s there was less automation so linen had to be pressed and folded by hand. I've no idea how we managed to supply the hospitals with enough linen and can only assume they weren't as busy as they are today.

Back then there were many small laundries dotted around at Mount Pleasant, Cefn Coed, Hill House, Swansea General and Neath General hospitals. In the early 1980s it was decided to shut these down and centralise laundry operations at one place – so was born the Central Laundry.

We all came over from the small laundries to have a look around the new plant before it officially opened. I remember how amazing and huge it all seemed and the fact that the toilets were inside (at Mount Pleasant there was a shared male/female toilet outside with a corrugated plastic sheet for the roof).

New, up-to-date machinery was installed and we couldn't get over the fact that machines were able to do so much of the work we used to have to do by hand. There were machines that pressed and folded all the linen - it was unbelievable.

After that we couldn't wait to move there and have these machines doing all the work. We all thought we were in for the life of Riley and within a few weeks Central Laundry had officially opened and we had transferred.

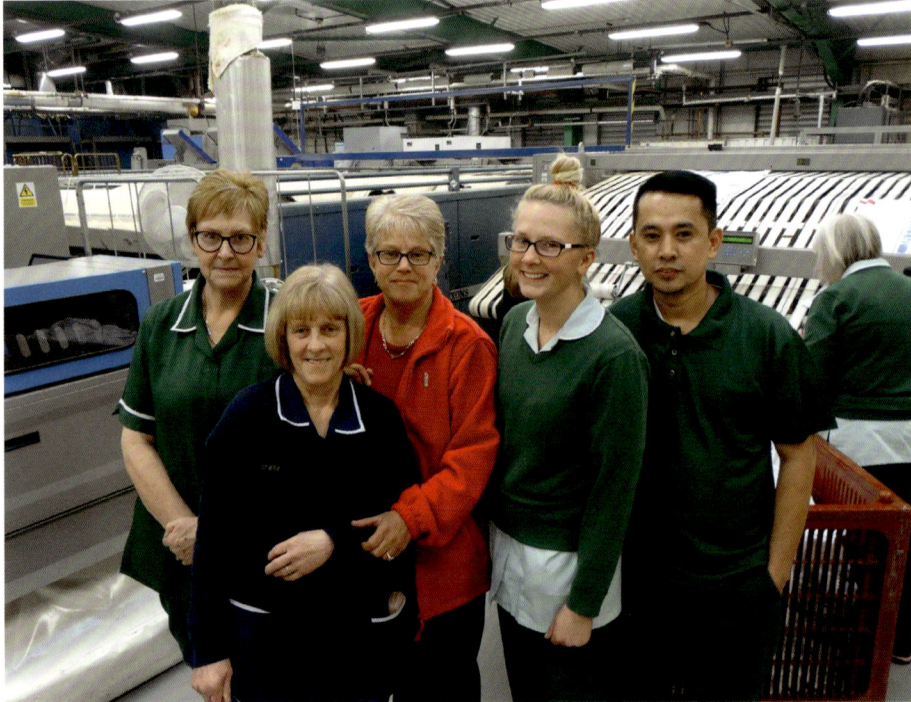

Some of today's central laundry staff: Linda Morgan, Sheila Courtney, Yvonne Watkins, Hayley Watts and Eric Valdeviezo.

Because there was so many staff the health board put on a bus to pick us all up each morning and take us home. This was great and we had bingo on the journey into work most days. But it wasn't so good for the health board though as our driver would wait for each person to get on the bus (even if they slept late). We rarely got to work on time, but we never lost any money as it wasn't our fault the bus was always late.

This next period proved very difficult. We had staff from a few different laundries all lumped together with everyone thinking their way of doing things was best, and it did take a good year before we began to think of ourselves as one team and a Central Laundry workforce.

After starting in the Central Laundry to say we were overstaffed would be an understatement as we now had machines to do all the work we previously had to do by hand. I think we were about 60 staff at the start, but as time went on colleagues who finished weren't replaced.

Although the machines were doing more of the work, the hospitals were getting larger, busier and wanting more linen so within a few years that life of Riley became a distant memory!

Machinery was now capable of doing labour intensive and heavy manual handling tasks. When we first started at Central Laundry we had individual washing machines and tumble dryers but the mid 1980s saw the development of the new all-singing, all-dancing washing machine called a CBW, a Continuous Batch Washer. In 1986 one of these incredible machines was purchased for the Central Laundry.

The one we currently have will drop a 50kg load of clean linen every three minutes.

In the 1980s many hospital services were put out to tender and lots of NHS laundries were shut down with their work taken over by outside companies.

In the 70s and early 80s the NHS laundries were far superior but this changed as private laundries invested more in machinery and somewhere in the fast-moving automation of plants the NHS laundries got left behind.

There are some private plants now washing millions of pieces of linen each week with fewer staff than it took us to wash 20,000 pieces back in the 1970s.

Now here we are in 2018, another year when the laundry team – like all staff working in the NHS – face tremendous challenges. And although I celebrate 41 years in the laundry this year, I am still waiting to have my life of Riley! **"**

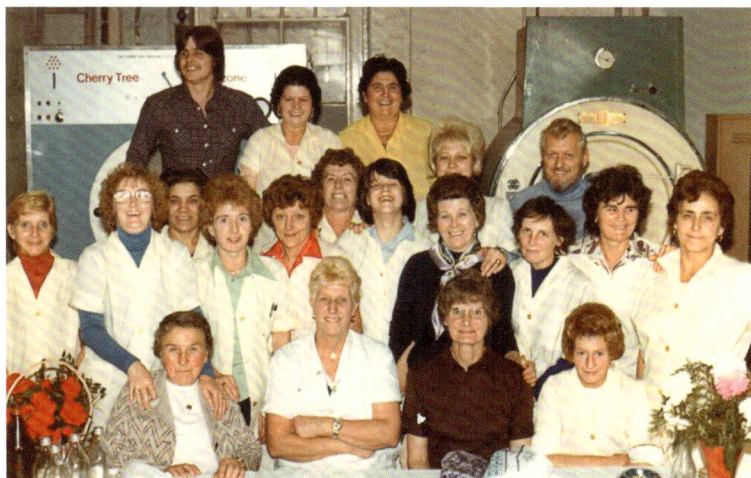

... and some of their counterparts from yesteryear.

Mike Cratchley

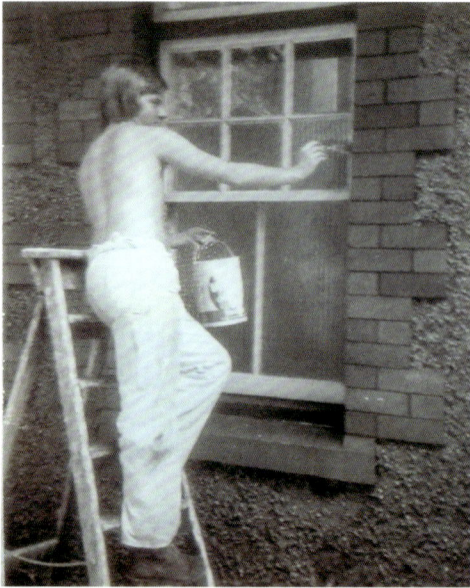

Mike in action at Convalescent Homes 26th June 1975 age 18

Estates officer **Mike Cratchley** clocked up 45 years working with the NHS before retiring in April 2017.

He first signed up as an apprentice painter and decorator in 1972 before he turned 16 and went on to become a building services officer.

Over the years his various roles in maintenance took him to all the hospitals and many of ABMU's clinics and health centres – some of which many colleagues might not remember.

"Stouthall convalescent home in Gower had the most beautiful gardens, as did Llwynderw House in West Cross," he recalled.

"My job has let me see different perspectives on life because it has brought me into contact with staff in every department.

"I am a great believer in first impressions - if a hospital looks well maintained, from a patient's perspective, it is going to give them some confidence in the service it offers. They can relax because they know they are going to be looked after. Those small things are all part of the bigger picture."

Mike, of Skewen, retired in 2017, and now he and wife Mary enjoy spending time with their family and six grandchildren.

He still has very happy memories of his years working in the NHS.

"Over my 44 years and 8 months in the NHS, I worked and liaised with a wide range of staff - from cleaners to surgeons - and every discipline in between. I enjoyed my time and my career in the NHS – but I was happy and ready to take early retirement."

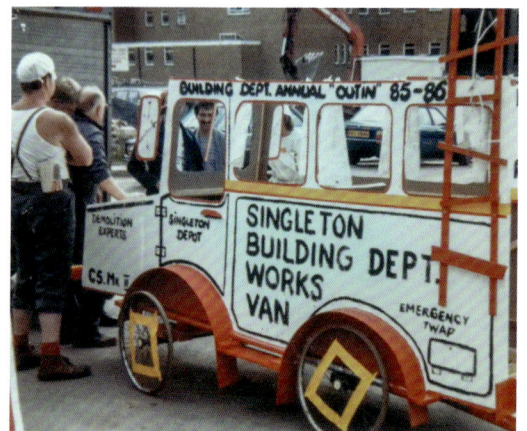

Taken in the early eighties. The Building Dept did many sponsored bed and pram pushes for Singleton.

As the son of a docker, it was presumed he would follow in his father's footsteps but Mike had the opportunity to stay on with the NHS after his apprenticeship ended.

"My father encouraged me and I progressed to charge hand and then foreman. But then I decided I wanted to get a lot more out of life and got my building qualifications eventually becoming an estates officer."

Over the years his various roles saw him carrying out in-depth building and engineering surveys of all properties owned by the then West Glamorgan Health Authority and was responsible for building maintenance issues for hospitals and ambulance centres throughout the region.

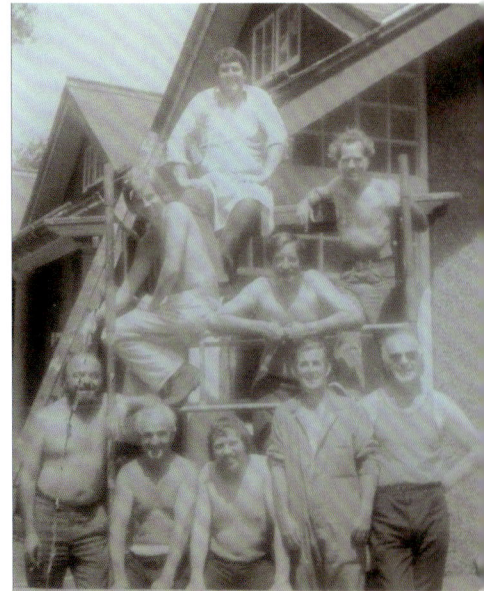
Maintainance team poses for the camera

"We had contractors dealing with every site, I really got to know everywhere very well.

"When Craig y Nos Hospital was open in the Swansea Valley we had to look after that. It was such a long way from Swansea and we only had one van then and if we had to go up there it meant the van was out of action all day.

"So when we had work to do up there the van used to deliver equipment and tools the day before then members of the team had to catch a bus up there to carry out the work and a bus home."

Mike added:

"Fairwood Hospital was always fantastic. Quite often when you would be working over there, because it was so close to Swansea Airport, you would get big RAF transporter planes on training exercises passing just a couple of hundred feet above the hospital. It was a spectacular sight."

Some more of Mike's memories ...

The Grey Lady

" By the late 1970s the wards at the old Swansea General Hospital had been closed and front part had been turned into offices. Working there one morning Doug the security man - a well-known hospital character – told us what had happened to him the night before.

At the time the hospital had a problem with break-ins and vandalism so Doug, who had two large pet Alsatians, volunteered to patrol the closed wards and the grounds during late evenings to deter thieves and vandals.

It seemed to work for a while until late one night, while out on patrol, Doug was walking down the main corridor when suddenly both dogs started whining, whimpering and crouched on the floor.

They both refused to move any further and while Doug was looking at the dogs he suddenly felt very cold and the hair stood up on the back of his neck. As the dogs still would not move he had to physically drag them away from the area.

He later told us that every night on patrol after this both dogs refused to go into that corridor again.

We were later told by a former matron at hospital that there had been sightings of a ghost who walked the wards during the night. It was thought it was the ghost of a ward sister who died in suspicious circumstances. She was dressed in the same type of uniform as Florence Nightingale and was called "The Grey Lady".

Doug was certain that the dogs saw the Grey Lady that night. **"**

Painting the outside of Singleton Hospital, summer 1984

" During the summer of of 1984 we painted the front, rear and side elevations of Singleton Hospital using cradles.

The cradles were approximately 12 feet long with guard rails all around and two electric motors on each end - enabling us to climb and descend.

This cradle was suspended from two cables on outriggers situated on the roof of the hospital and the cables were 10mm thick (the width of your little finger). The motors were powered via a very long cable that reached to the top of the hospital roof.

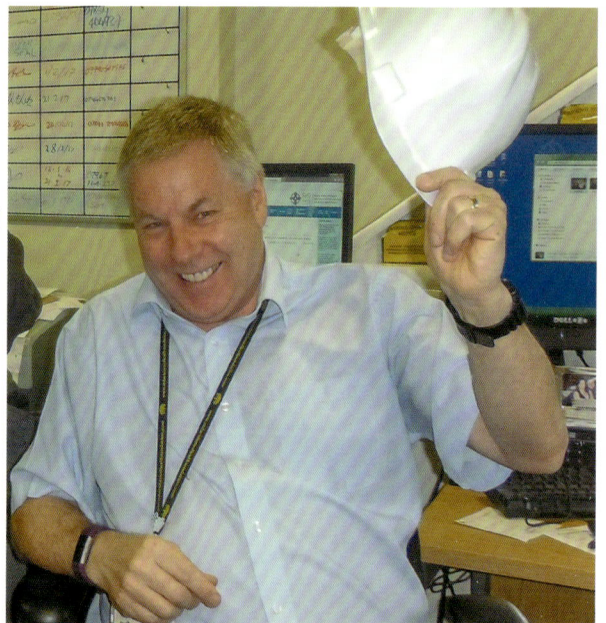

Mike shortly before his retirement.

We had been given only an hour of training before embarking on this mammoth task (it was fortunate we weren't afraid of heights as the building is over 100ft.) We were constantly told by our over-zealous boss at the time that the paint specification had to be adhered to as it was a costly job (even though the work was carried out by the hospital decorators rather than painting contractors).

I explained many times to him that I was a fully qualified decorator and supervisor and we would adhere to the specification. He said he would be fully inspecting our work after every drop - a group of windows from top to bottom.

After the completion of the first drop I took him up in the cradle to just below the very top.

He looked very frightened as I stated that he should not look down, only at the platform we were standing on.

He did the fastest inspection I have ever seen and said he was ready to return to terra firma. As we were descending the cradle lurched and jumped and was followed by a loud bang with sparks flying everywhere.

It turned out one of the patients opened a window to see what was going on, this in turn snagged the cable, causing it to snap with sparks flying as it was still live.

This led to the cradle lurching and jumping before grinding to a halt.We were stuck 75ft up without power and unable to move.

We hadn't been trained in emergency descents as the cradle company didn't think it necessary. We remained in this position for around three hours as the cradle company representative had to come from Manchester to instruct us on using the emergency descend brakes.

Needless to say our overzealous boss never inspected any further work, leaving us to get on with the job (and get a fantastic suntan during our summer heatwave!). 99

Brian Williams

Brian Williams is now an estates engineer at Cefn Coed
Hospital but he started out as a porter at Mount Pleasant
Hospital back in the early 1980s

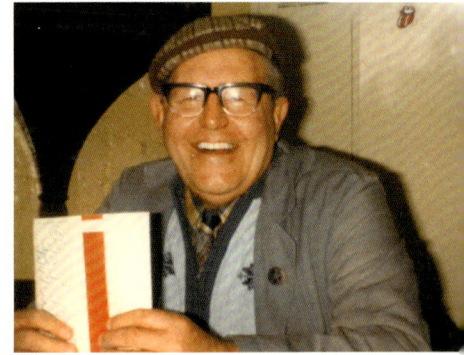

*"The porters' Christmas party was notorious. They were
held in the porters' mess and the porters used to start
brewing wine for it in September in loads of demijohns.*

Porter Bob Pratt
enjoys one of the parties

*"We used to buy shorts and beers and doctors, nurses
and all staff groups would come.. In the end management closed it down
on the grounds it wasn't fair to the other staff who had to work that night."*

Brian said the porters were also very fond of a four-legged member of their
team, pet pooch Nobbie.

*"Nobbie would be there 24 hours a day and used to follow the porters on
jobs.*

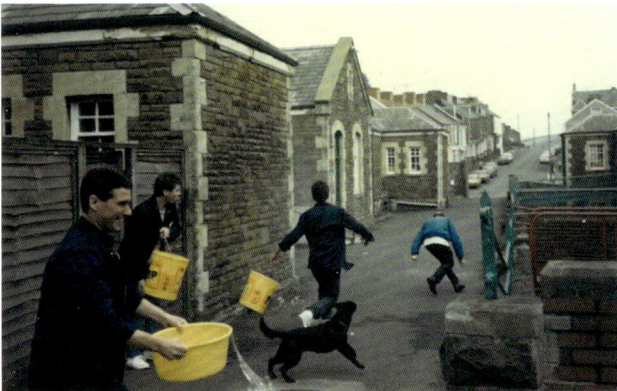

Nobbie chasing staff

*"At night if they had to go to the
mortuary they used to send the dog
in first as the porters would be too
scared.*

*"Every lunch time the porters would
all go to the Mountain Dew Inn, just
up the hill in Mount Pleasant and
the dog would go.*

*"If they were ever too busy and couldn't get there by about 2pm there
would be a call from the landlord saying 'Nobbie's here, can you send
someone to get him please?' The dog would go on his own anyway!"*

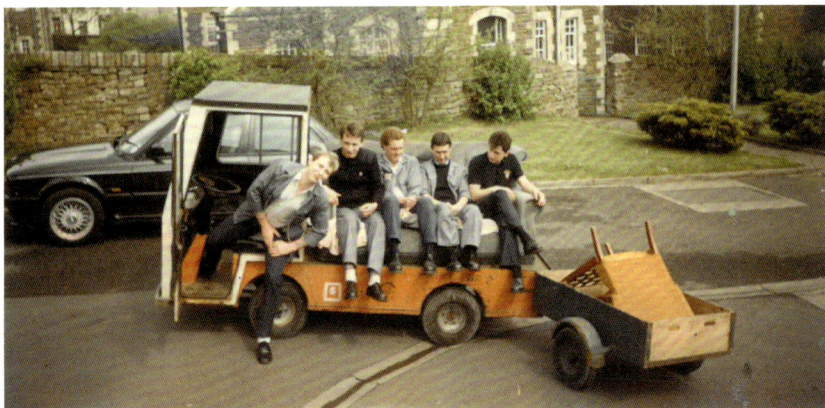

Russell Williams, Brian Williams, Tony Snell, Tony Mort, Mark Walsh

Margaret James

When Margaret James finished her final shift as a receptionist at Swansea's Central Clinic she wasn't just leaving a workplace she was also saying goodbye to her old home.

She was just a teenager back in 1968 when her father Irfon Morgan took up his job as caretaker of the building in Orchard Street and moved his family into its top floor flat.

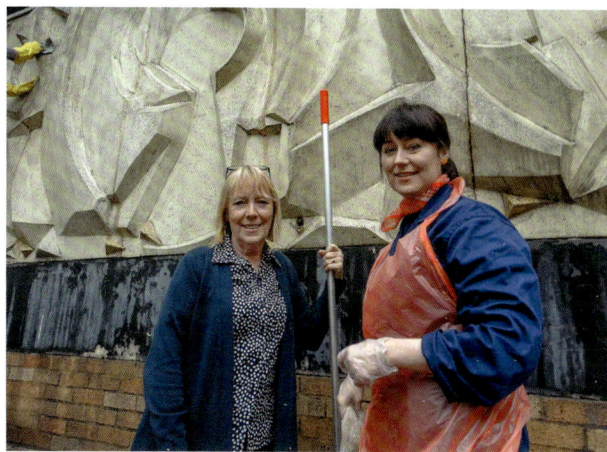

Margaret and daughter Catrin clean the Central Clinic mural

"I remember living there with my mum and dad very well, it was a lovely flat, very roomy and we were very happy," said Margaret who retired last year from her dual roles as receptionist with the Community Dental Service and Community Mental Health Service.

Margaret first began working for the health service back in 1969 but didn't have far to go to work. Her job saw her manning the reception desk at Central Clinic.

"It was so easy, I just rolled down the stairs and straight to work. My mum Gwennie worked for Swansea Council then and was based in the building too so all three of us were working under the same roof."

Her father was a familiar figure around the building until he sadly died in the flat a few months before he was due to retire.

Margaret, who now lives in Fforestfach, eventually went on to work in child health and several other departments before leaving in 1978 to have her daughters Catrin and Nerys. But she was back at Central Clinic by 1989 and has been there ever since.

"I have loved working here. The flat is now offices but I never go up there. I like to remember it as it was."

The building also holds a special place in the heart of her daughter Catrin. She was the artist whose original Guerrilla Restoration project was the inspiration behind a high-profile clean-up of the distinctive mural artwork on the building's facade by ABMU's Heritage Group.

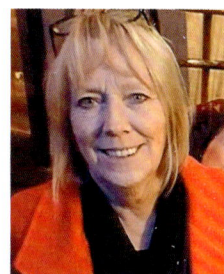

After a 49-year association with the building Margaret *(right)* has very fond memories.

"Central Clinic has always been my home from home. It's been a huge part of my life and I will miss it. I have made many friends and have many happy memories."

Robert Redfern

Although he spent most of his working life in Morriston Hospital, Robert Redfern enjoyed a remarkable career that even took in Vietnam too.

Neurosurgeon Mr Redfern qualified in 1977 and came to Morriston in 1992, remaining there until his retirement earlier this year.

He became a very popular figure with patients and staff alike, but his many achievements were not just confined to the operating theatre.

He took an active interest in charitable causes and, away from the NHS, will be known to many from his year as High Sheriff of West Glamorgan.

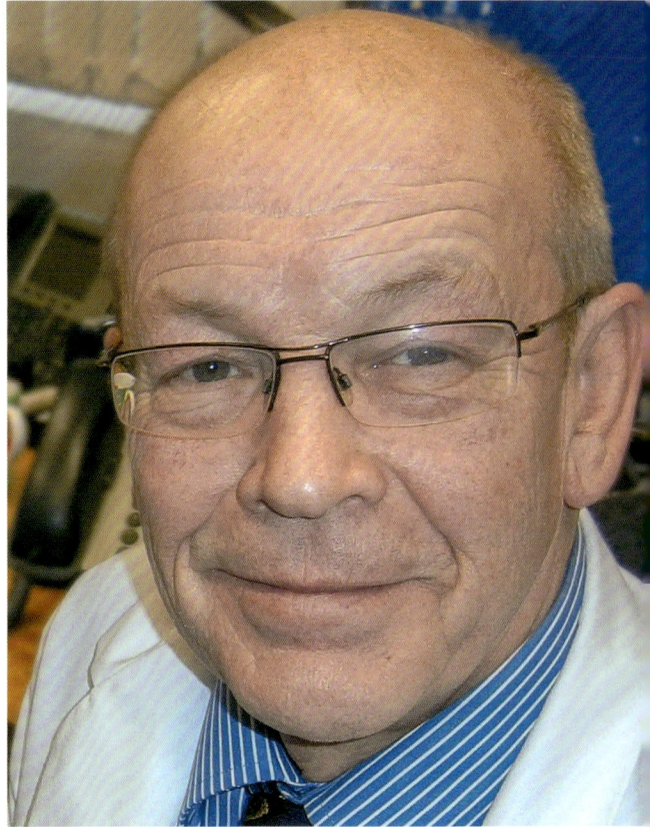

Looking back on his time in the NHS, Mr Redfern said: *"There have been a number of very big changes.*

"Since I qualified in March 1977, there have been technical advances in terms of the equipment, in radiology and in drug therapies.

"All of these have improved outcomes for patients.

"There have been improvements in throughput too. If someone had a back operation years ago, they would have been in bed for 10 days.

"Now we are getting them out of bed after they recover from anaesthetic and most of them are going home the next day.

"I've had to adjust to the changes that have taken place, and it has been very rewarding to do so."

Looking beyond his work as a neurosurgeon, Mr Redfern took an active role supporting the Ann Conroy Trust.

This is a small but active charity that helps fund research and provide support and education for people living with Chiari Malformation, Syringomyelia and associated conditions.

In 2009 he became involved in voluntary educational work in Vietnam, through the Foundation for International Education in Neurology Study.

He made five annual visits, paying for his own flights and accommodation, to share his knowledge and experience with Da Nang Hospital.

Following his first visit, Mr Redfern said: "I was not insured to operate, so I couldn't take part in any surgery – but I was able to advise and offer guidance.

"As a result I was able to ensure a lot of patients avoided unnecessary procedures or serious complications."

Mr Redfern set up the Swansea Vietnam Fund, which helped pay for small pieces of equipment for the Vietnamese hospital, including drill bits, a new computer and bone biopsy equipment.

Additionally, the fund sponsored a visit by its head of neurosurgery department, Dr Ngoc Ba Nguyen, to Morriston Hospital.

Today it continues to support Swansea medical students who wish to pursue a career in the neurosciences to undertake a period of elective study in Vietnam.

In 2015, Mr Redfern became High Sheriff of West Glamorgan, an independent and non-political appointment that lasts for one year.

Duties include attendance at Royal visits in the county, and support for High Court judges. Supporting the Crown and the judiciary remains a central element of the role.

Mr Redfern retired from the NHS at the end of March this year. He said:

"I had been thinking about it for a while.

"You have to retire at some stage and I decided I would give myself another two years after I finished my time as High Sheriff.

"I have a family, I have non-NHS work and I have hobbies and interests outside of work – including becoming a magistrate – so I have plenty to keep myself busy."

Memories of Cefn Coed

How would you feel if you had to live at hospital as well as work in it?

Back in the 1940s, living at Cefn Coed hospital was just another part of the job for a team of around 15 catering staff.

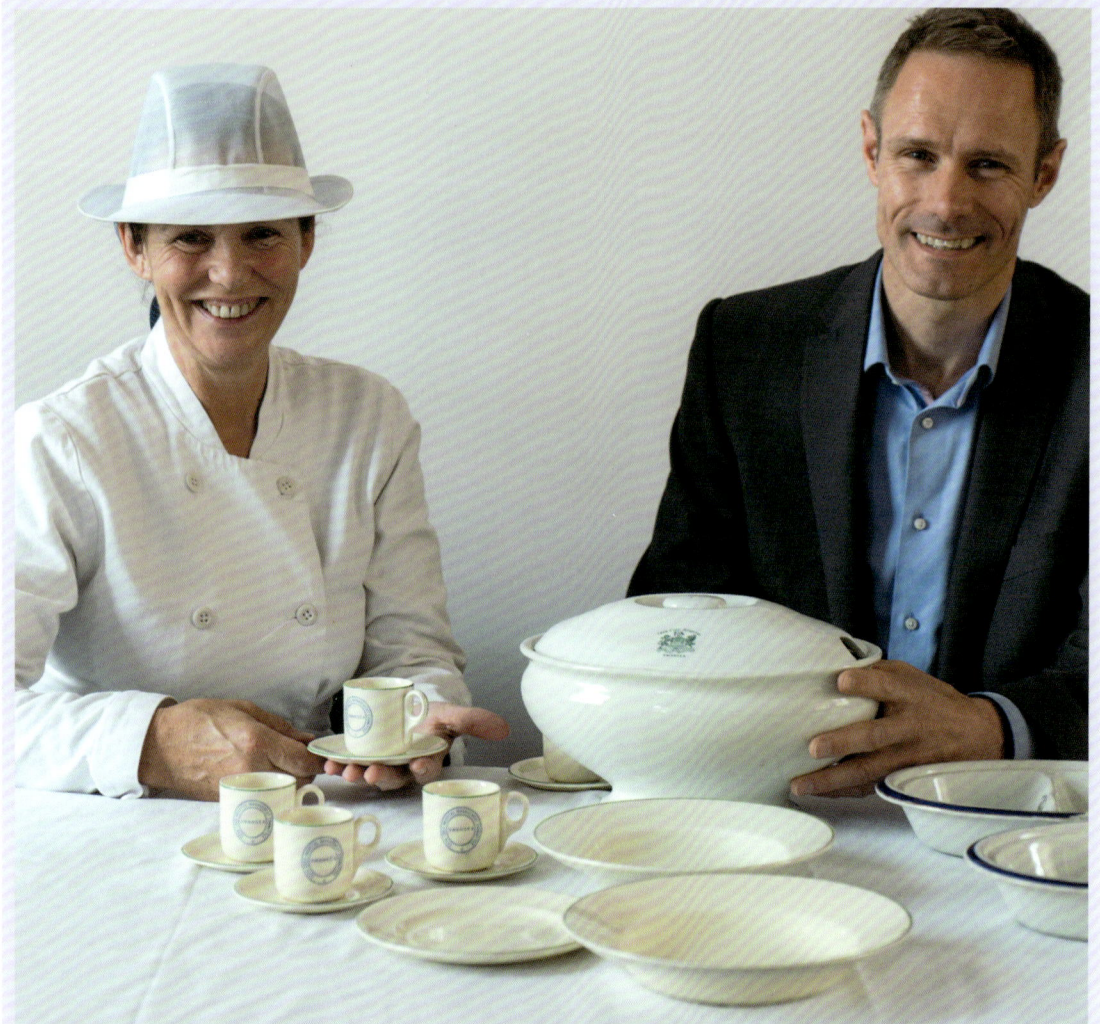

Heritage Officer Martin Thomas and hospital cook Tina Maddrell with some of the Cefn Coed crockery collection she kept safe. Service changes meant it was no longer needed. Tina did not want to throw it away - and has presented it to the health board's Heritage Group.

One member of staff was just a teenager when she started working at – and living in — the hospital said:

"Back then there were around 700 patients to cook for, as well as the staff. We used to have these large ovens and the food we cooked was really good quality.

"Breakfast could include porridge, fried eggs and bacon, and we had these big steamers for kippers.

"For lunch we'd make a treat once-a-week of fish and chips.

"We had a baker and a butcher at the hospital so we had fresh bread and meat. We'd put the food in the trolleys and in the early days the patients would come down and take them to the wards.

"We worked hard and had one day off a week."

She added:

"Every so often the patients would give the hospital a big clean. You'd see some of them in the corridors on their hands and knees. To be fair, the place was spotless.

"The staff and patients also had an annual sports day up on the green. We'd have egg and spoon races and stalls, all the traditional stuff. I've got some really good memories, it was an enjoyable time."

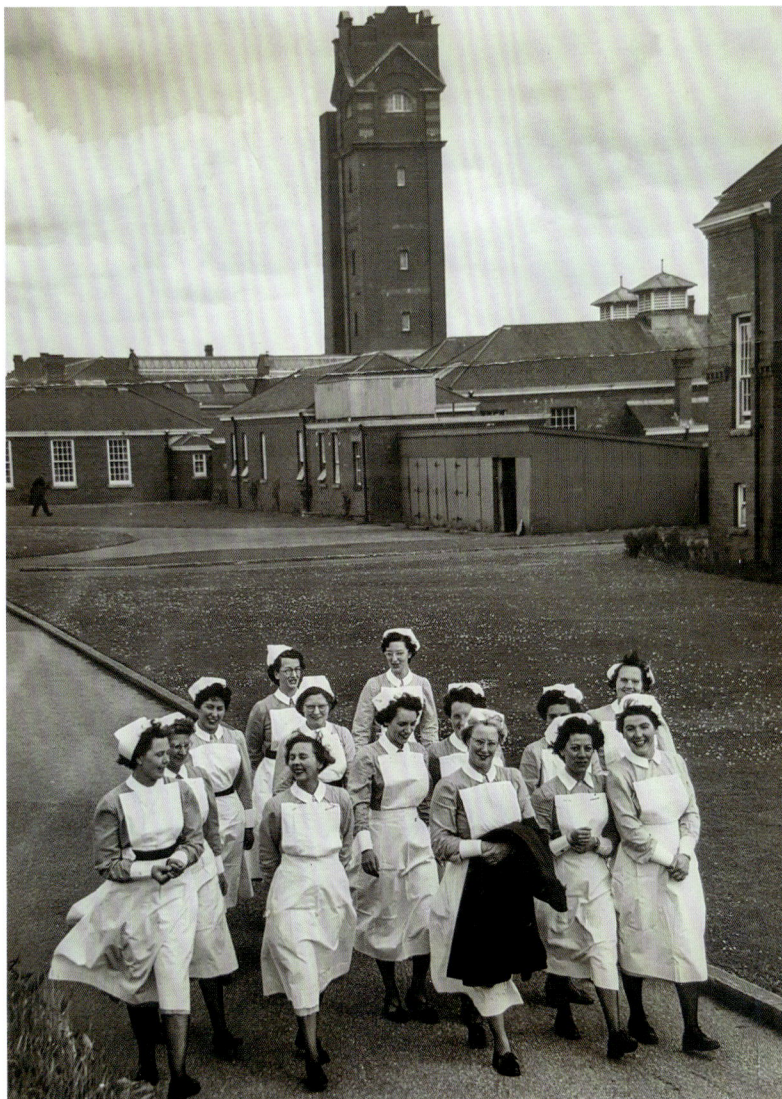

Nurses out and about at Cefn Coed Hospital.

Dr Kim Harrison

Consultant chest physician Dr Kim Harrison witnessed many changes during 39 years working in the NHS.

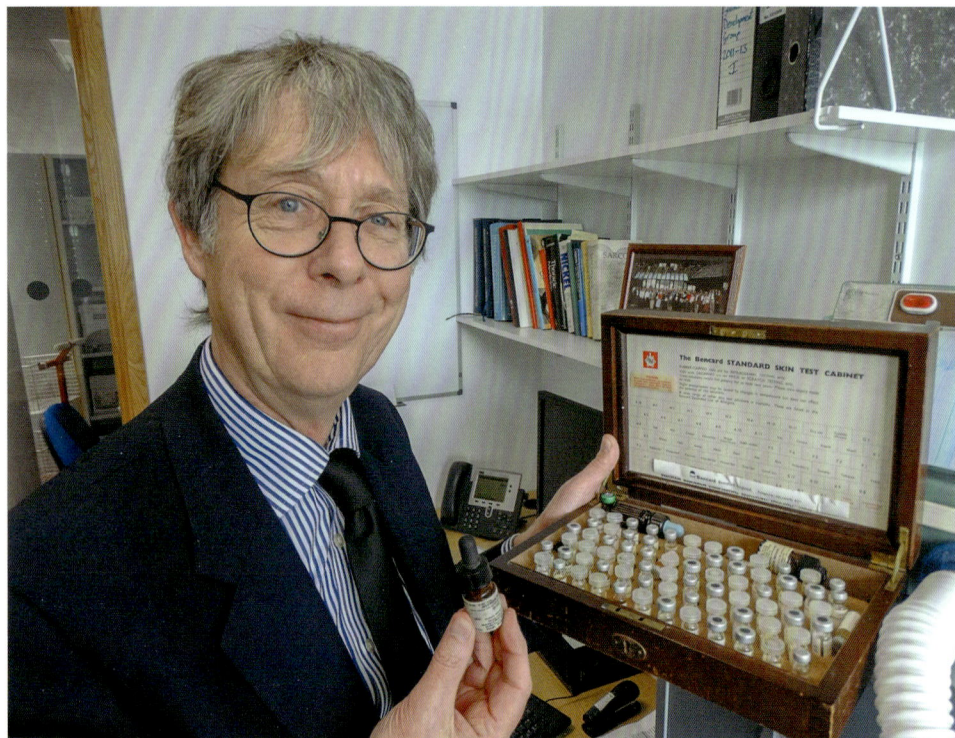

Dealing with chest conditions brought him into contact with many patients who had paid the price for a lifetime working in heavy industry across South Wales.

"We are seeing less pneumoconiosis related to mining as that industry declines however the legacy of asbestos is still prevalent and exposure to it can have lasting implications for people's health," he said.

Dr Harrison came to Swansea in 1994 to work as consultant chest physician and set up the Respiratory Unit at Morriston Hospital where he was based until his retirement earlier this year.

He also worked with consultant cardio-thoracic surgeon Aprim Youhana to develop the thoracic surgical service at Morriston.

"But we were very much re-establishing the services and building on work previously done by such esteemed surgeons as Cyril Evans at Morriston."

Alongside Mr Youhana, consultant oncologist Kath Rowley and palliative care consultant Sue Closs, Dr Harrison was also responsible for setting up the first lung cancer multidisciplinary team in Swansea.

Growing up in Lancashire, Dr Harrison had an inspirational careers master, who encouraged his ambition to become a doctor.

It was during his time working in the East End of London that he says he developed his passion for chest medicine.

On arriving at Morriston, Dr Harrison initially developed the chest clinic, bronchoscope service, the Lung Function laboratory and facilities for sleep studies.

"At the time sleep apnoea wasn't widely accepted as a disease. We had to produce better evidence. It has lots of social implications so it is only right and proper to investigate it thoroughly."

Dr Harrison was also instrumental in finding funding for the first respiratory nurse specialist and the lung cancer nurse specialist posts at Morriston.

More recently, he set up the interstitial lung disease clinic at Morriston Hospital, which he runs with a group of specialist nurses for patients with a wide range of lung conditions.

Following his retirement Dr Harrison is still pursuing his passion for research and will be continuing to work on projects investigating blood clotting abnormalities in people with lung disease with Prof Adrian Evans in the Haemostasis Biomedical Research Unit at Morriston and with colleagues at Swansea University's College of Engineering focusing on the effects of exercise on people with IPF.

Dr Harrison added:

"When I came here to Swansea, I knew the service for chest diseases was something that could be improved and now it has developed into something I can feel very proud of."

And if he needed a reminder of how his field has developed Dr Harrison didn't have to look far – a Vitalograph Spirometer for measuring lung function dating back 30 years sat near his desk and he still has a kit, in pristine condition, for testing asthma patients' allergies dating back to the late 1960s *(pictured right)*.

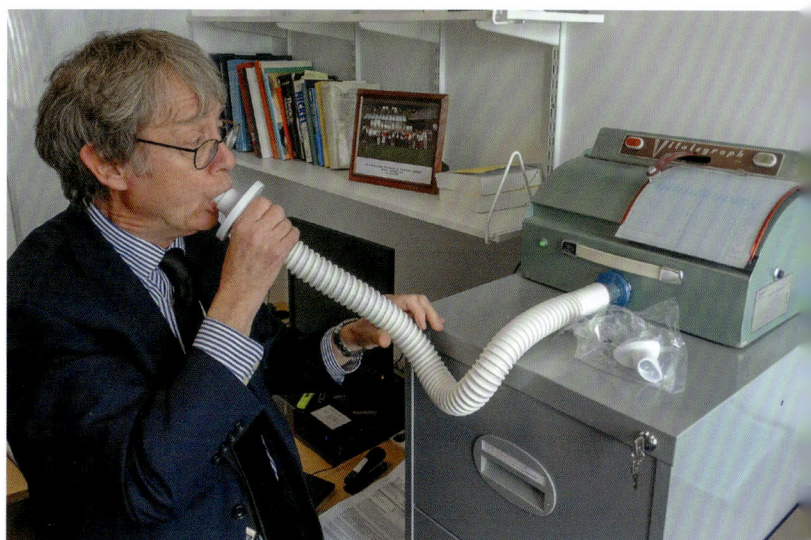

The way we were

The following pages are a collection of photographs from our past

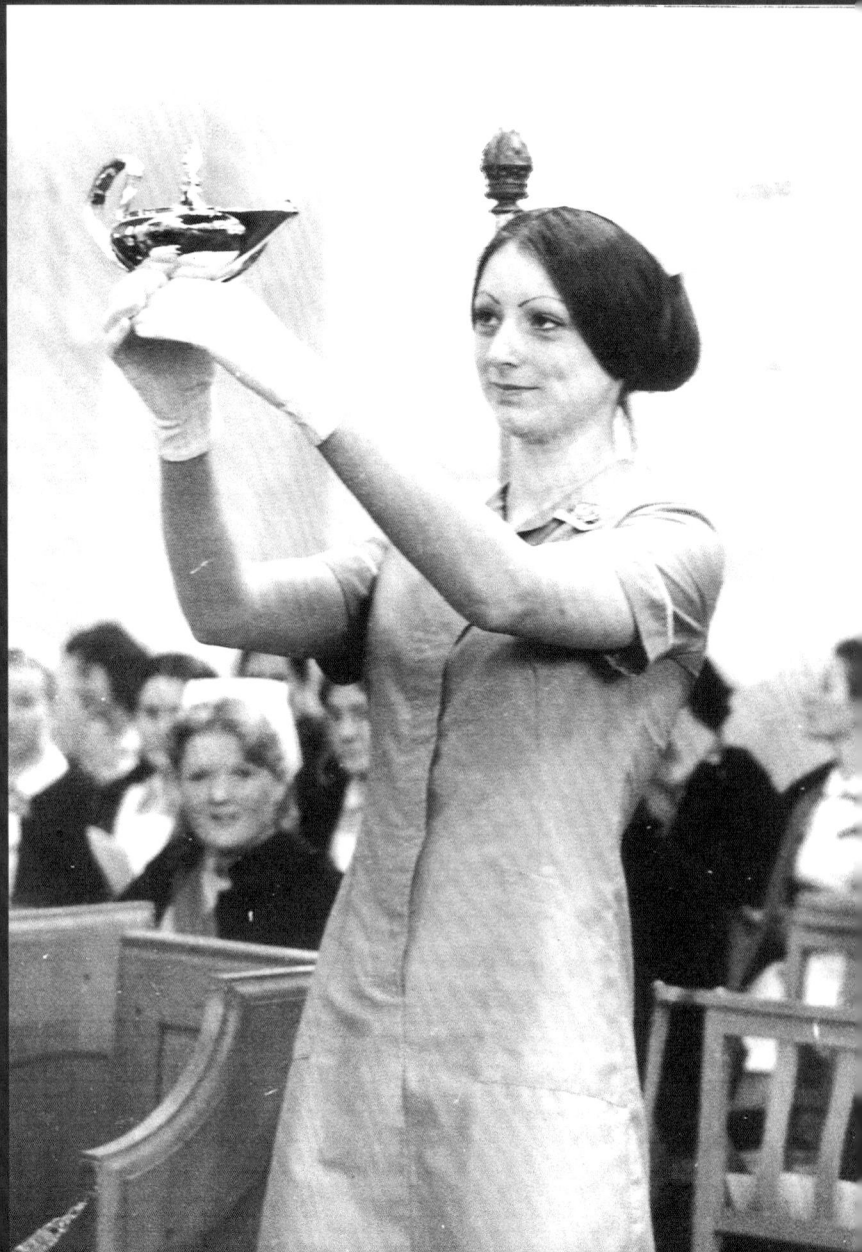

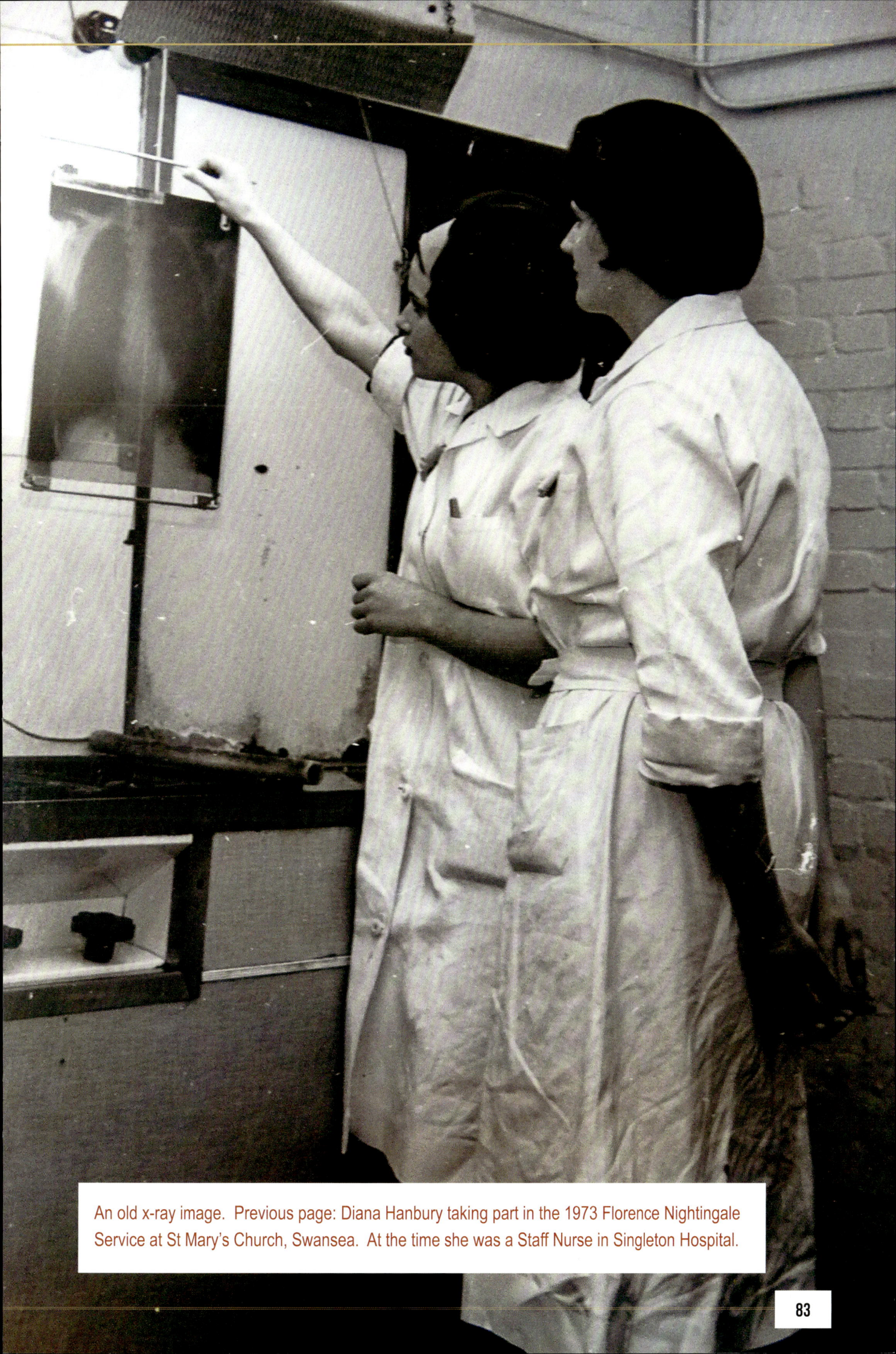

An old x-ray image. Previous page: Diana Hanbury taking part in the 1973 Florence Nightingale Service at St Mary's Church, Swansea. At the time she was a Staff Nurse in Singleton Hospital.

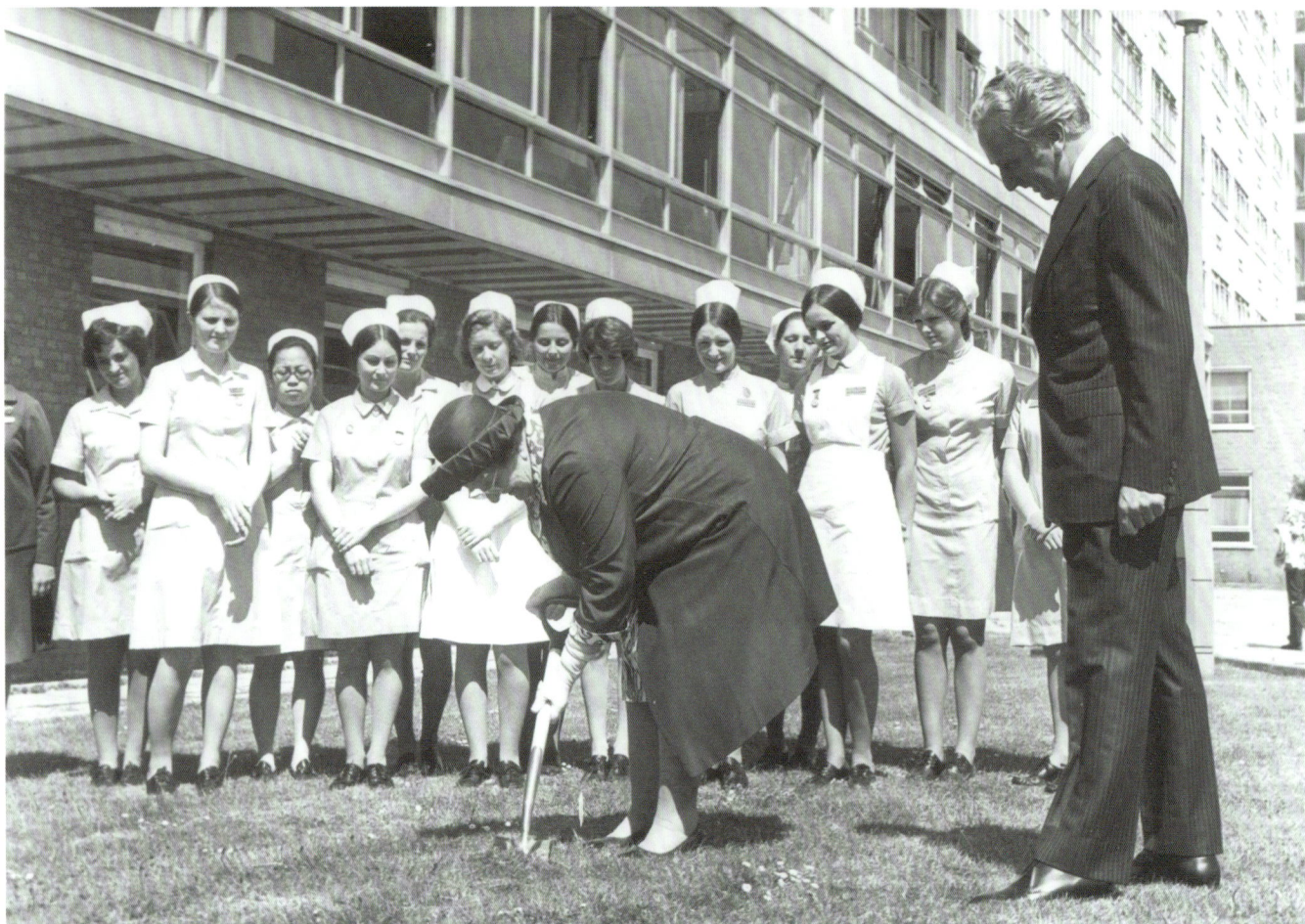

Mrs Olwen Morgan, wife of Swansea businessman JP Morgan, at the ceremony to start work on Singleton Hospital's Chapel. Mrs Morgan would go on to give her name to the palliative care centre at Morriston Hospital

Below - historical pictures predating the NHS

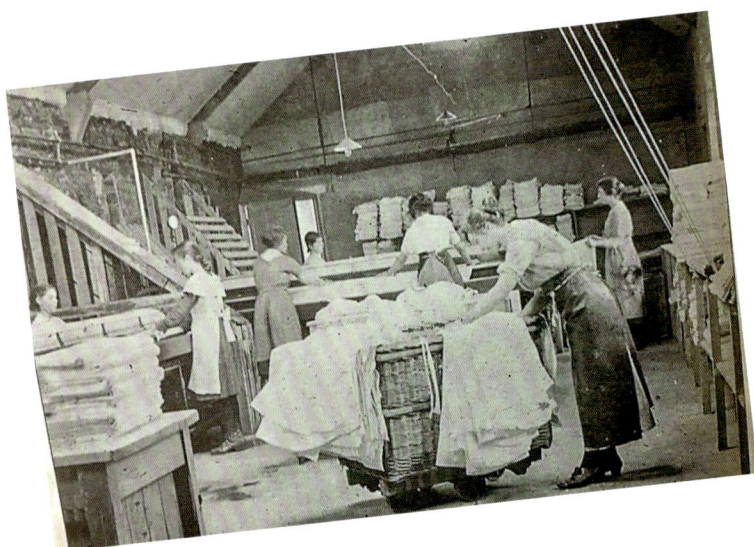

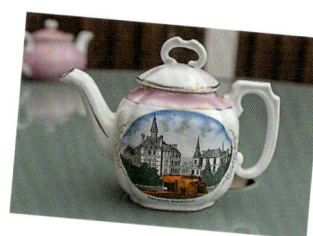

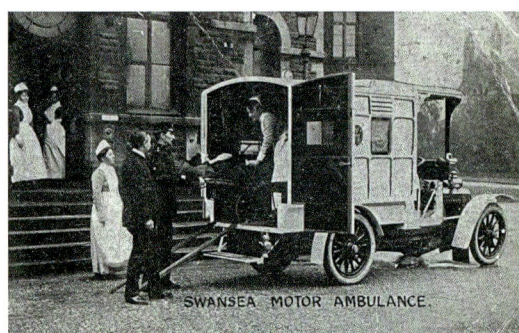

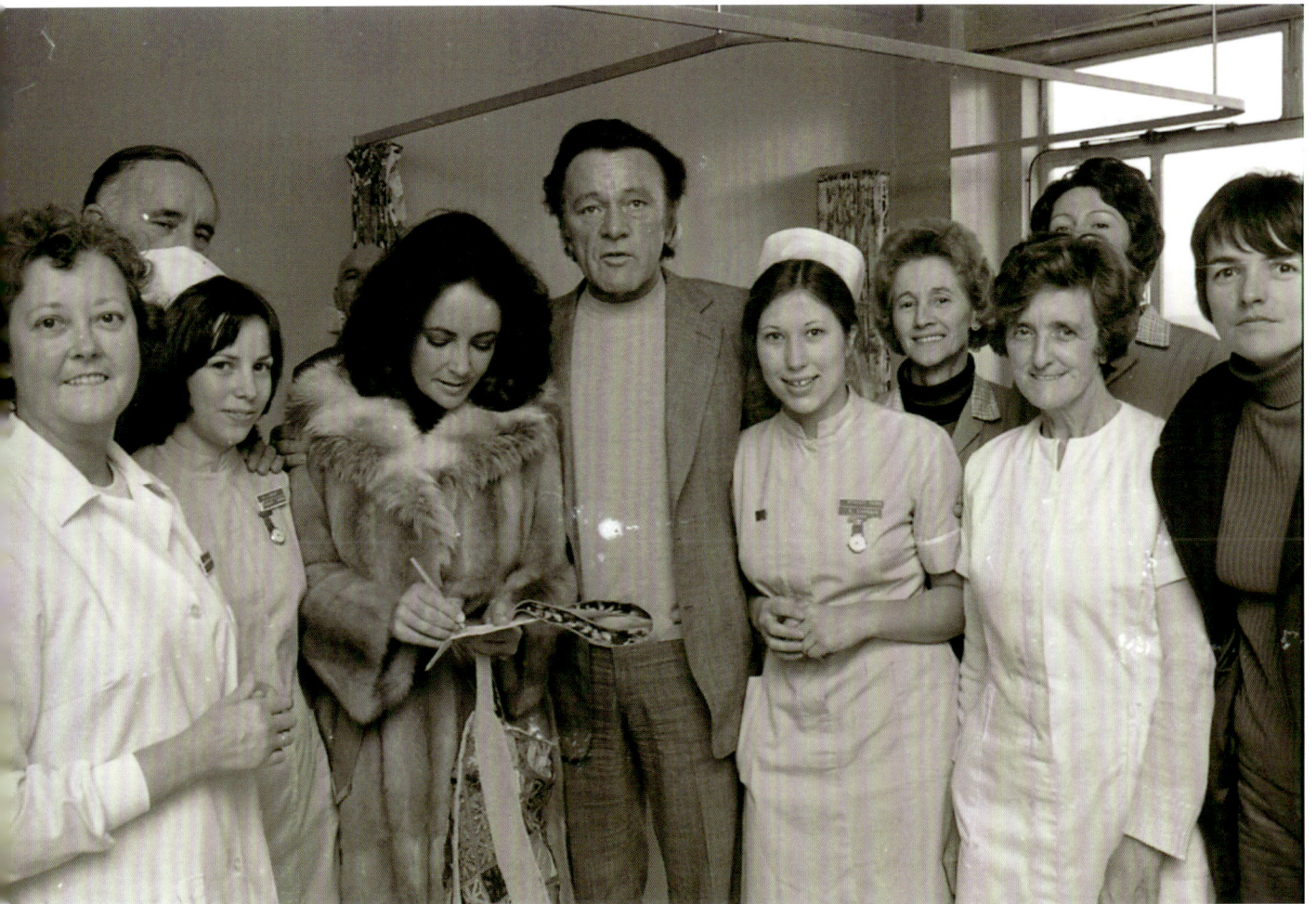

...ollywood's most famous couple, Elizabeth Taylor and Richard Burton, meet up with a group of Swansea nurses

...elow - Singleton Hospital students, 1980s

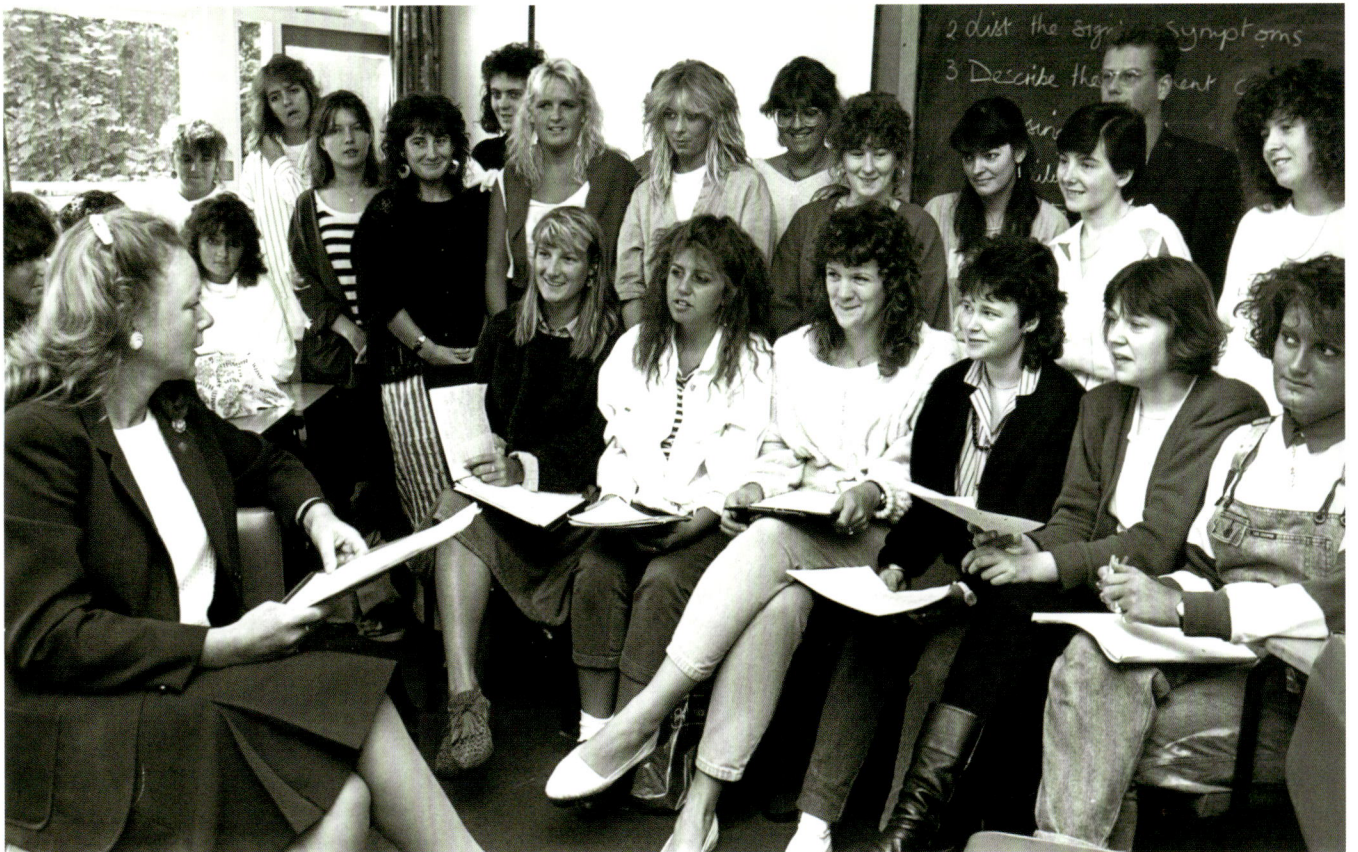

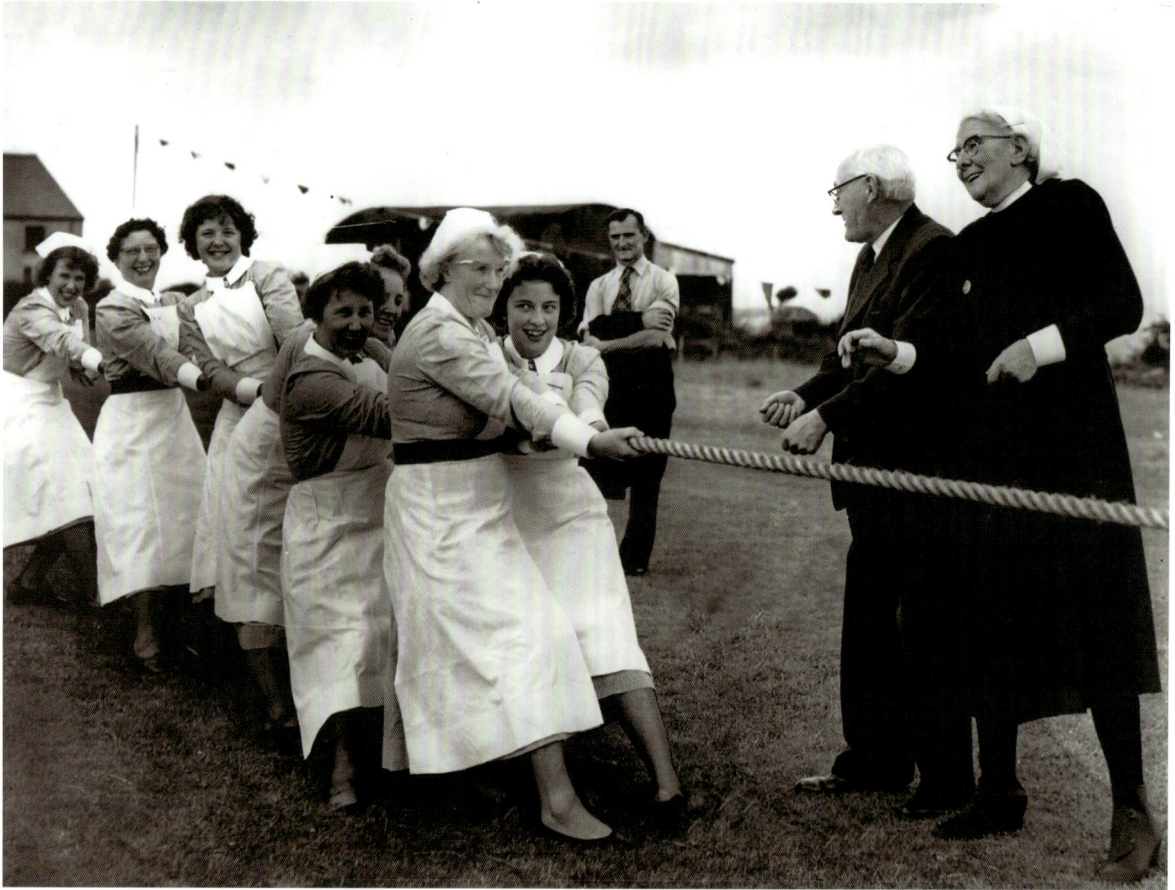

Cefn Coed Hospital staff enjoy a tug of war, July 1960

Below - Cefn Coed staff cricket team

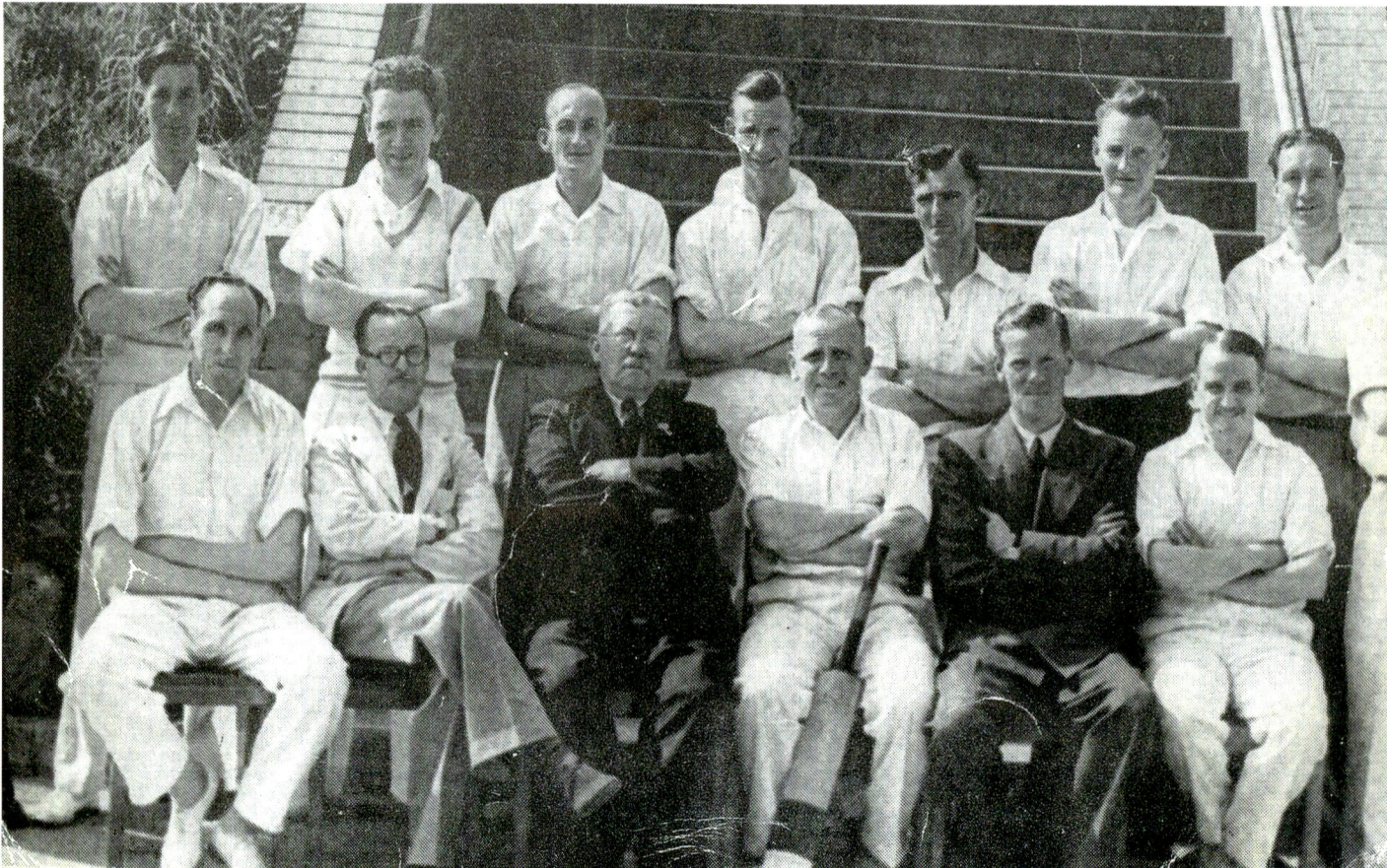

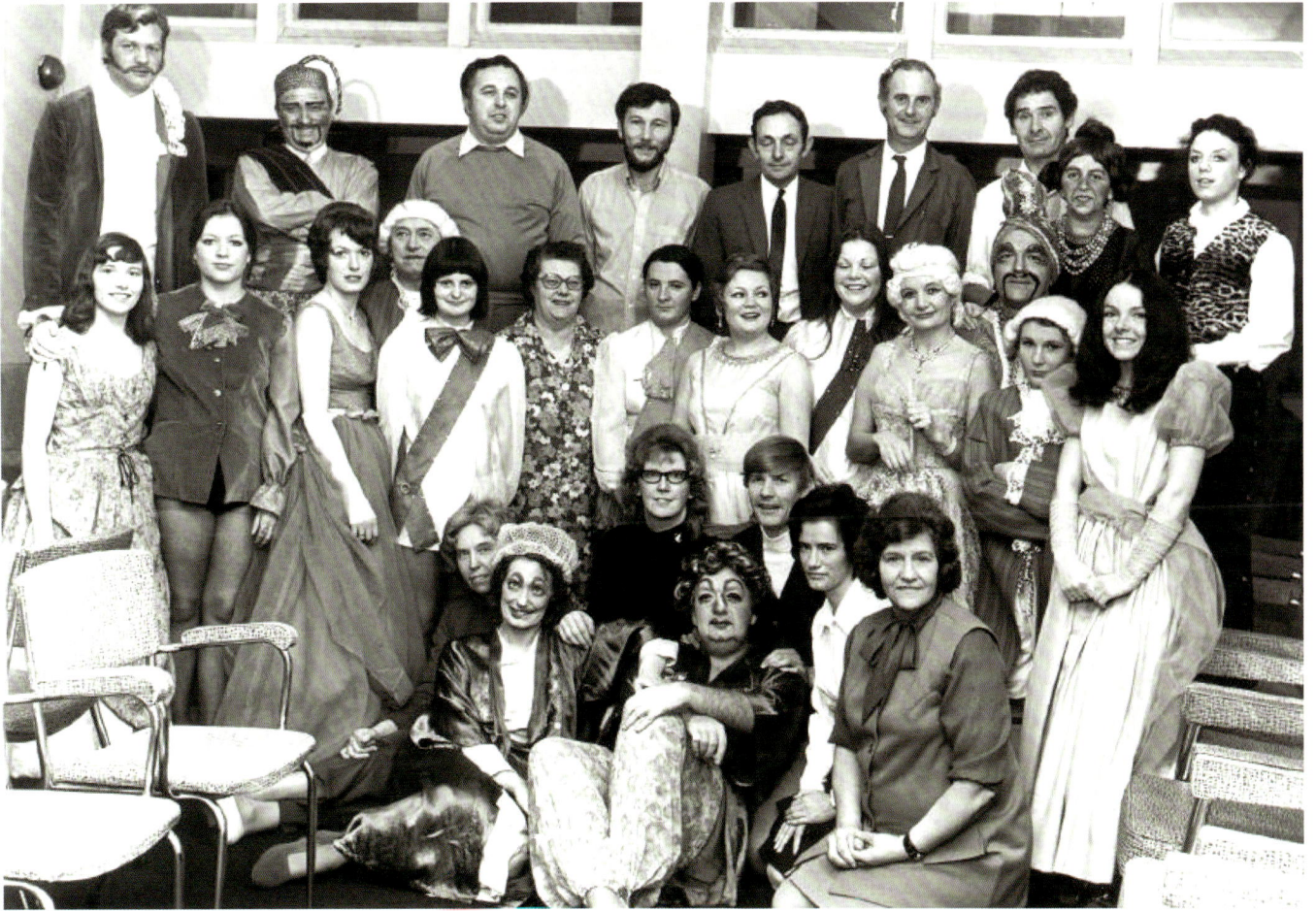

Members of Singleton Hospital Dramatic Society in its early days

Below - Parc Beck nursing students pay attention

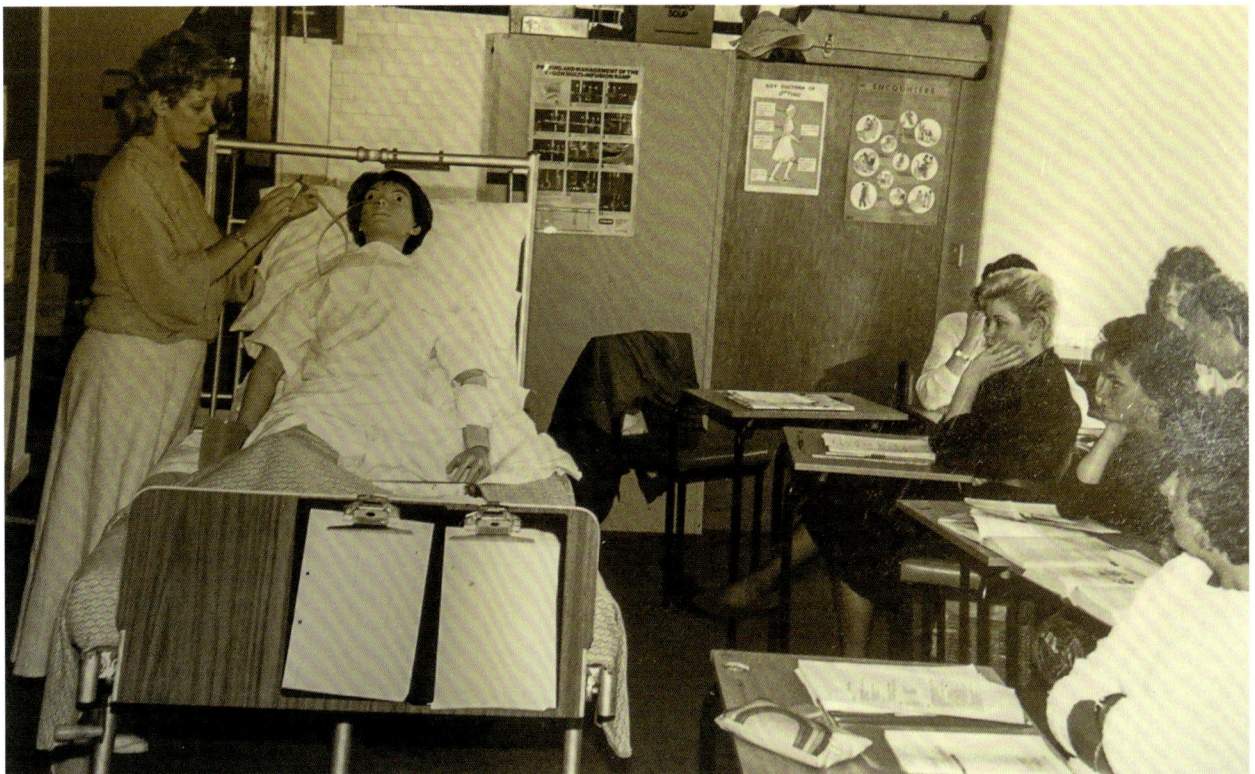

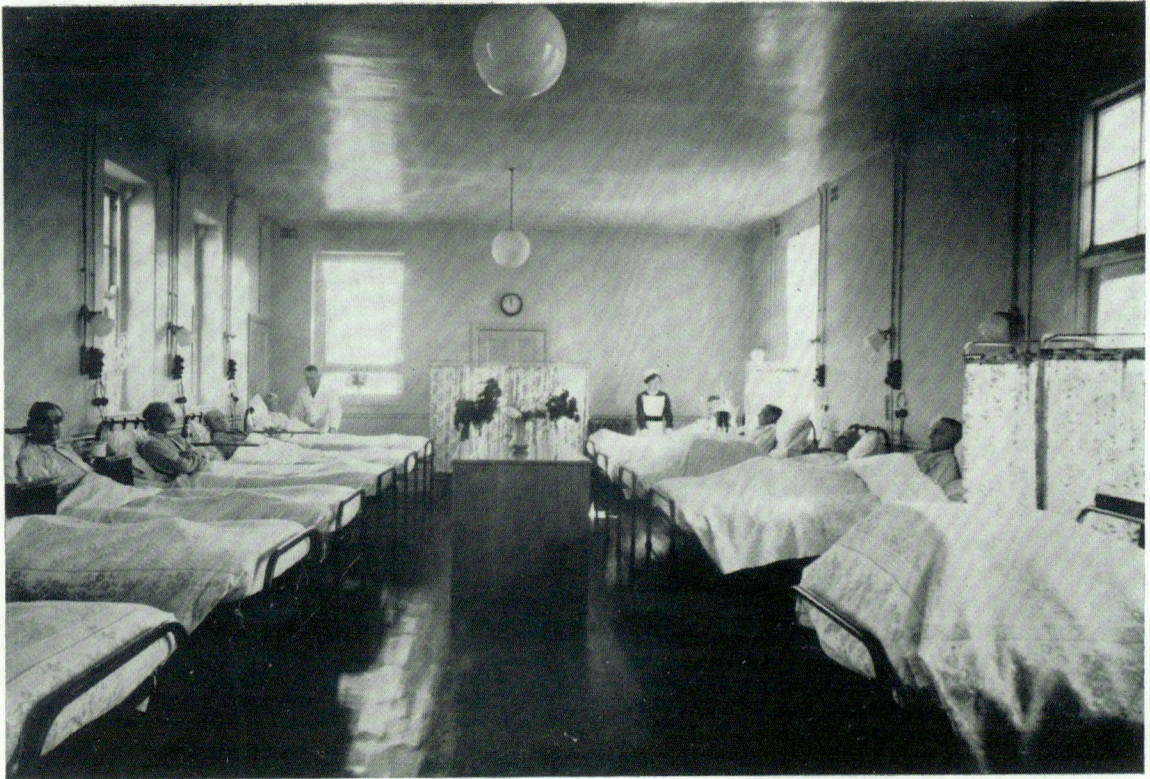

BRYNTIRION HOSPITAL.   MALE WARD.

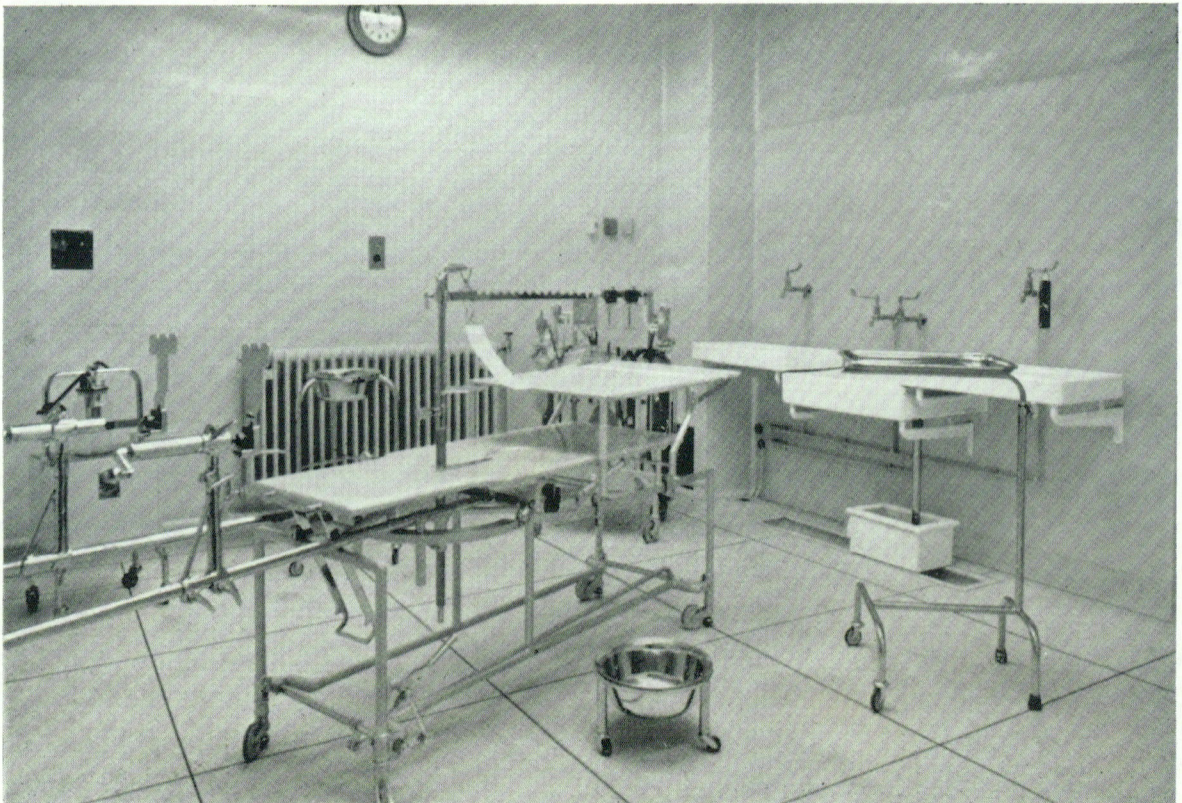

LLANELLY HOSPITAL.   FRACTURE THEATRE.

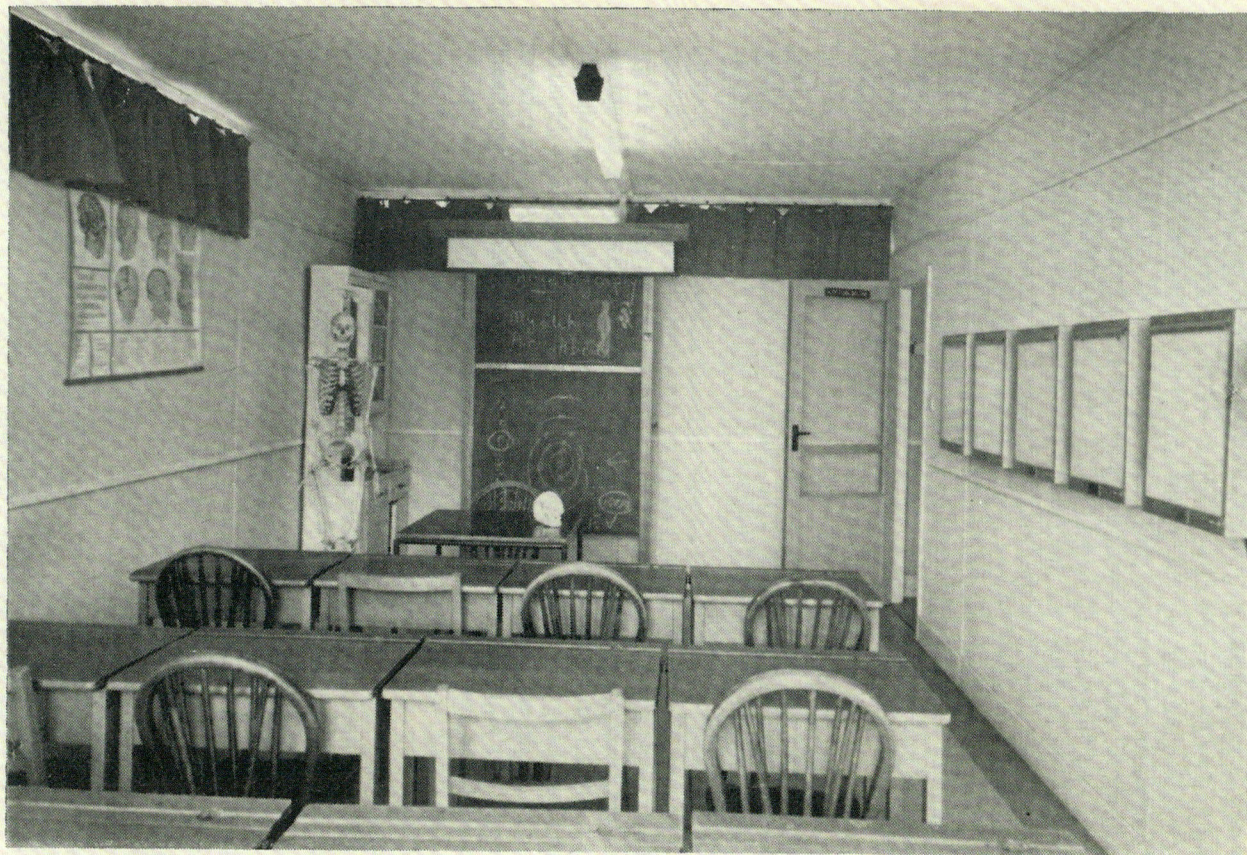

Lecture Room, School of Radiography, Morriston Hospital.

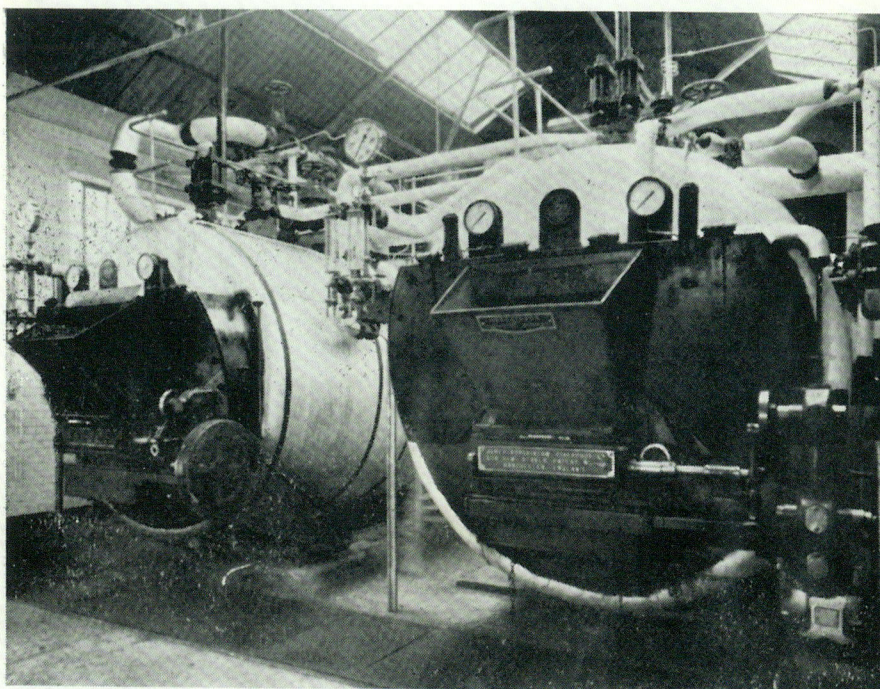

LLANELLY HOSPITAL. SUPER ECONOMIC BOILERS FITTED WITH AUTOMATIC LOW RAM STOKERS.

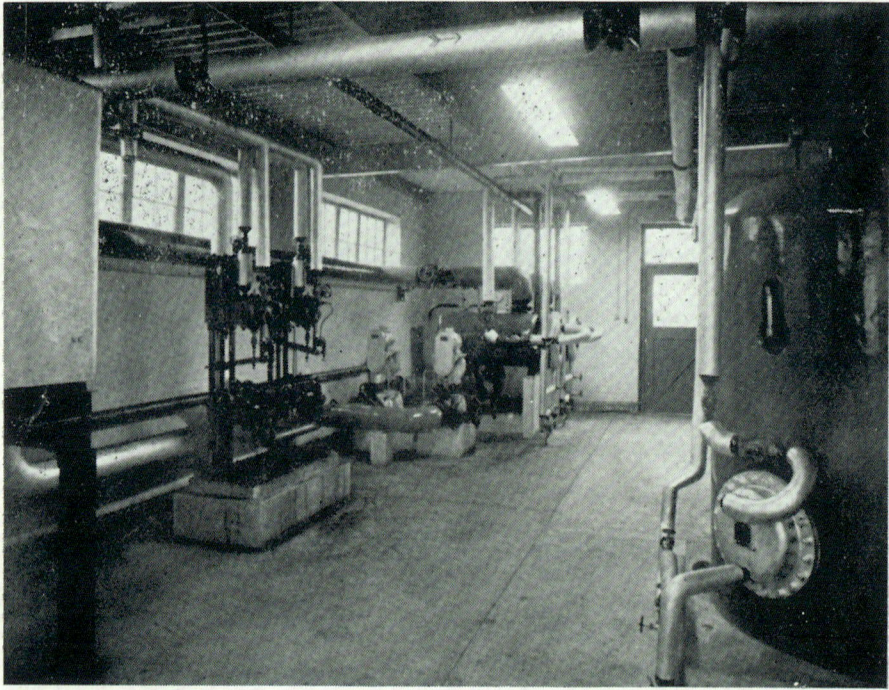

LLANELLY HOSPITAL.   PUMP AND CALORIFIER ROOM.

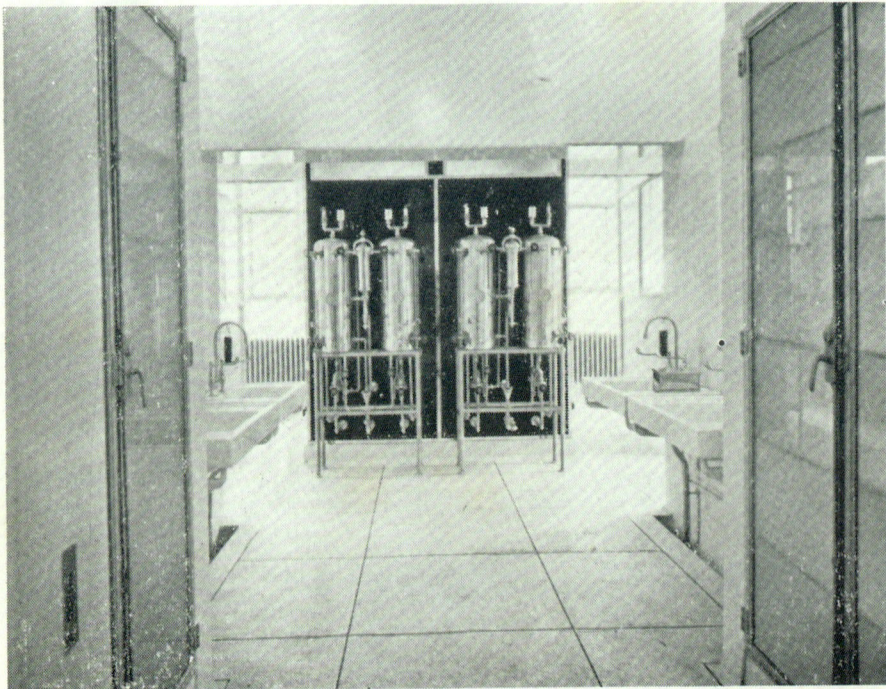

LLANELLY HOSPITAL.   THEATRE STERILISING ROOM.

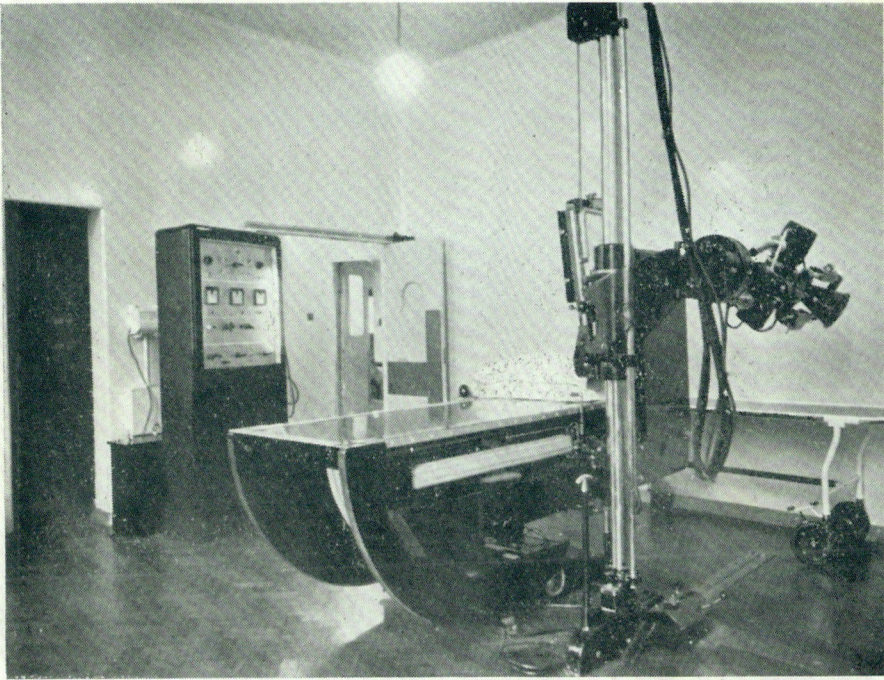

LLANELLY HOSPITAL.   ONE OF THE X-RAY
                                      DIAGNOSTIC ROOMS.

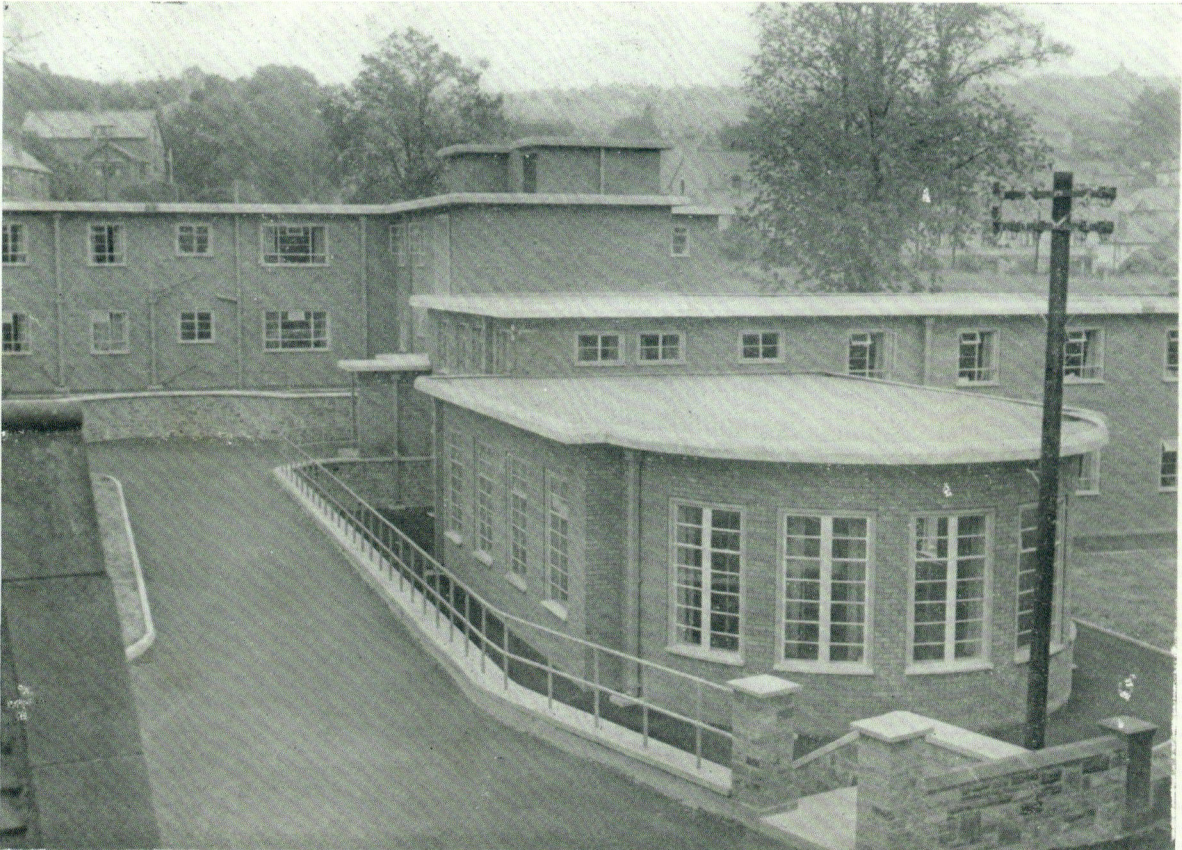

NURSES HOME.   PARC BECK, SKETTY

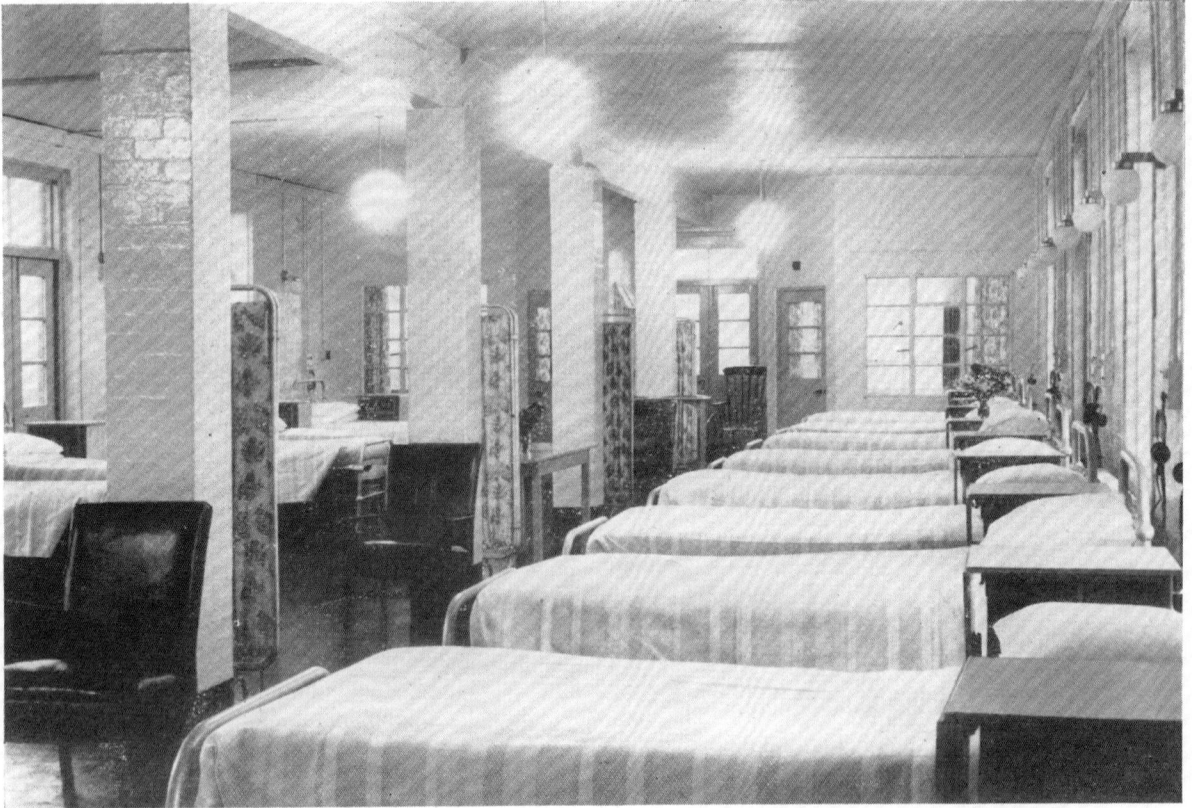

MORRISTON HOSPITAL.   RECONSTRUCTED WARD,

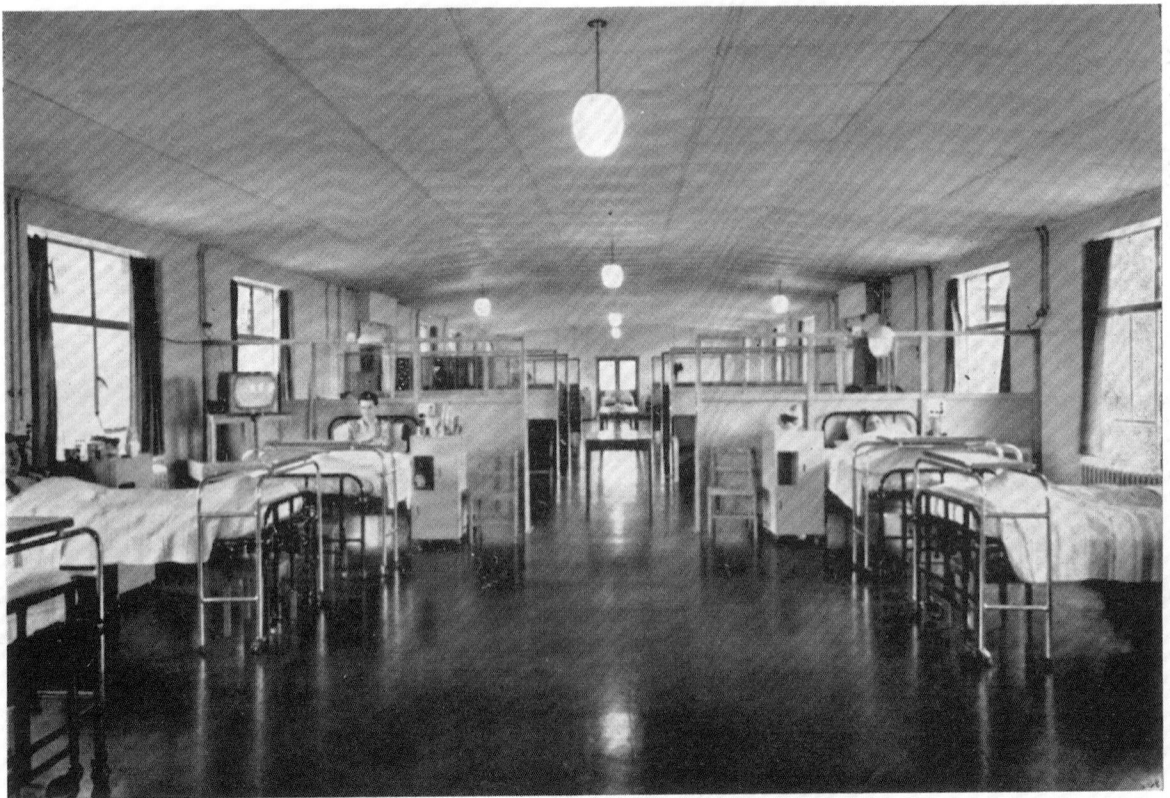

MORRISTON HOSPITAL.   CHEST WARD,

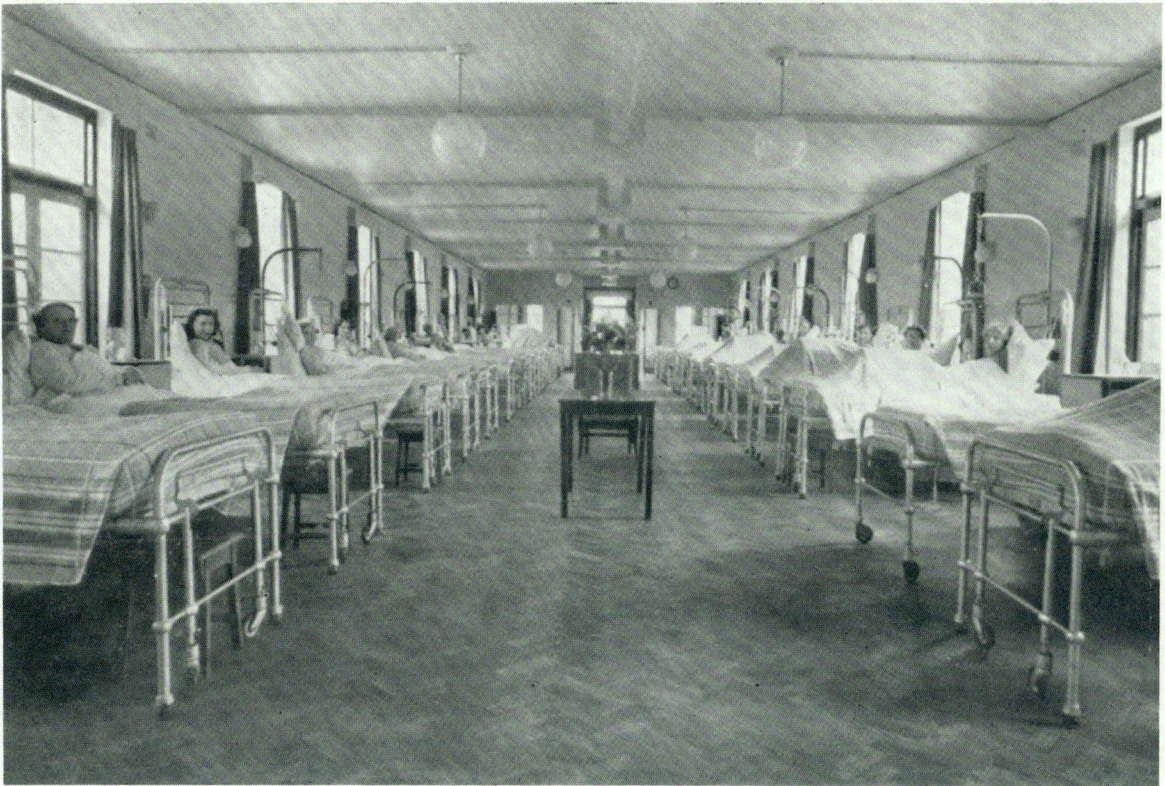

MORRISTON HOSPITAL.   WARD 2—RECONSTRUCTED SHOWING REMOVAL OF CENTRE PILLARS.

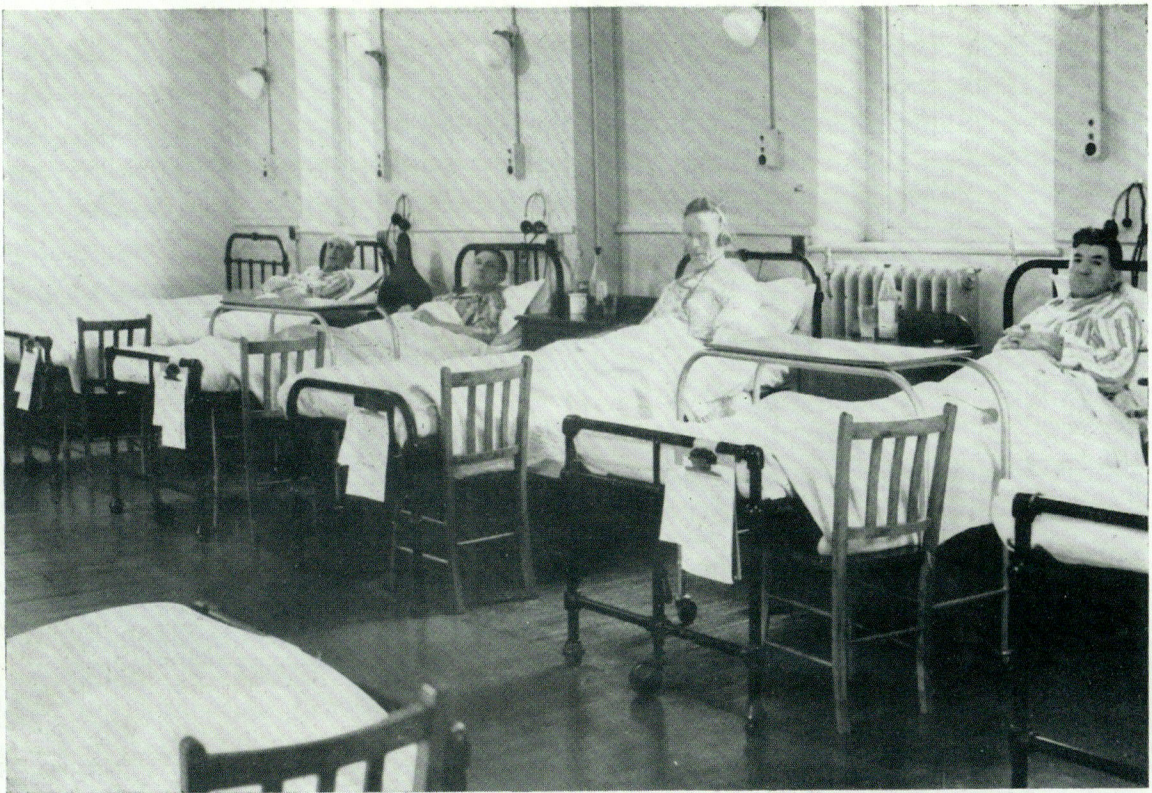

MOUNT PLEASANT HOSPITAL.   MALE SURGICAL WARD.

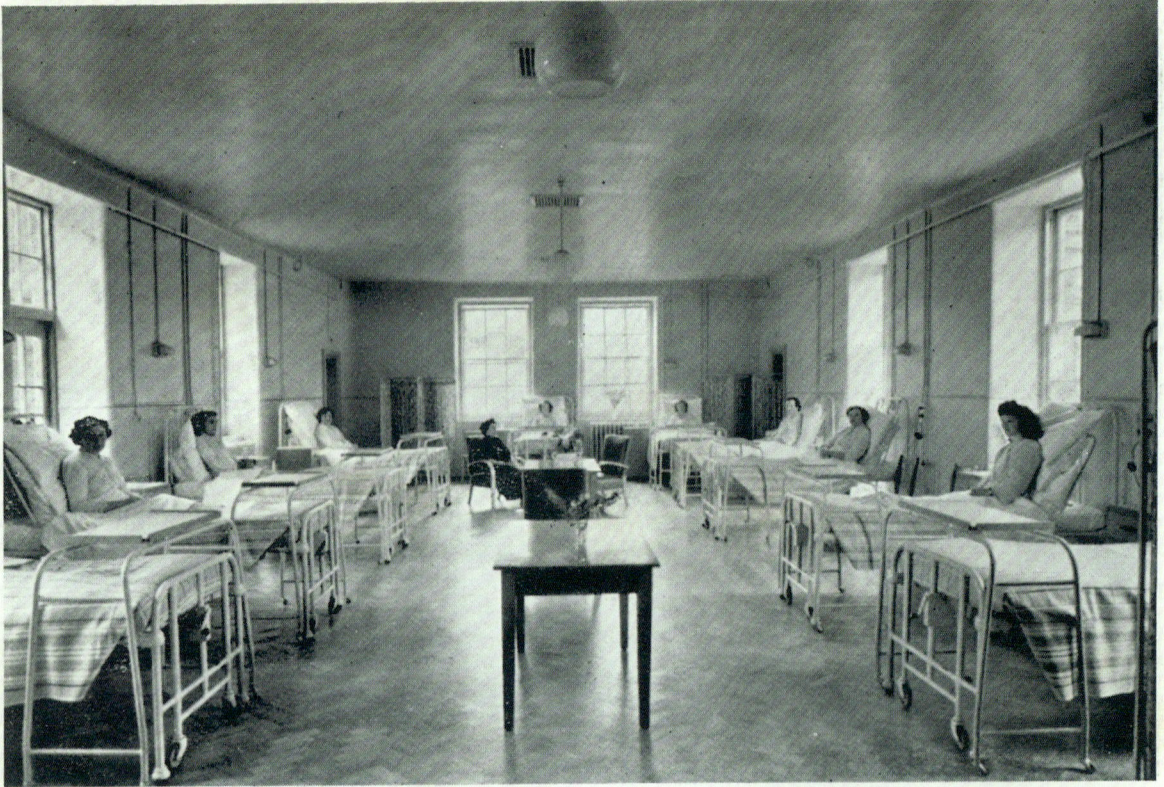

MOUNT PLEASANT HOSPITAL.   ONE OF THE NEW MATERNITY WARDS.

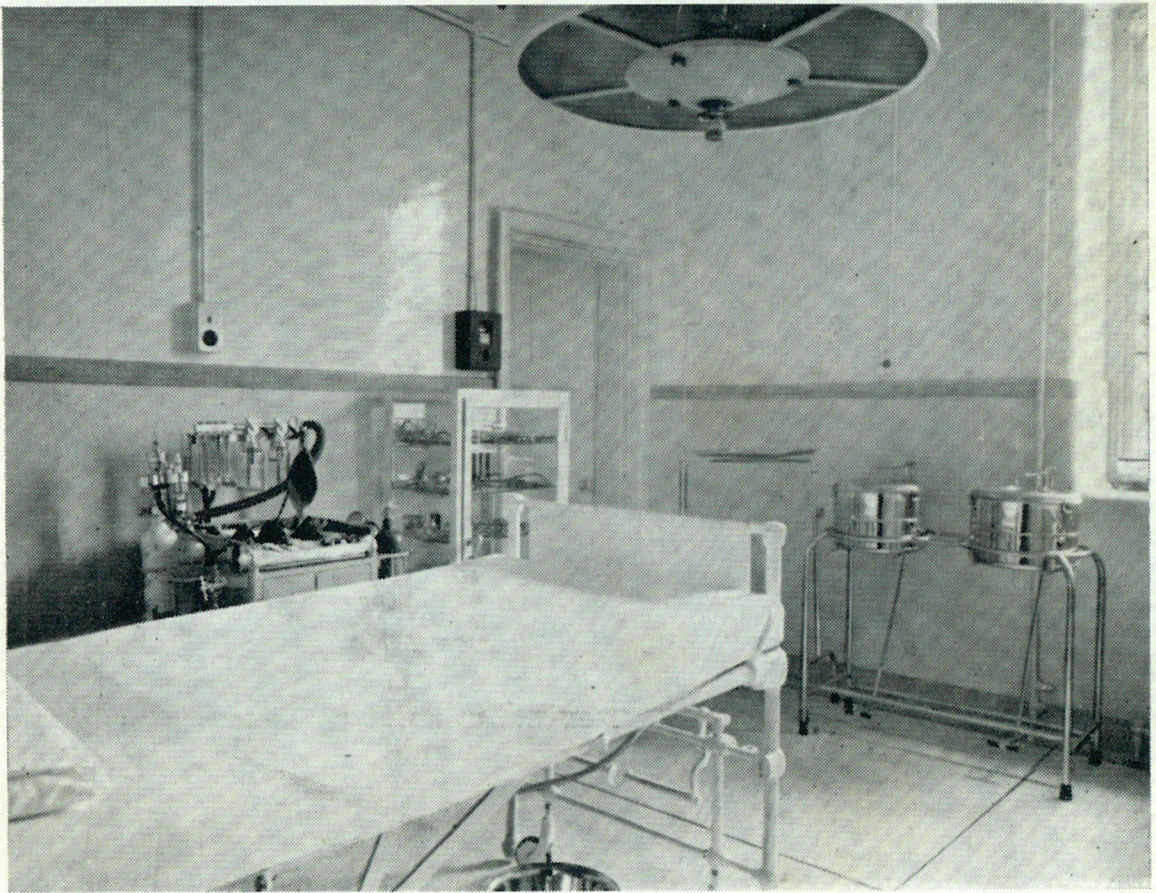

MOUNT PLEASANT HOSPITAL.   OPERATING THEATRE, MATERNITY UNIT.

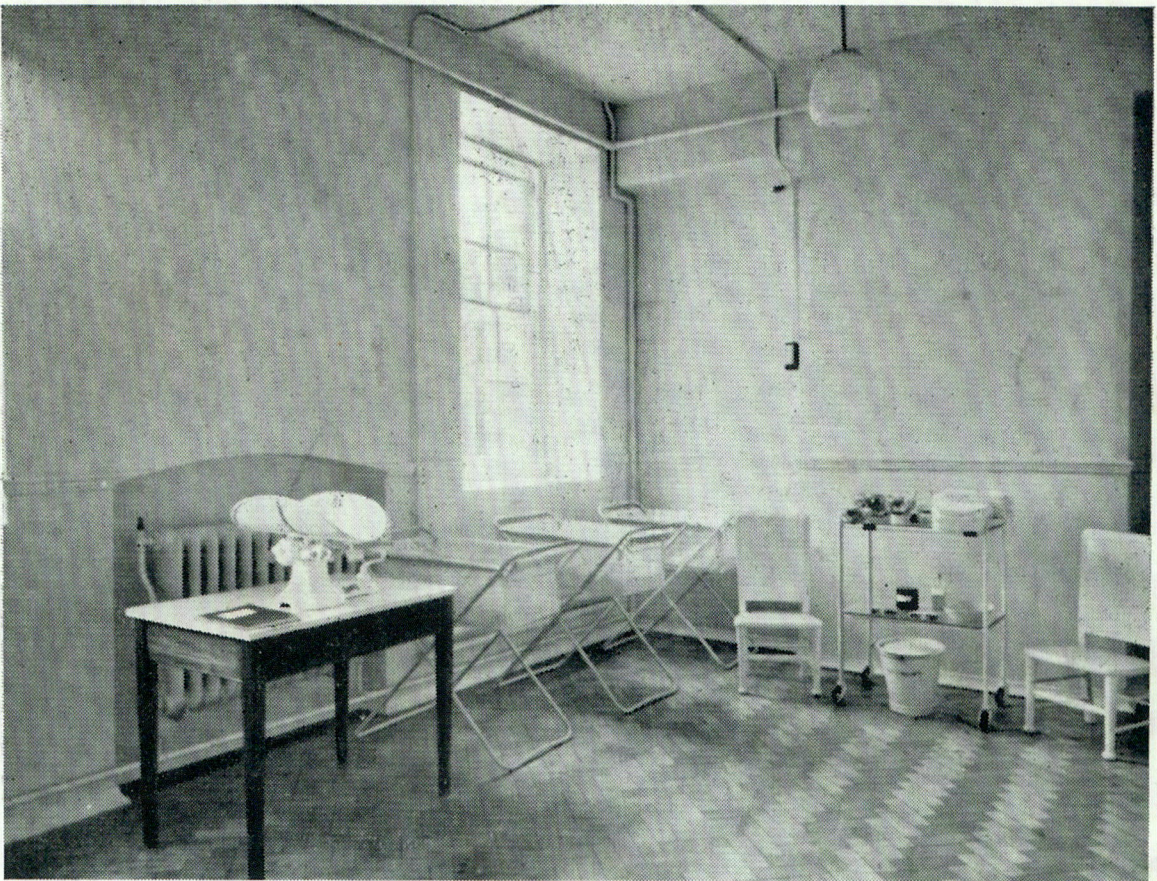

MOUNT PLEASANT HOSPITAL.   CORNER OF NURSERY.

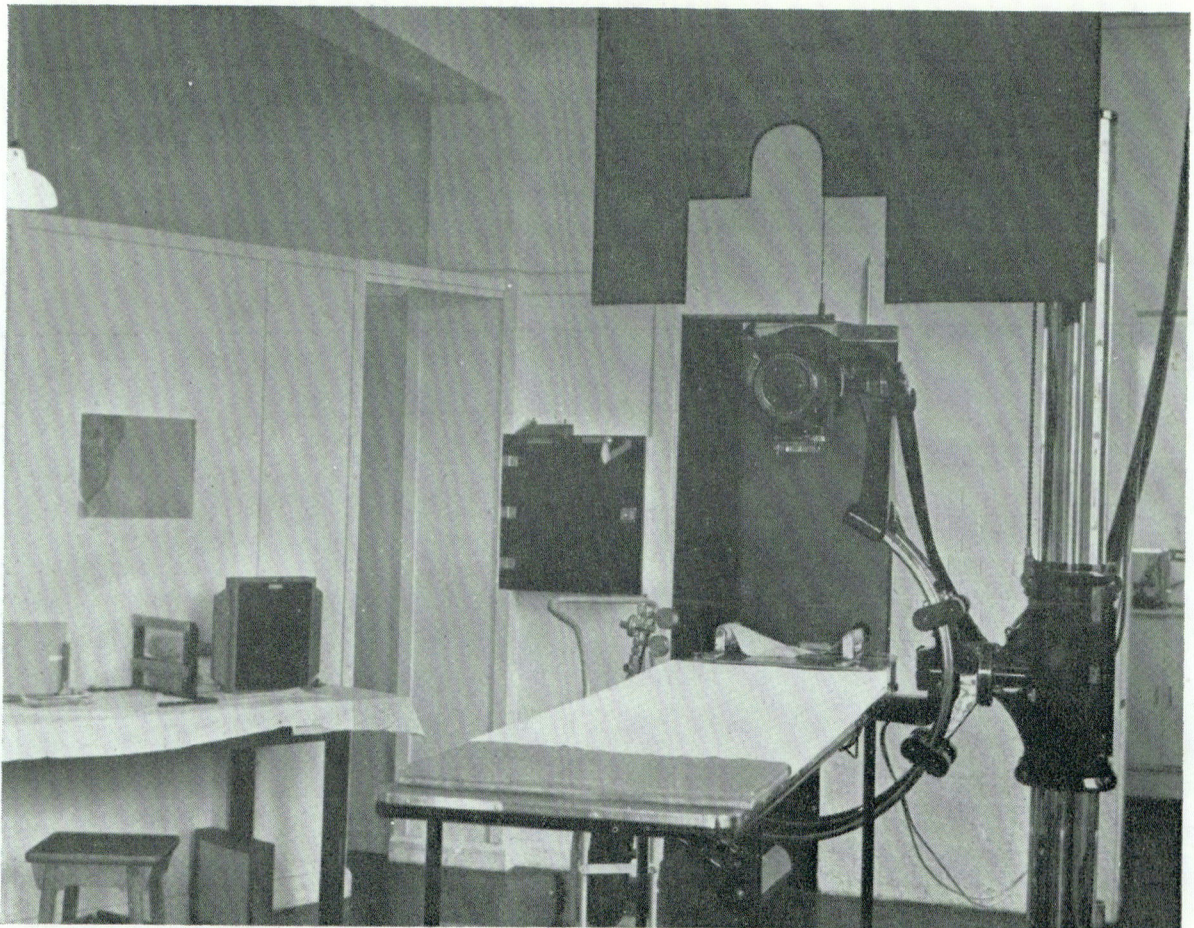

NEW X-RAY DEPARTMENT   MORRISTON HOSPITAL

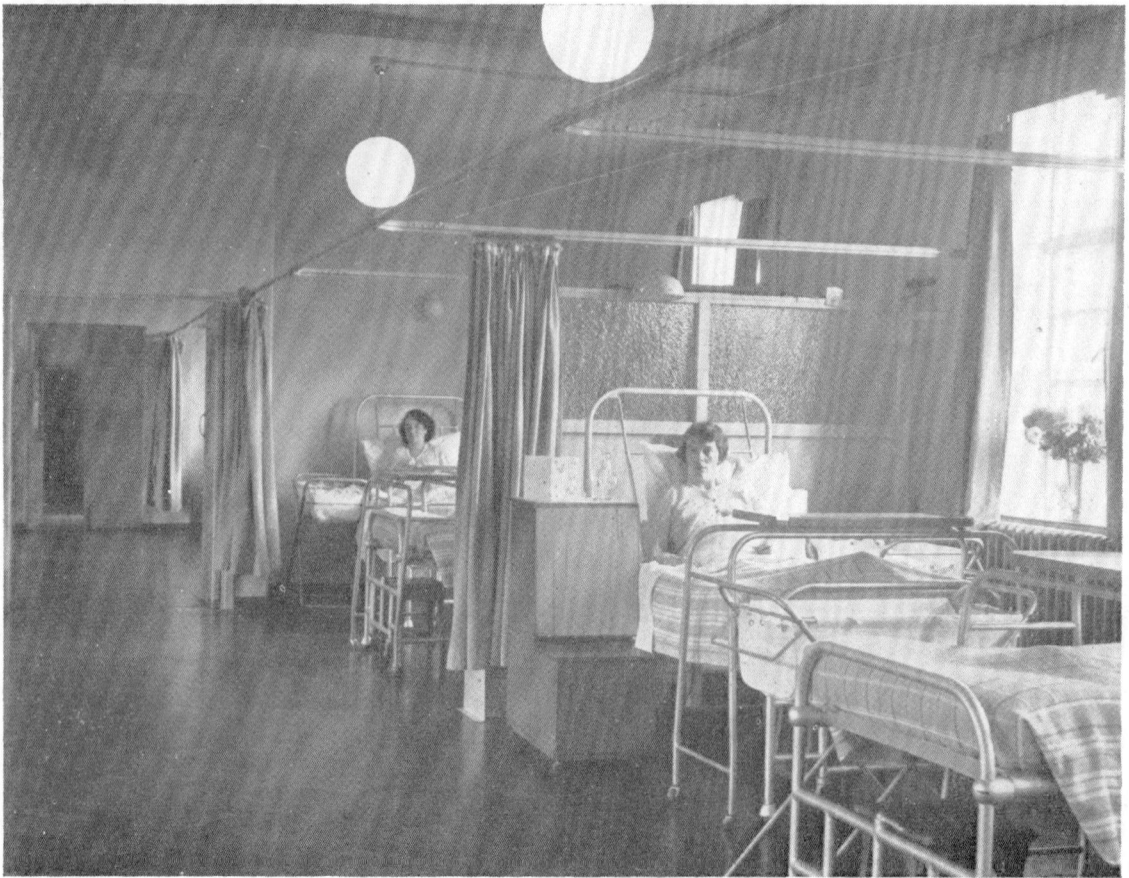

WARD 12   MORRISTON HOSPITAL

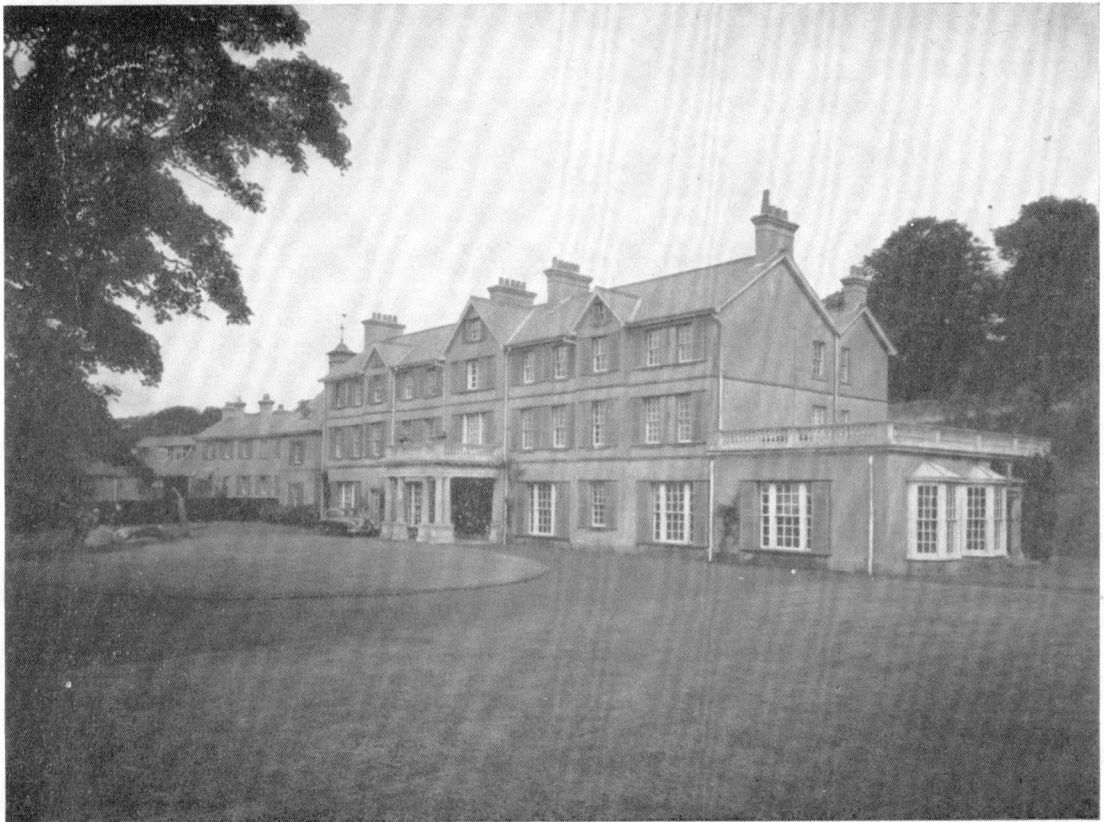

CILYMAENLLWYD HOSPITAL

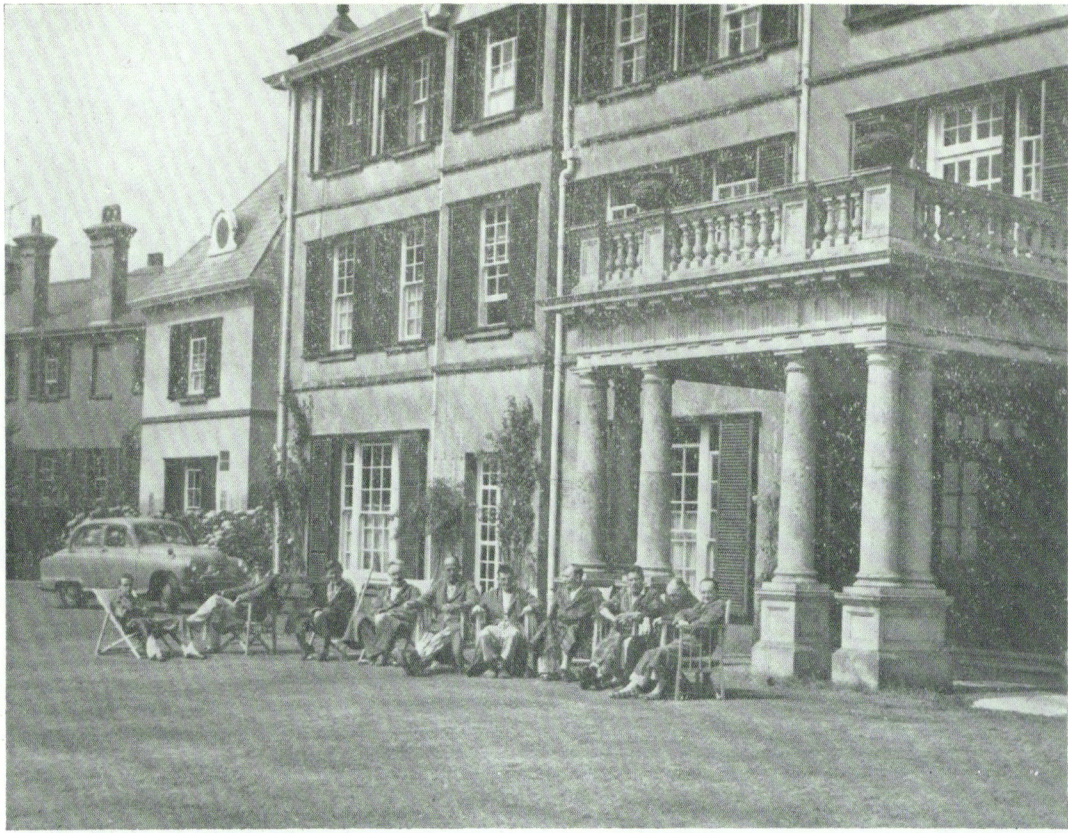

ENTRANCE   CILYMAENLLWYD HOSPITAL

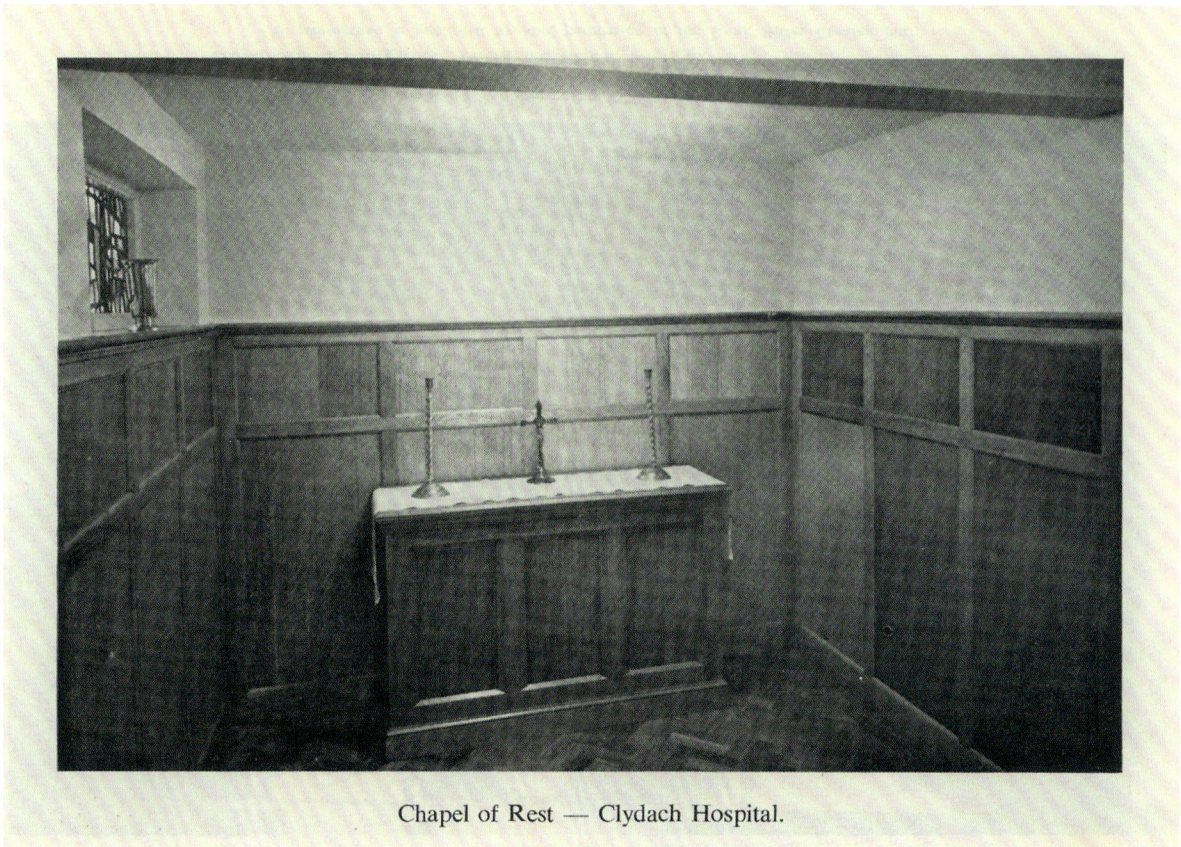

Chapel of Rest — Clydach Hospital.

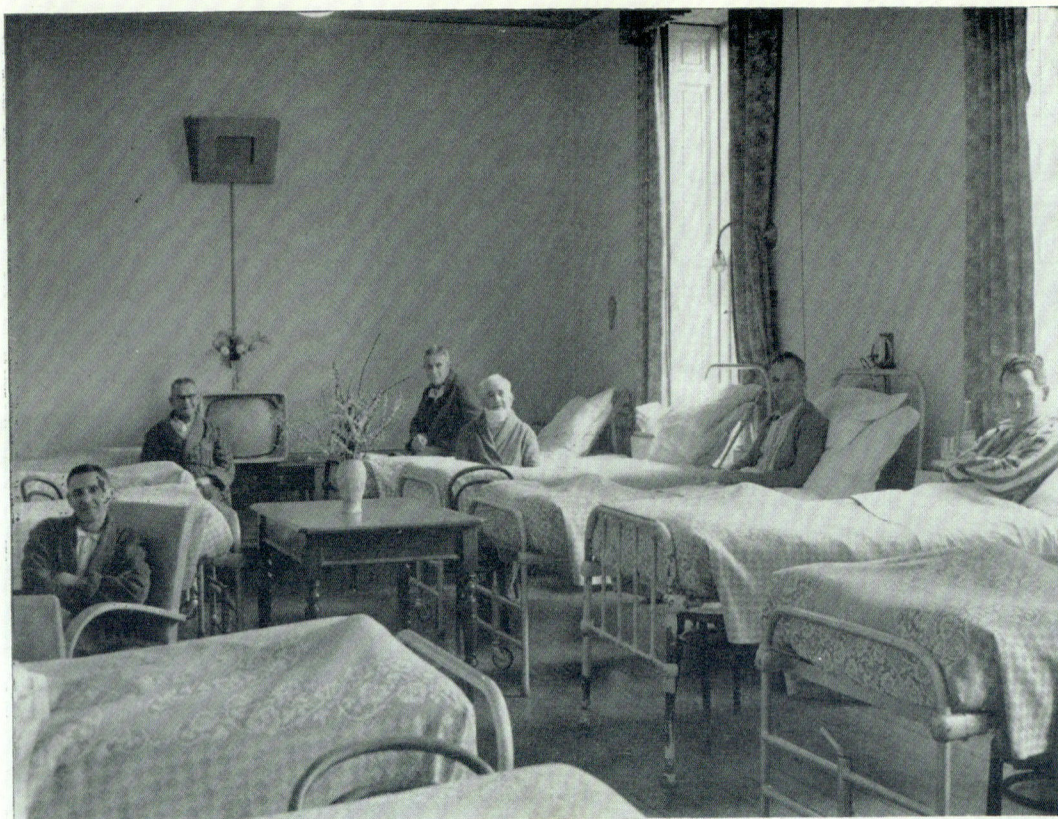

MALE WARD   STOUTHALL HOSPITAL

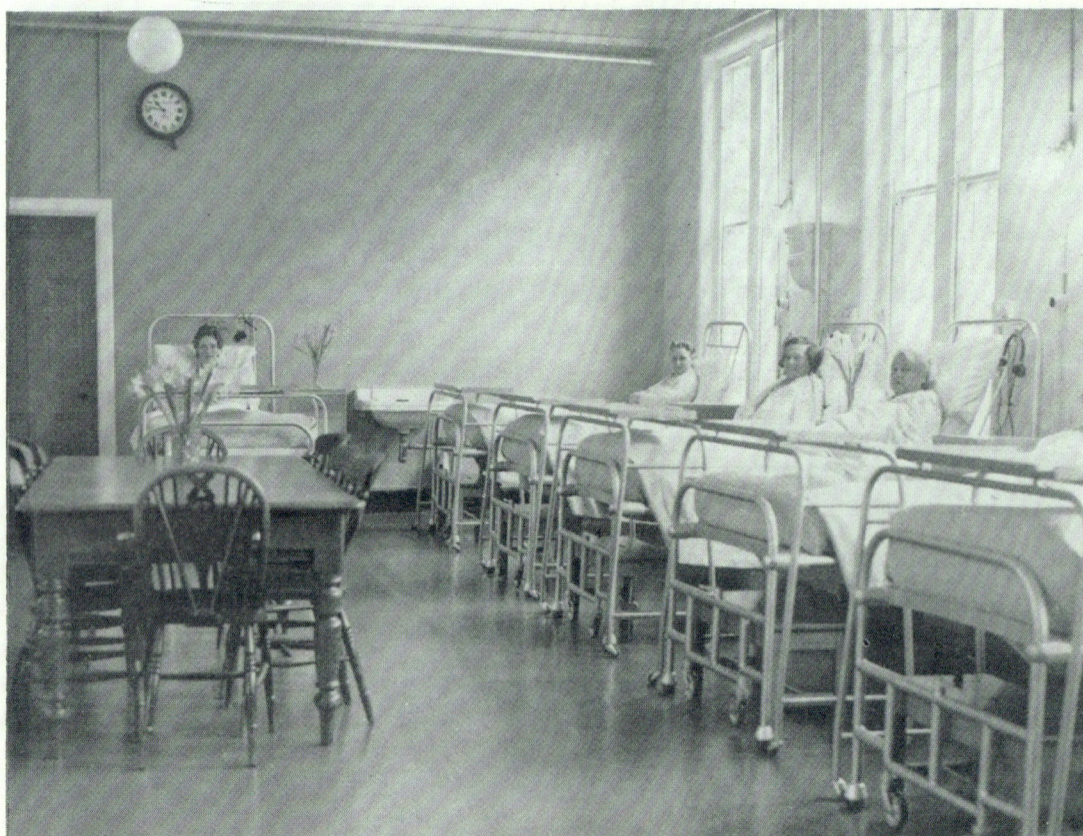

FEMALE WARD   CONVALESCENT HOME, SWANSEA

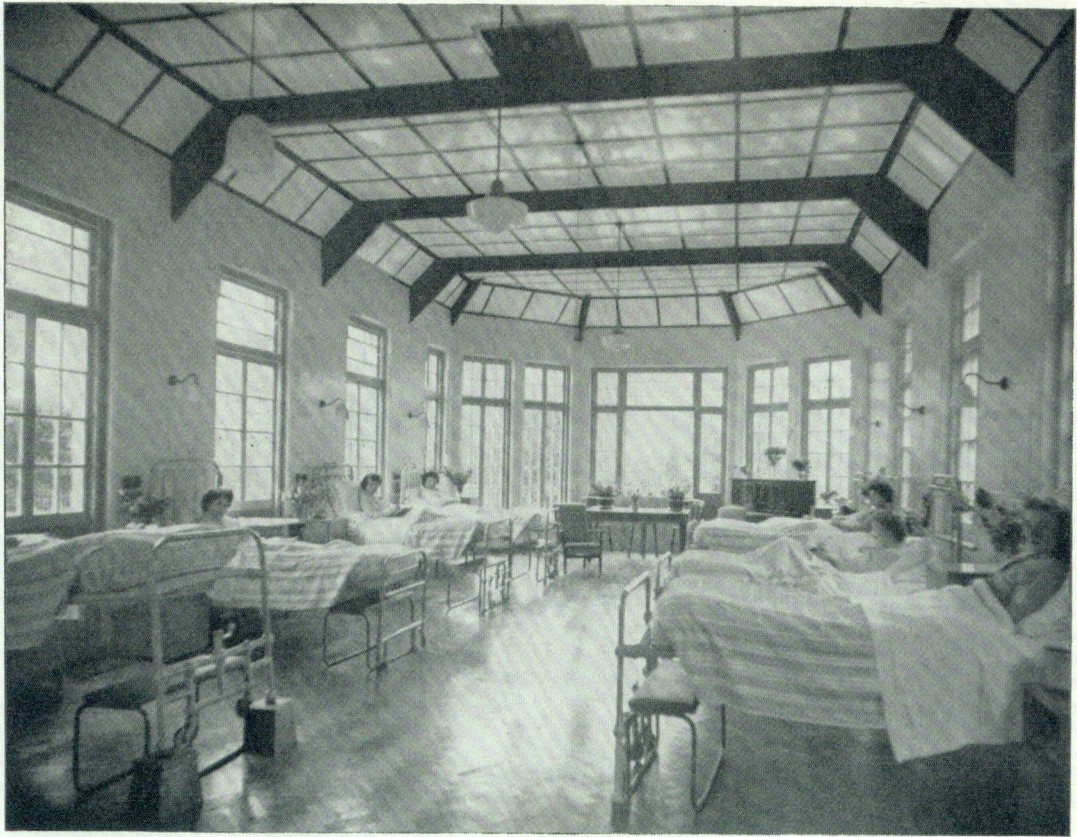

FEMALE WARD   ADELINA PATTI HOSPITAL

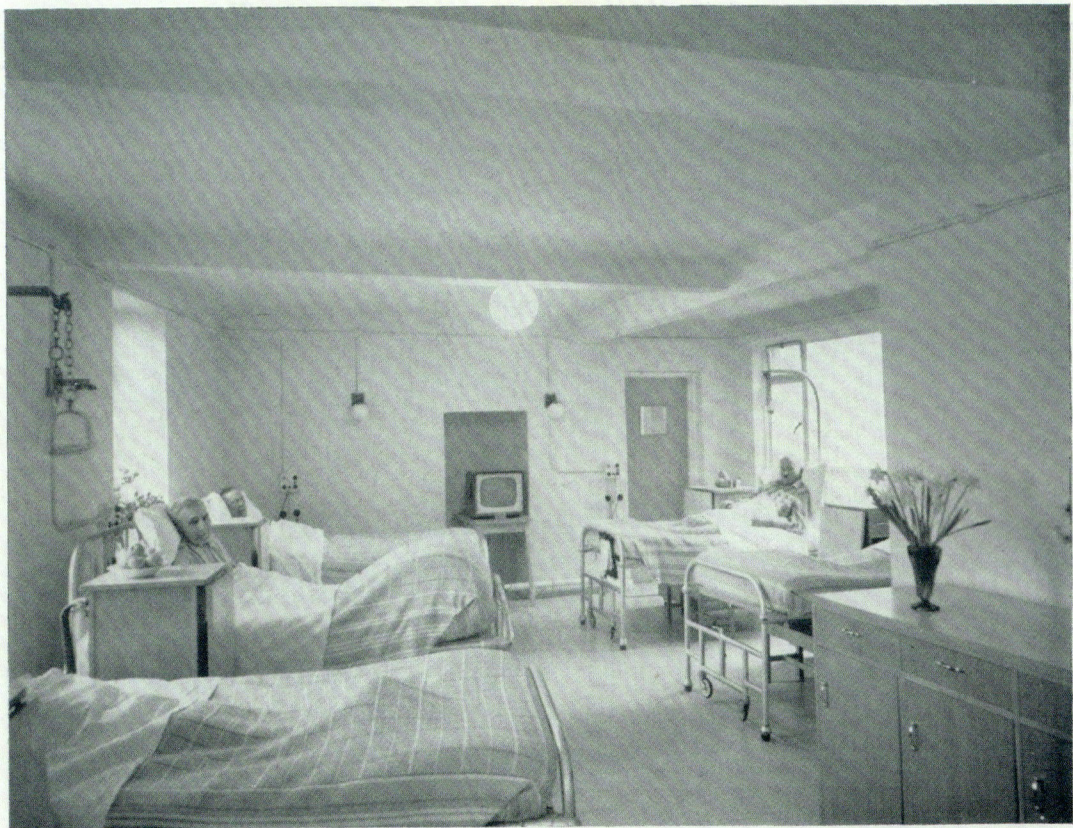

RENOVATED WARD   BRYNTIRION HOSPITAL

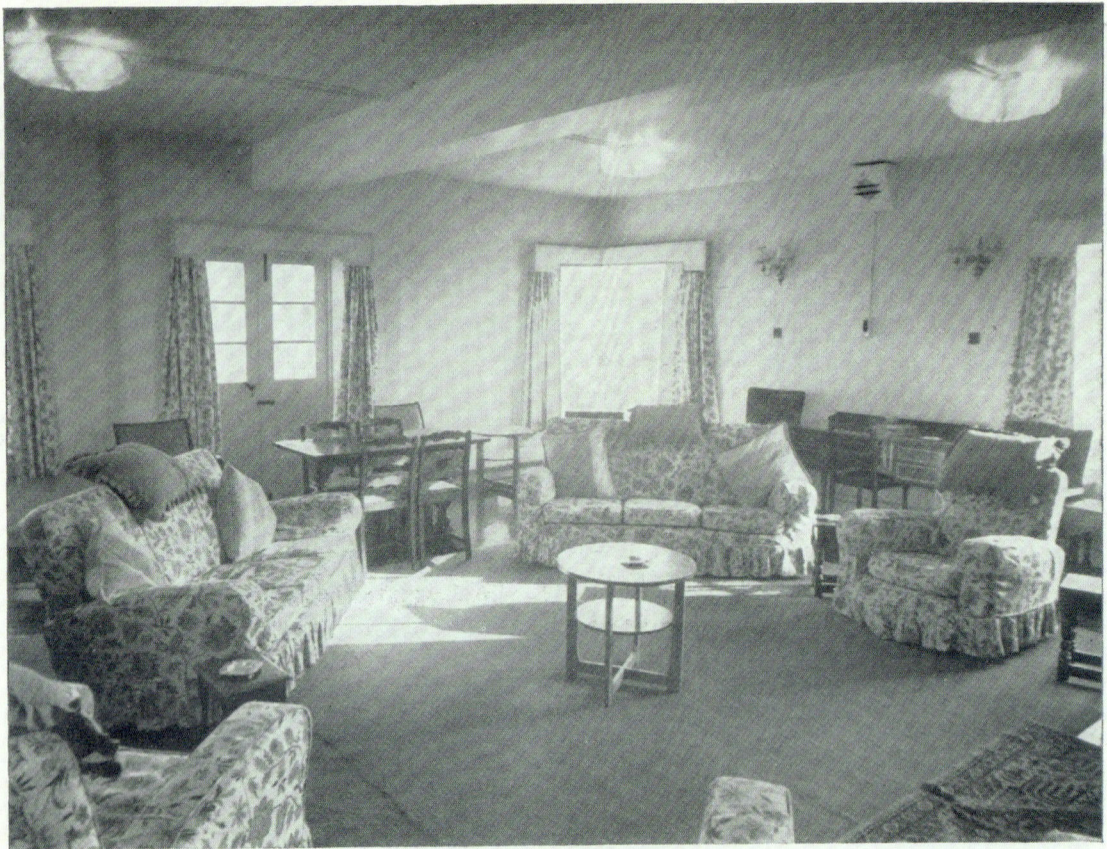

SISTERS' HOME

MORRISTON HOSPITAL

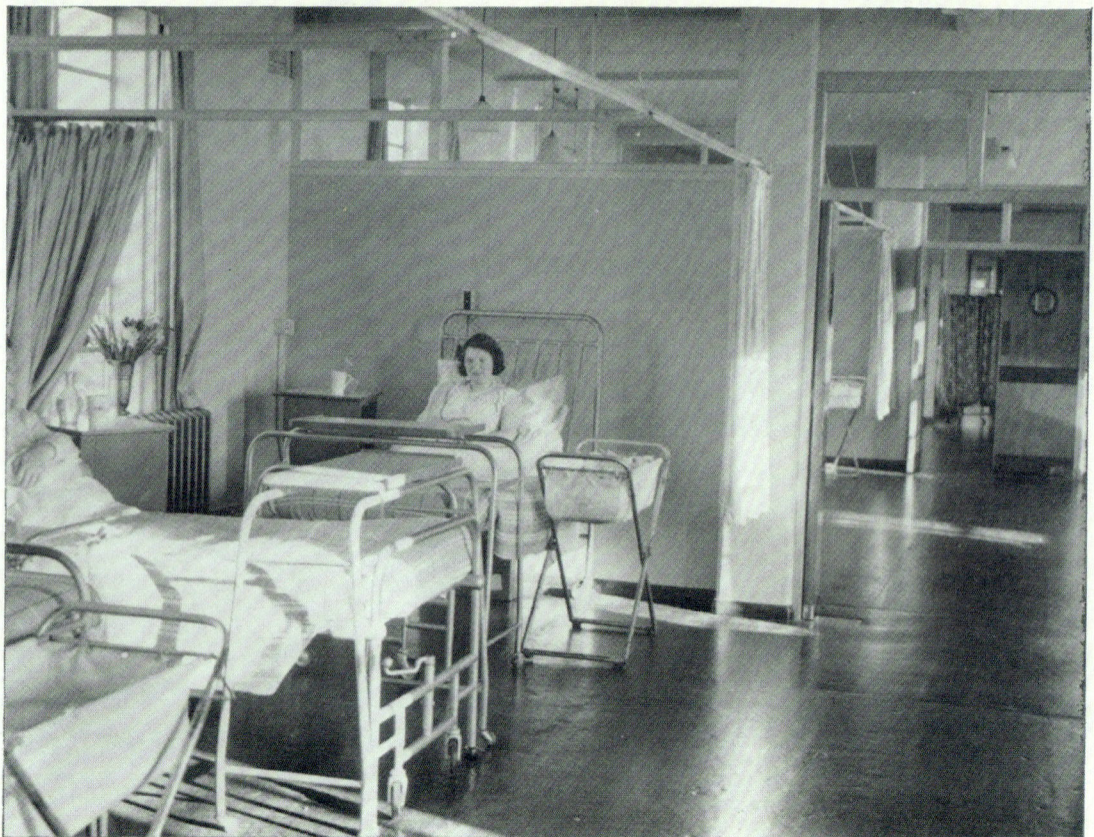

WARD 10

MORRISTON HOSPITAL

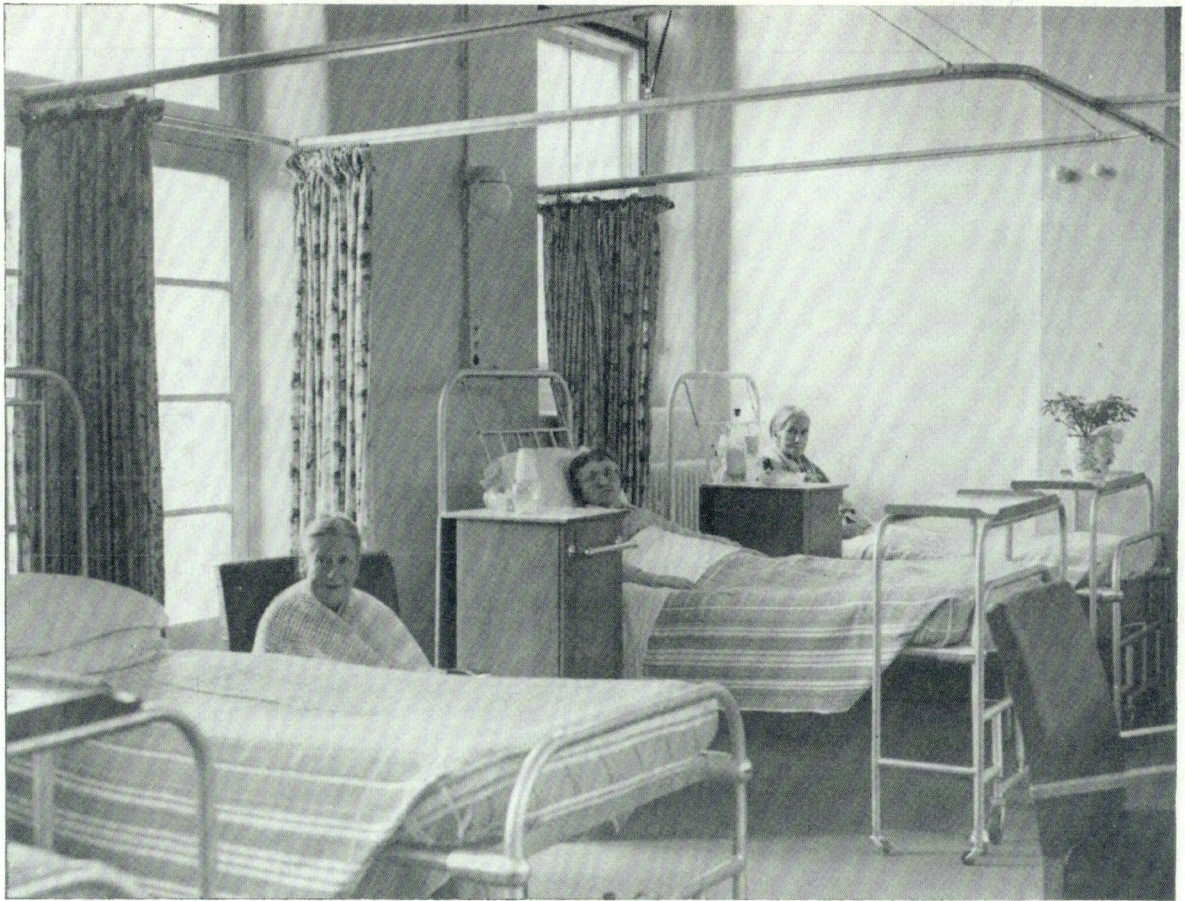

FEMALE WARD   GELLYNUDD HOSPITAL

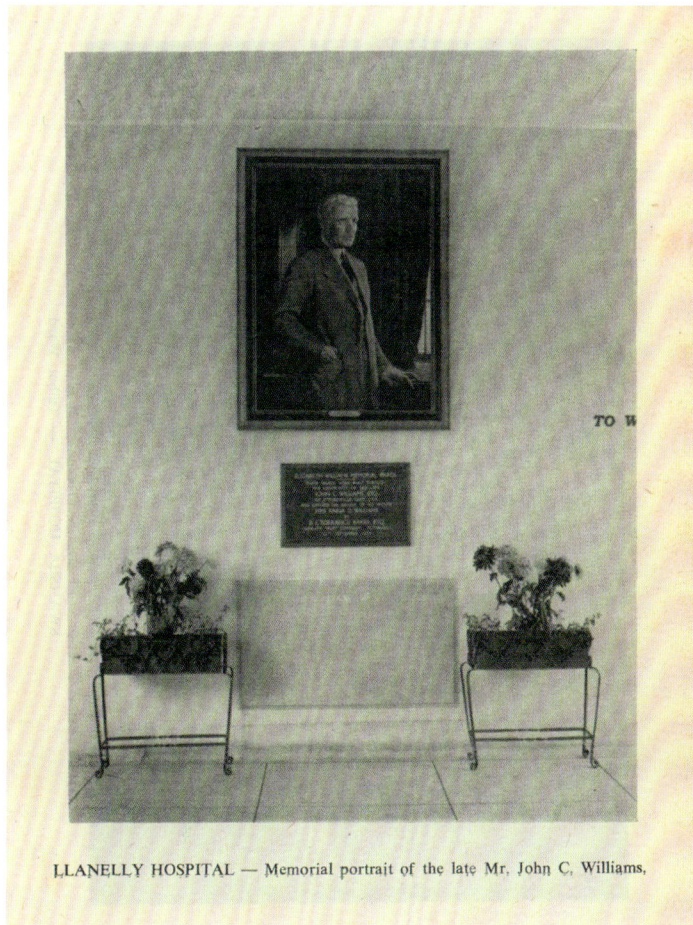

LLANELLY HOSPITAL — Memorial portrait of the late Mr. John C. Williams,

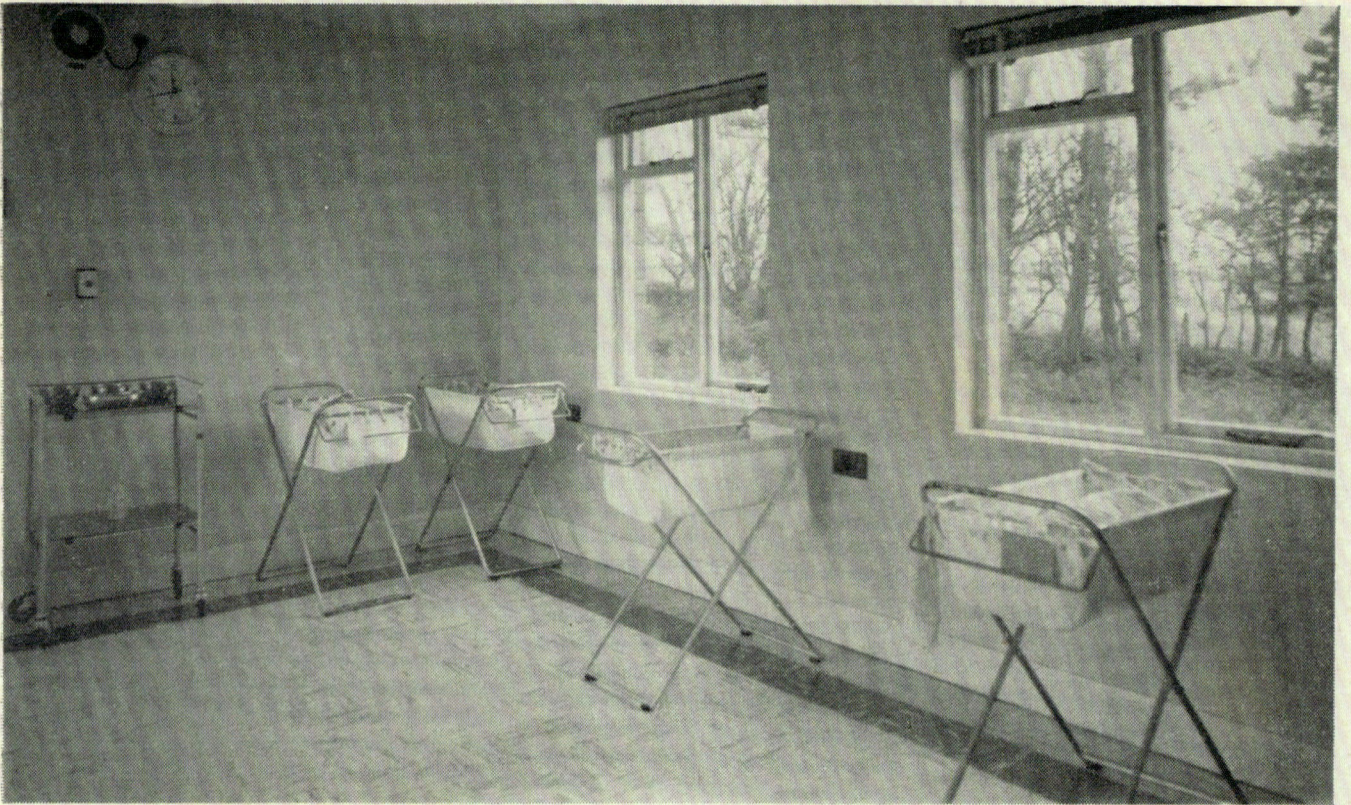

FAIRWOOD MATERNITY HOSPITAL — Nursery.

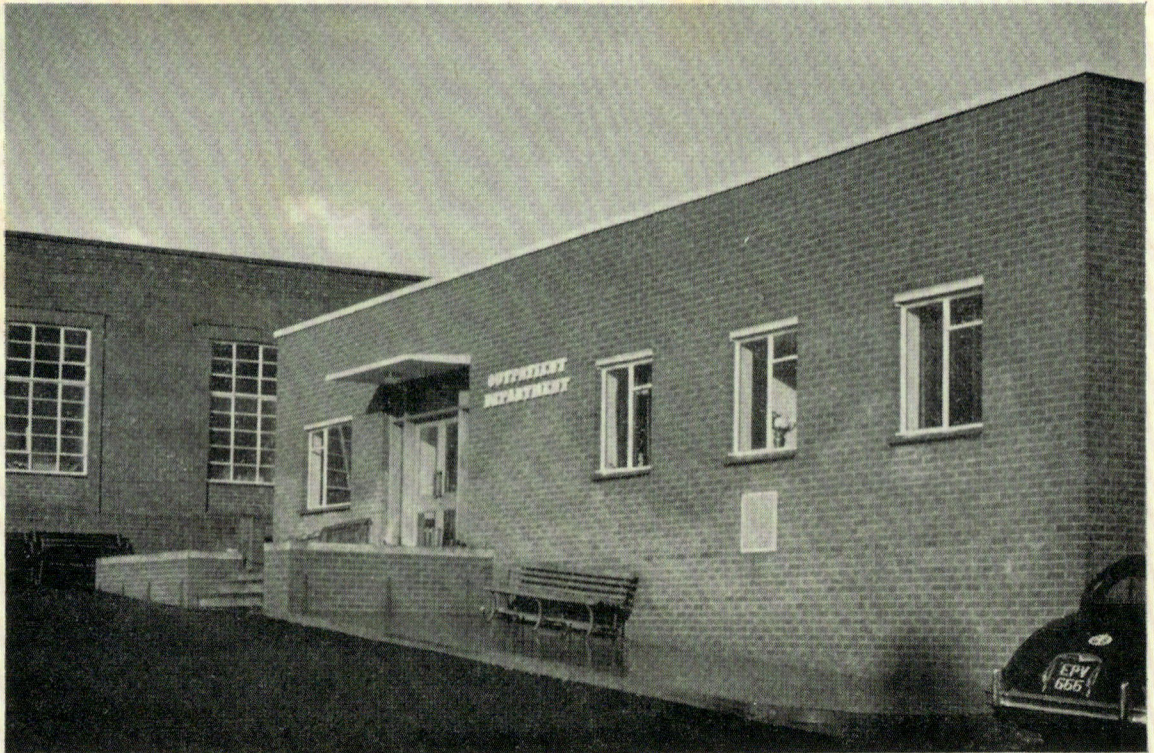

MORRISTON HOSPITAL — Outpatient Department.

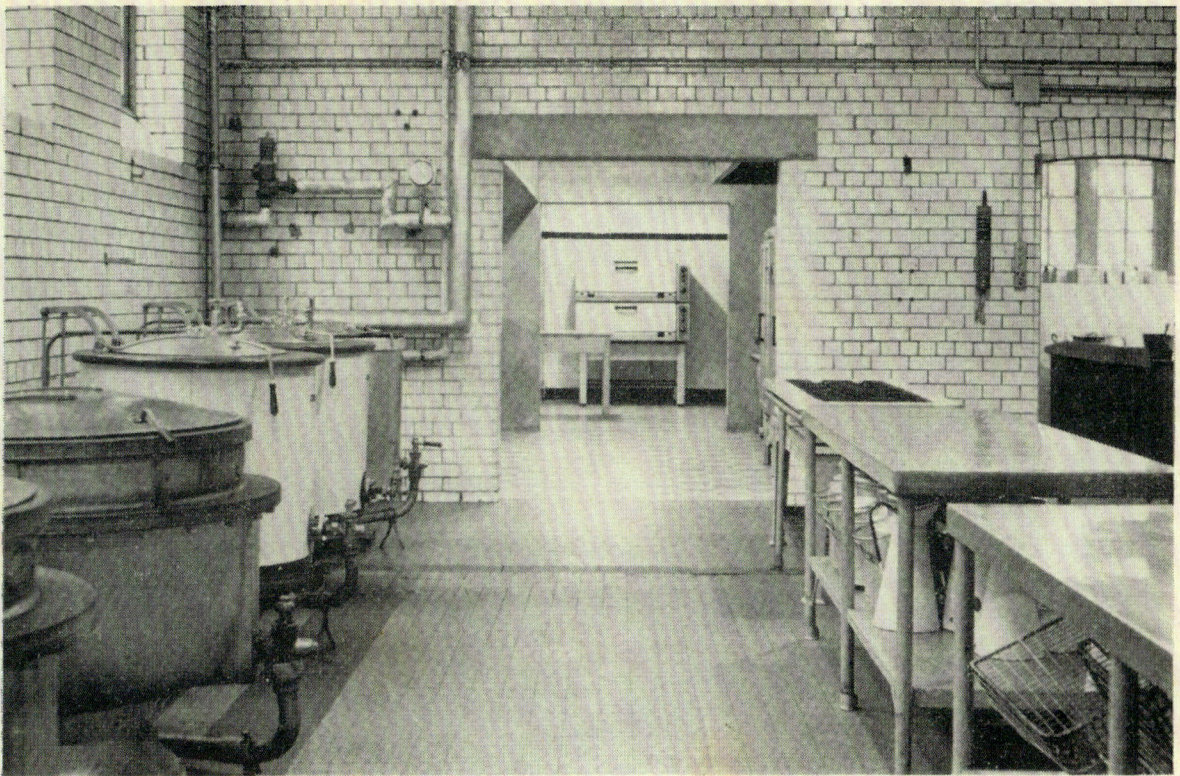

MOUNT PLEASANT HOSPITAL — Kitchen.

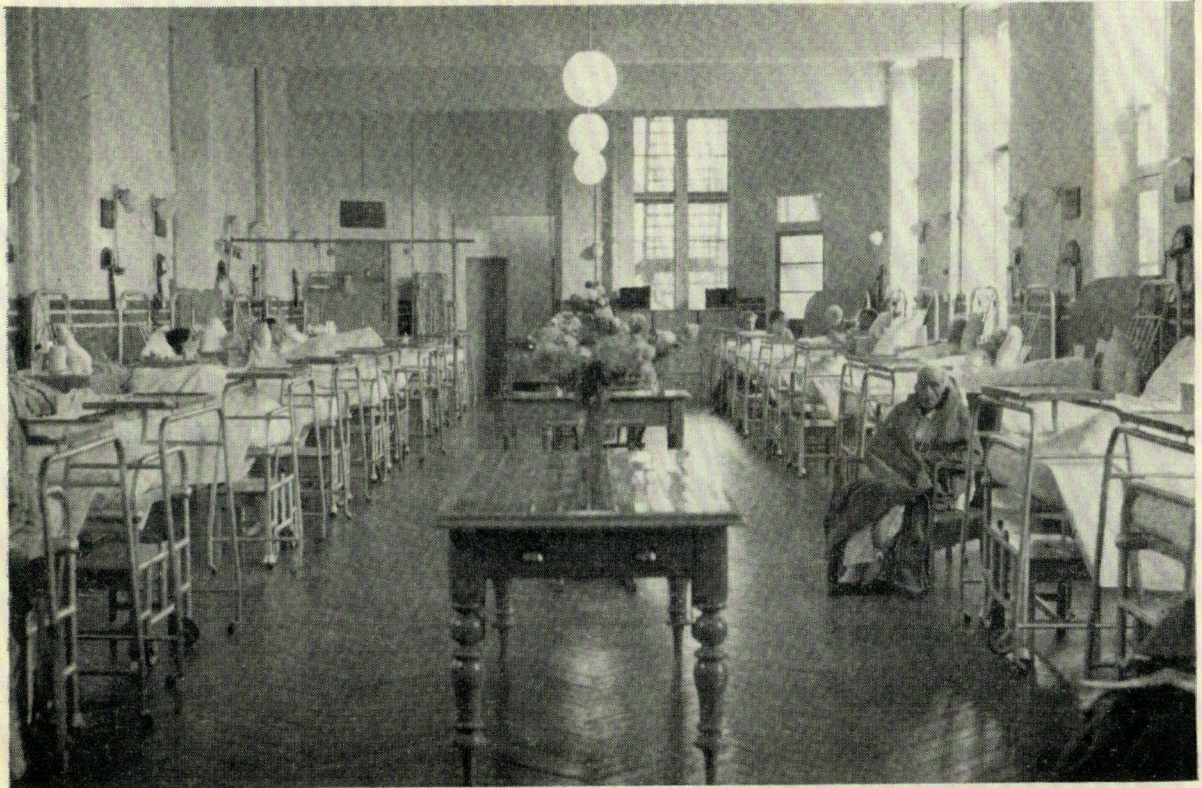

SWANSEA HOSPITAL — Talbot Ward.

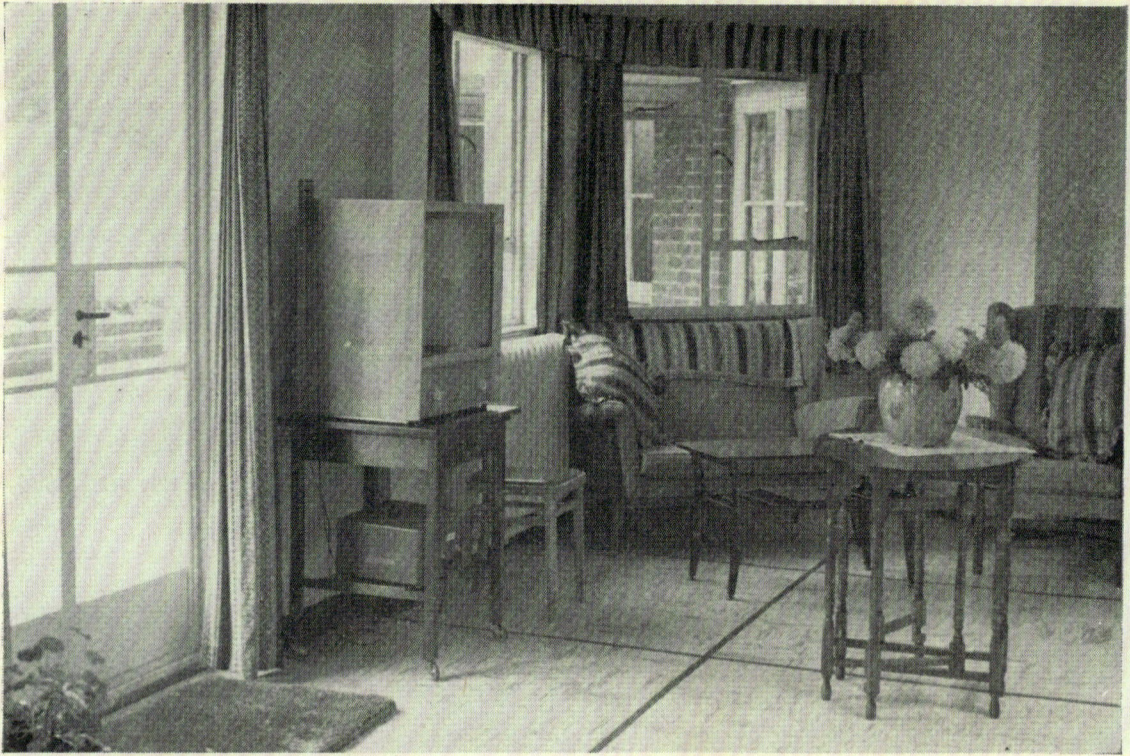

CLYDACH HOSPITAL — Dayroom.

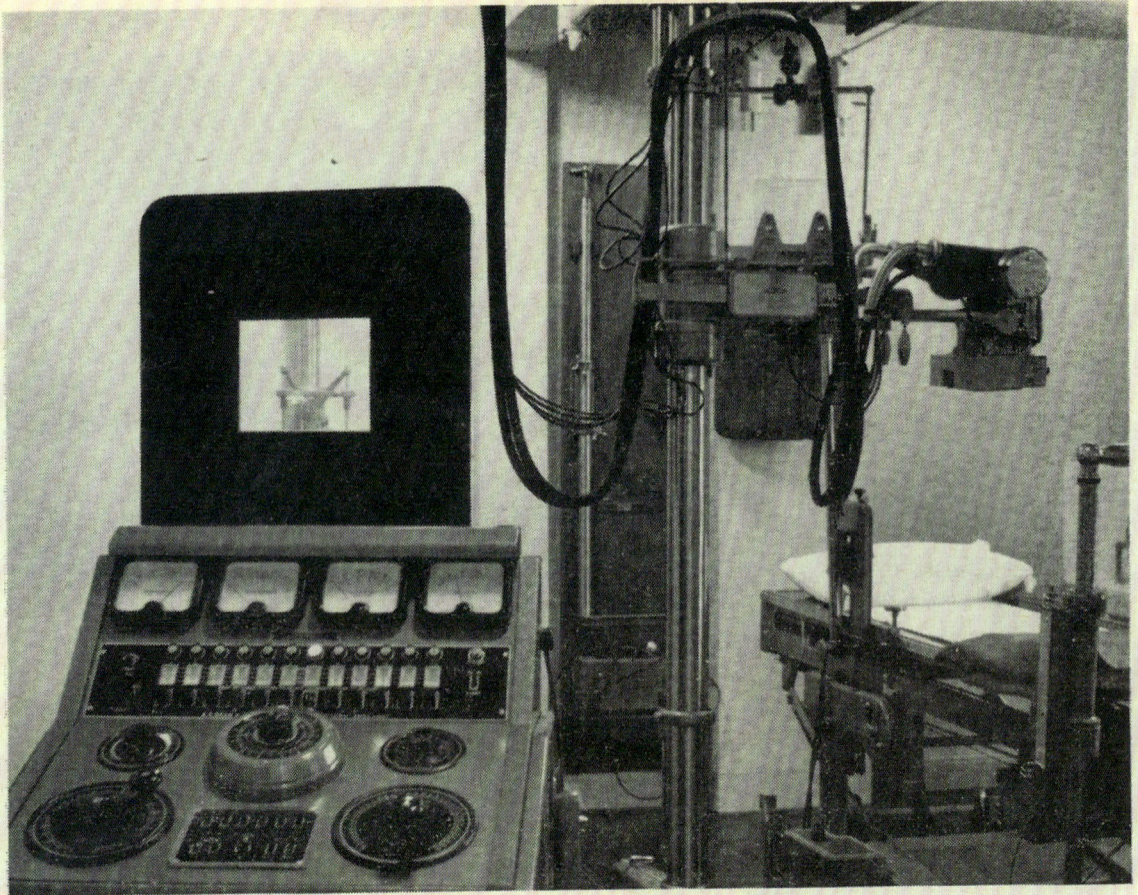

LLANELLY CHEST CLINIC — New X-ray Set.

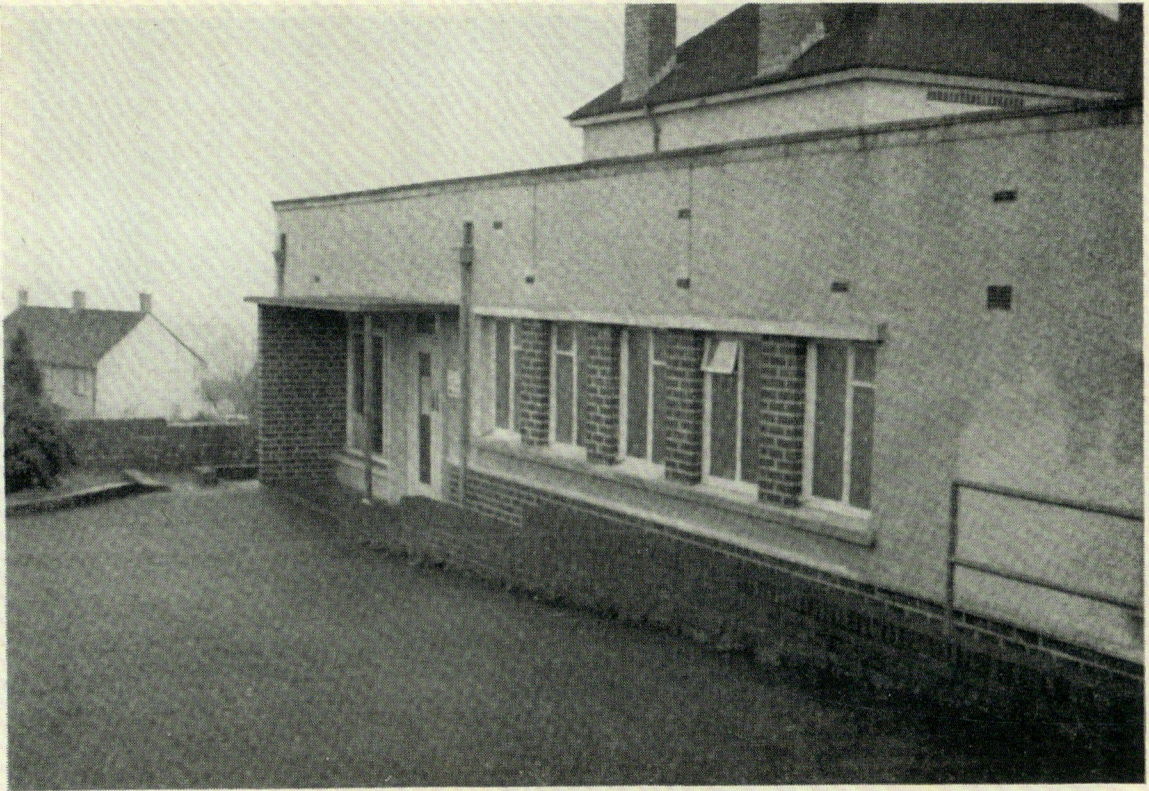

LLANELLY CHEST CLINIC — Exterior

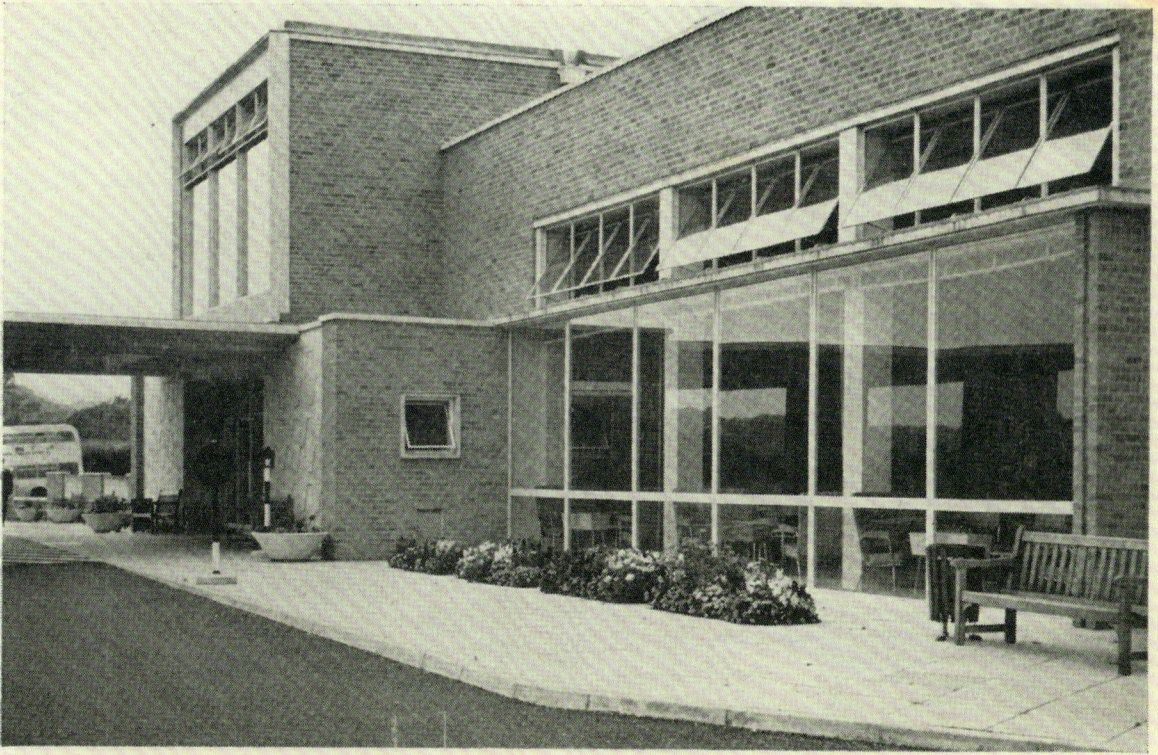

MAIN ENTRANCE—New Out-patient Department, Singleton

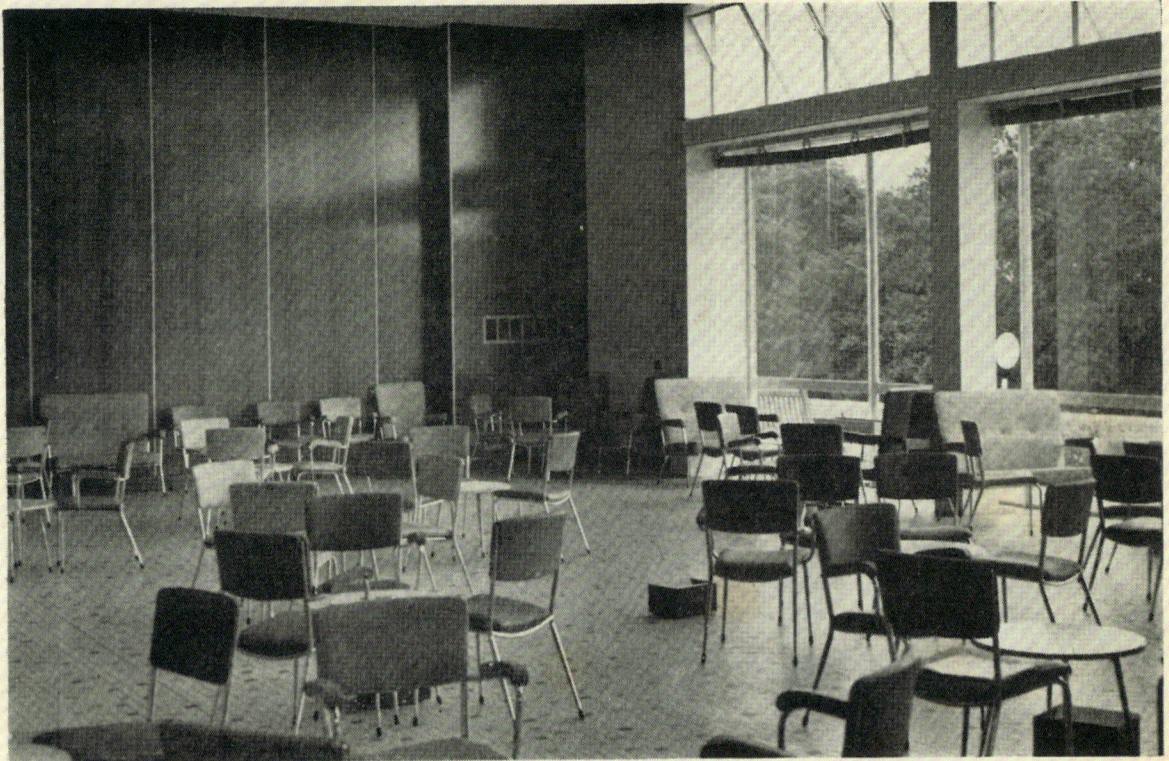

WAITING HALL—New Out-patient Department, Singleton

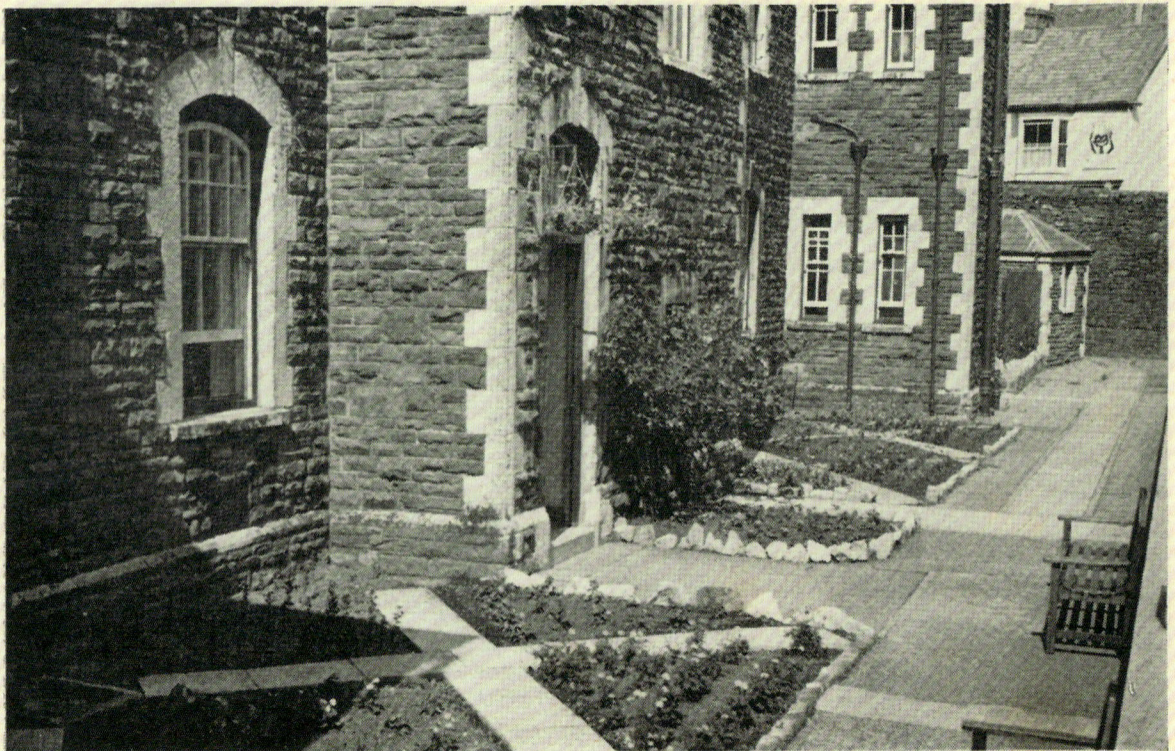

EXTERIOR—Mewslade Ward, Mount Pleasant Hospital

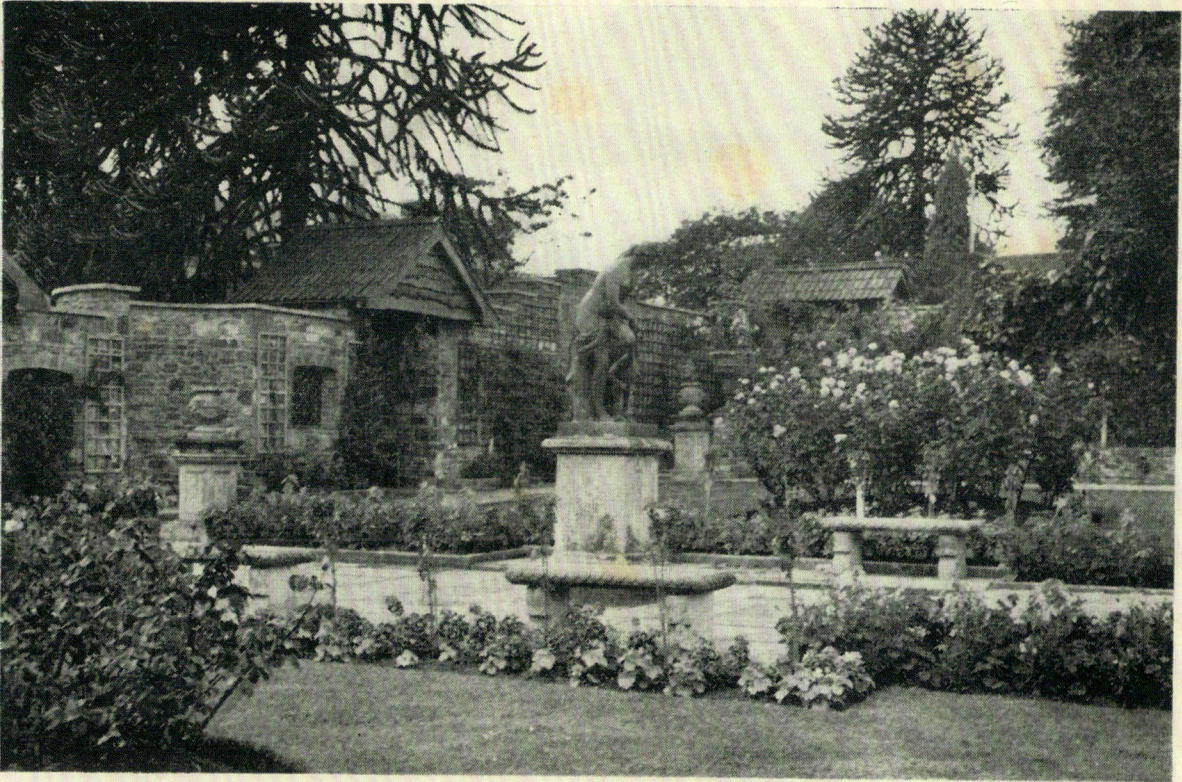

ORNAMENTAL GARDEN—Morriston Hospital

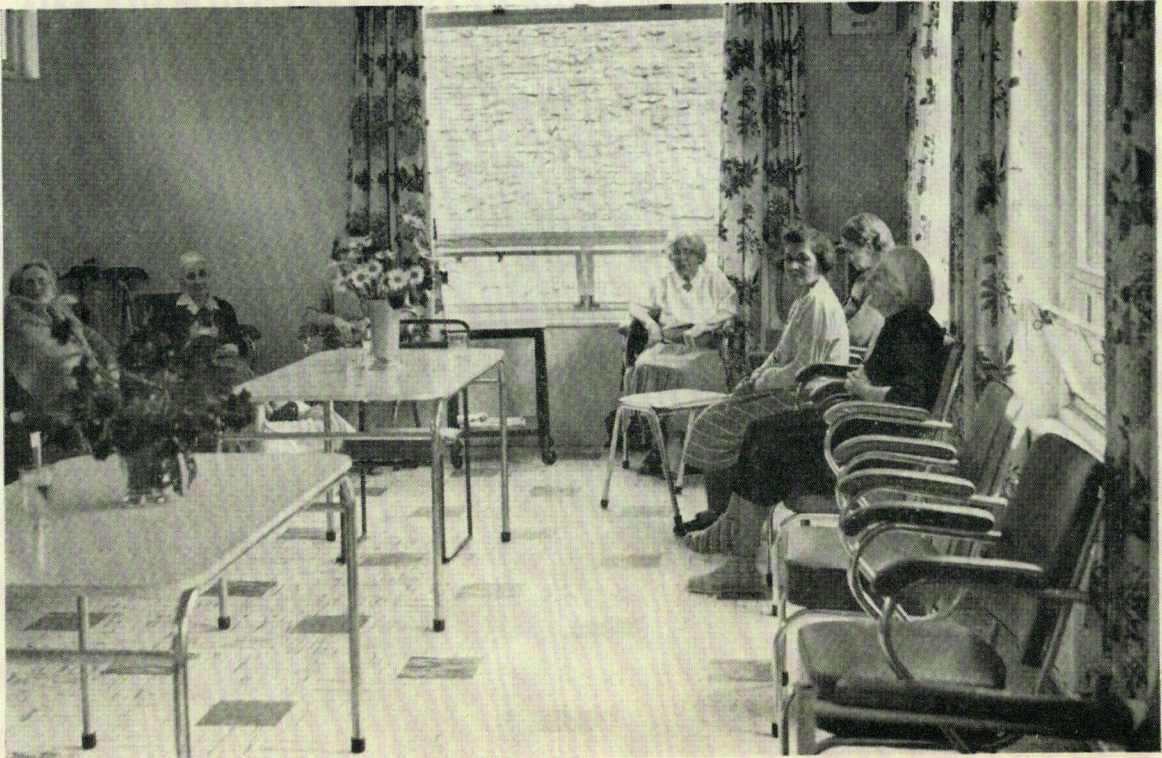

NEW DAY ROOM—Mewslade Ward, Mount Pleasant Hospital

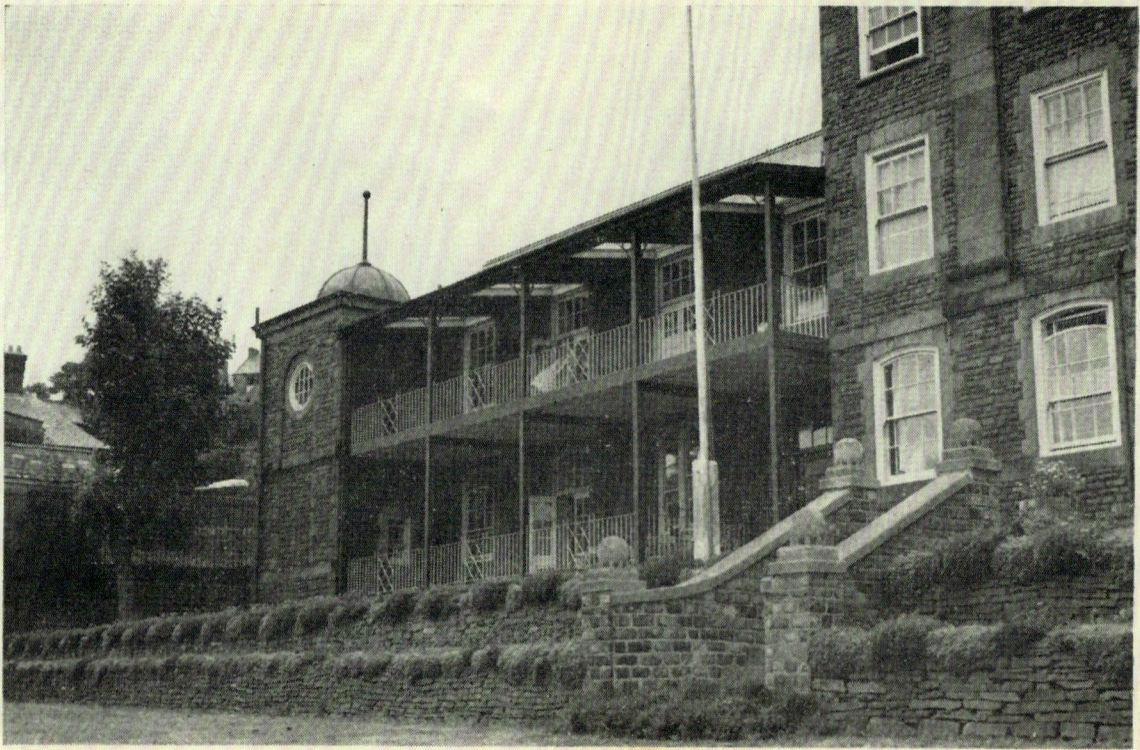

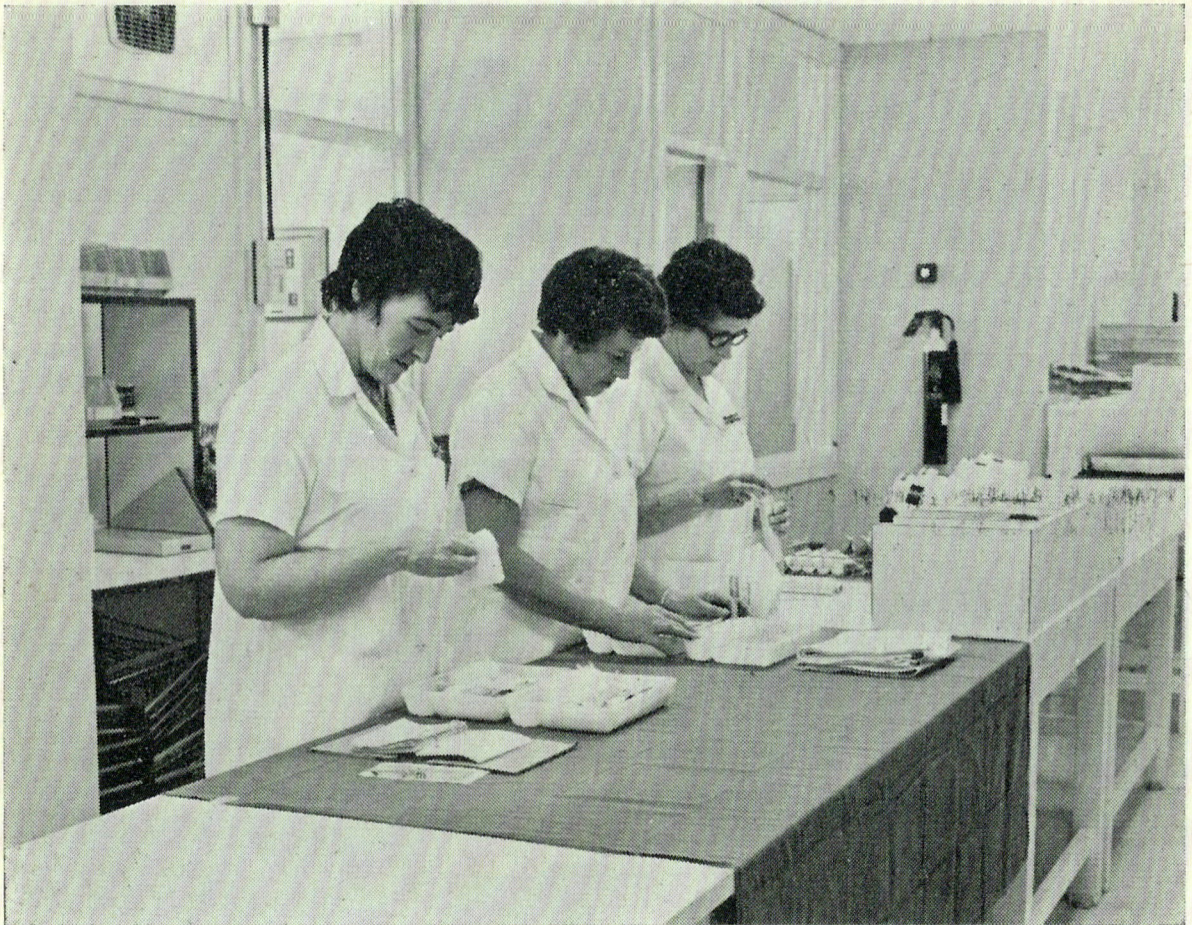

C.S.S.D. Assistants producing Comprehensive Packs for ward use.

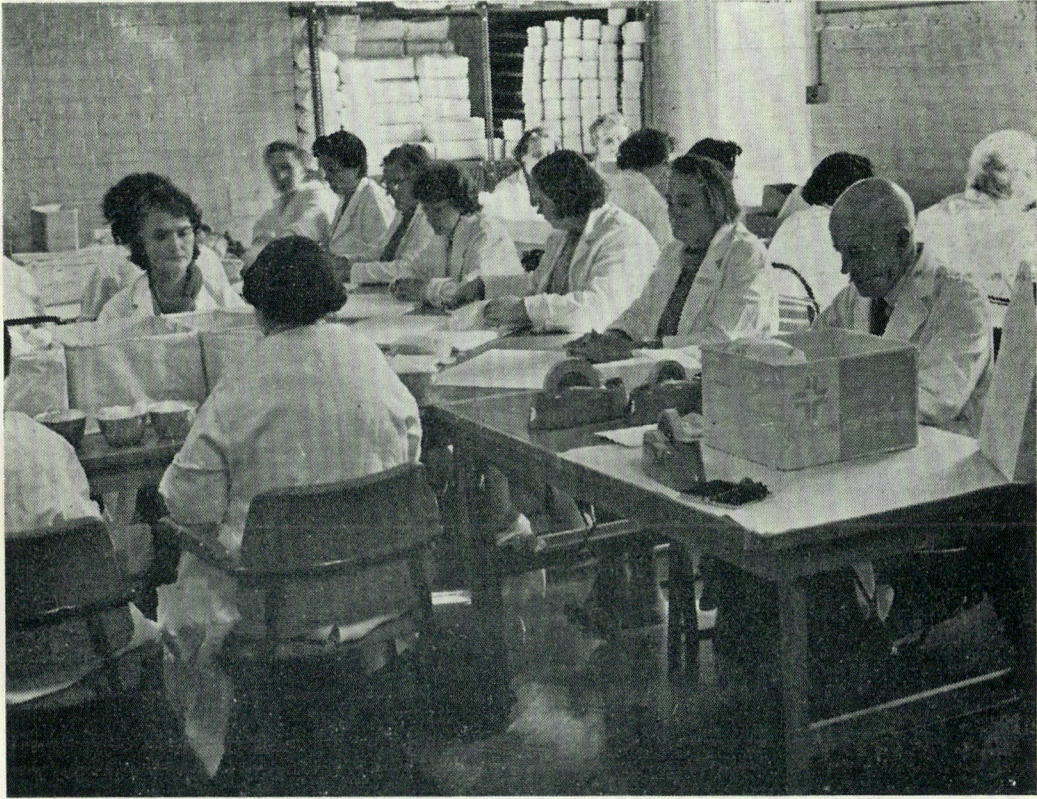

Industrial Therapy Patients producing simple basic packs.

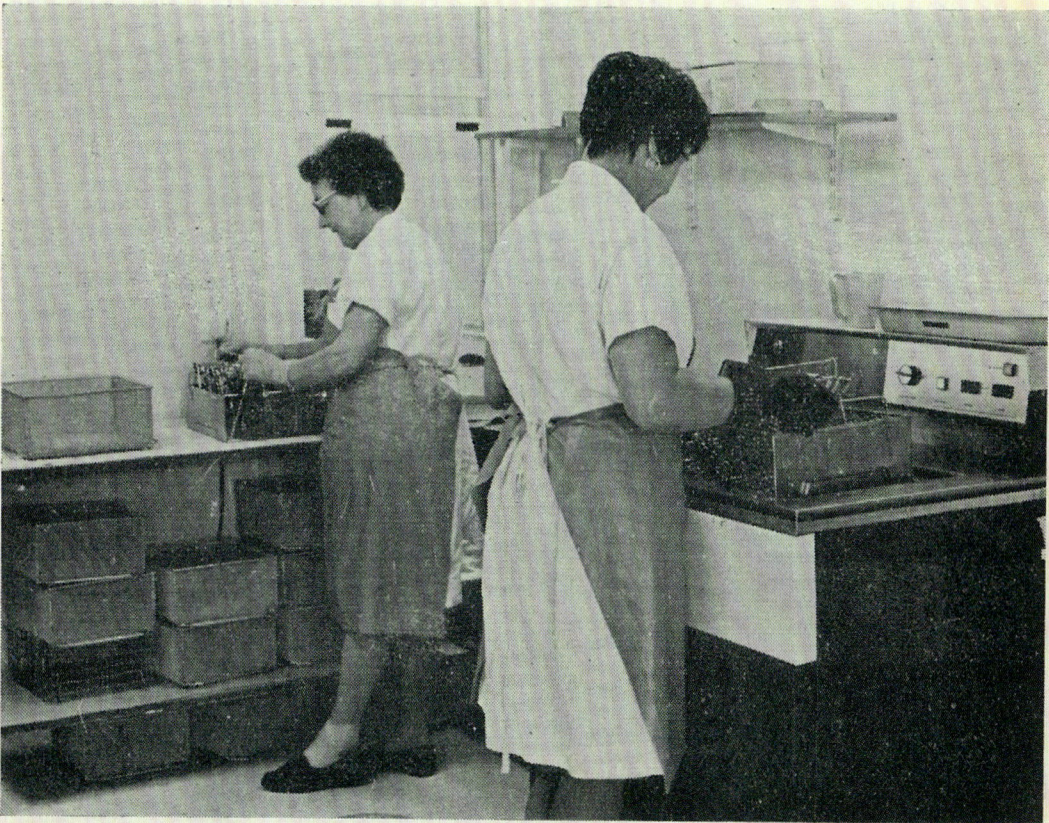

Major Operating Theatre Instruments being sorted and washed.

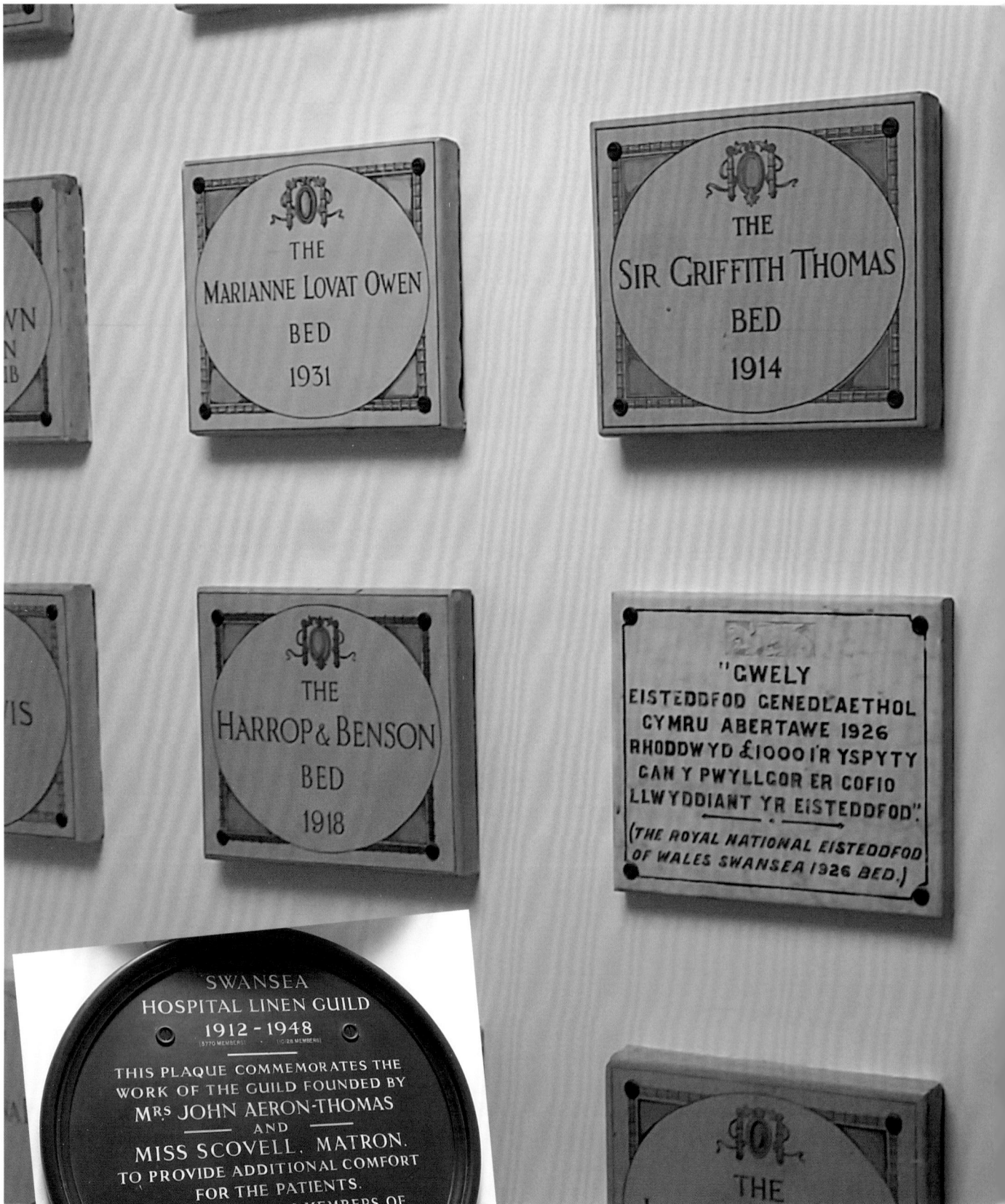

THE
MARIANNE LOVAT OWEN
BED
1931

THE
SIR GRIFFITH THOMAS
BED
1914

THE
HARROP & BENSON
BED
1918

"GWELY
EISTEDDFOD GENEDLAETHOL
CYMRU ABERTAWE 1926
RHODDWYD £1000 I'R YSPYTY
GAN Y PWYLLGOR ER COFIO
LLWYDDIANT YR EISTEDDFOD"

(THE ROYAL NATIONAL EISTEDDFOD
OF WALES SWANSEA 1926 BED.)

SWANSEA
HOSPITAL LINEN GUILD
1912 - 1948
THIS PLAQUE COMMEMORATES THE
WORK OF THE GUILD FOUNDED BY
MRS JOHN AERON-THOMAS
AND
MISS SCOVELL, MATRON.
TO PROVIDE ADDITIONAL COMFORT
FOR THE PATIENTS.
DURING 36 YEARS, MEMBERS OF
THE GUILD IN SWANSEA AND
DISTRICT HAVE CONTRIBUTED
£55,000 FOR THIS
PURPOSE.

THE

THE
ALICE DAVIES
BED
1928

THE
ALDERMAN EV.
BED
1920

THE
WILLIAM JONES
(Master Mariner)
BED
1930

IN MEMO
OF
ELIZABETH A
A TRIBUTE OF
FROM HER
ALFRED EDWARD

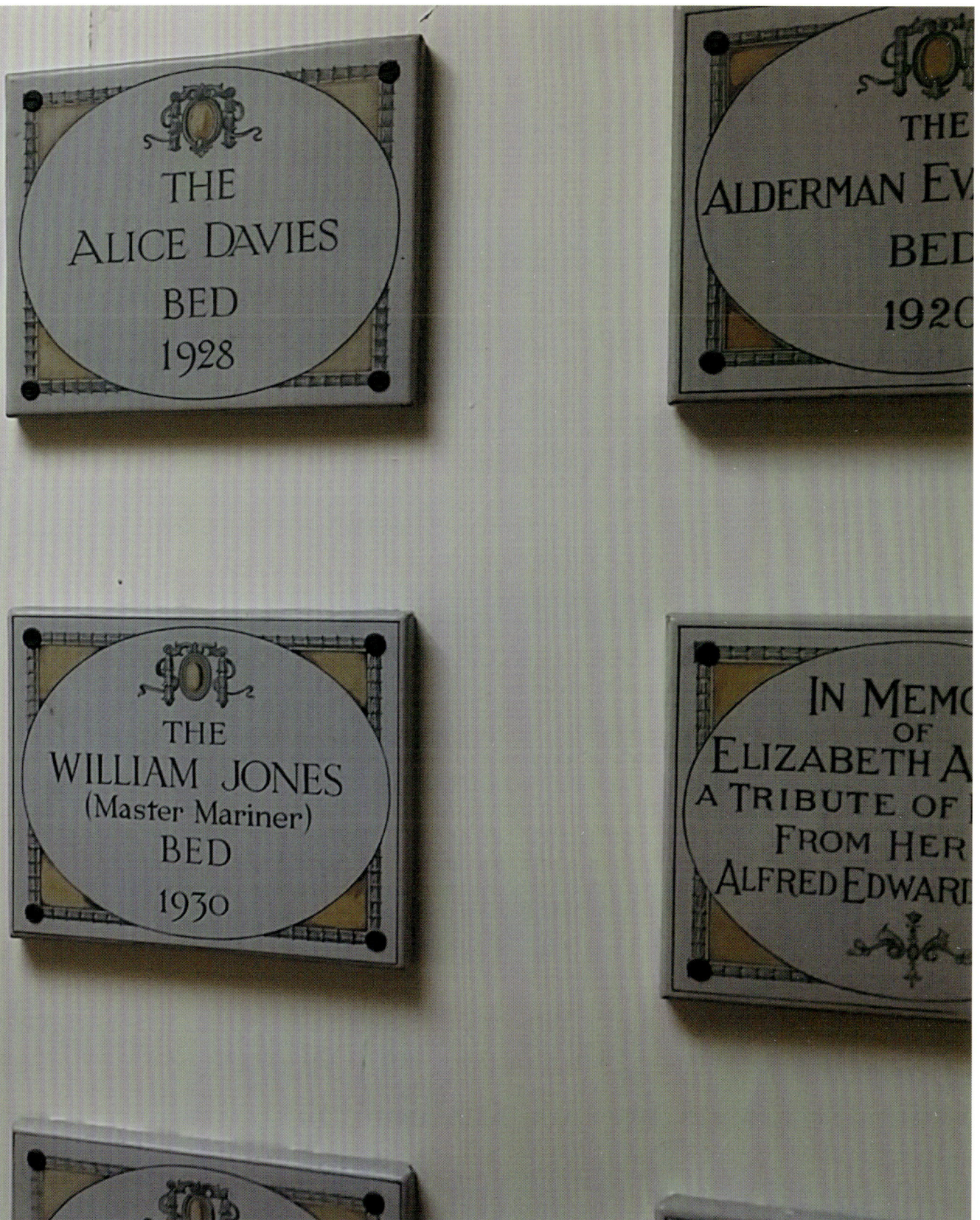

Some of the bed plaques on display at Singleton Hospital, and (left) one of the plaques, celebrating the work of Swansea Hospital Linen Guild

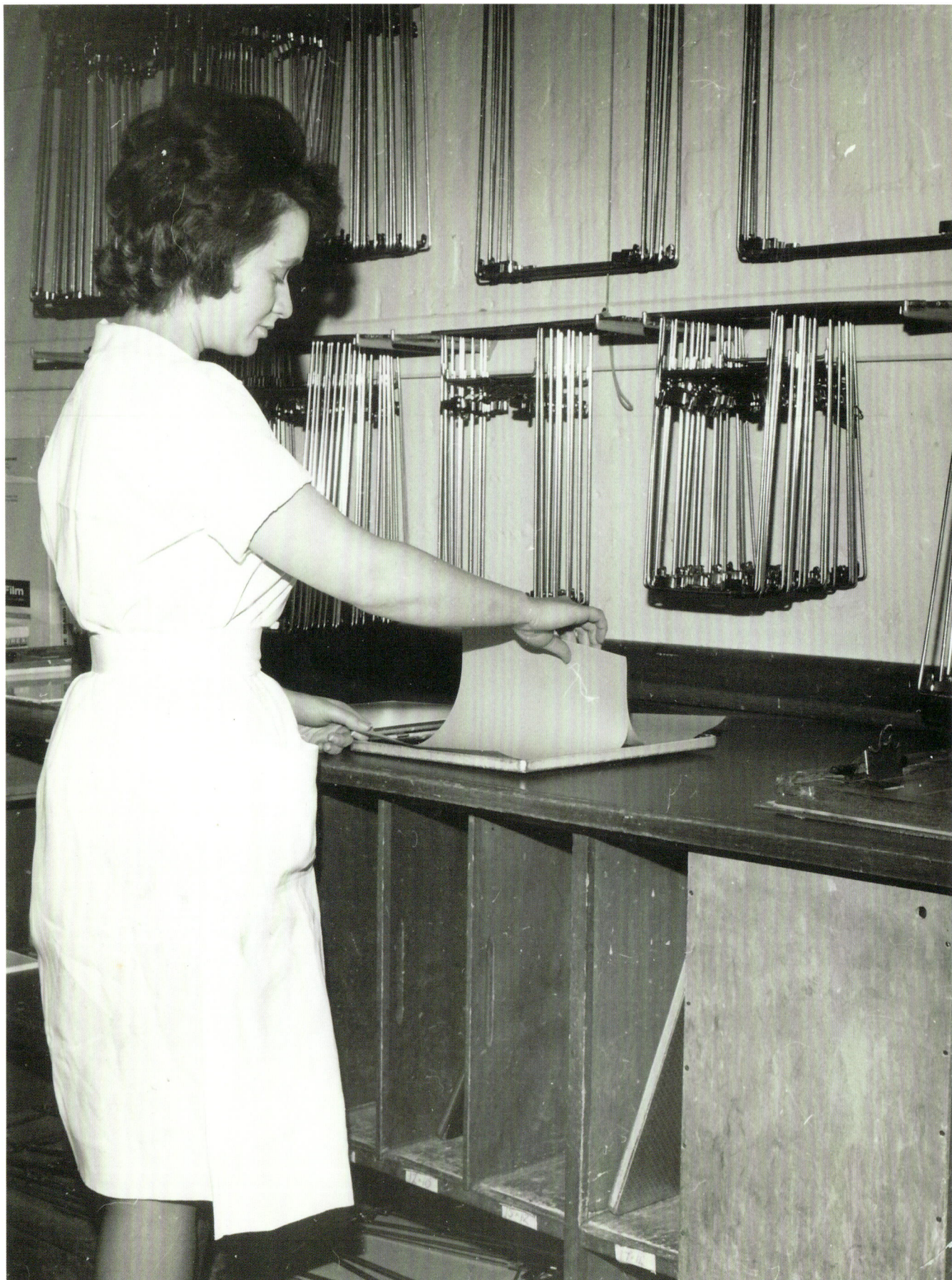

Processing x-rays

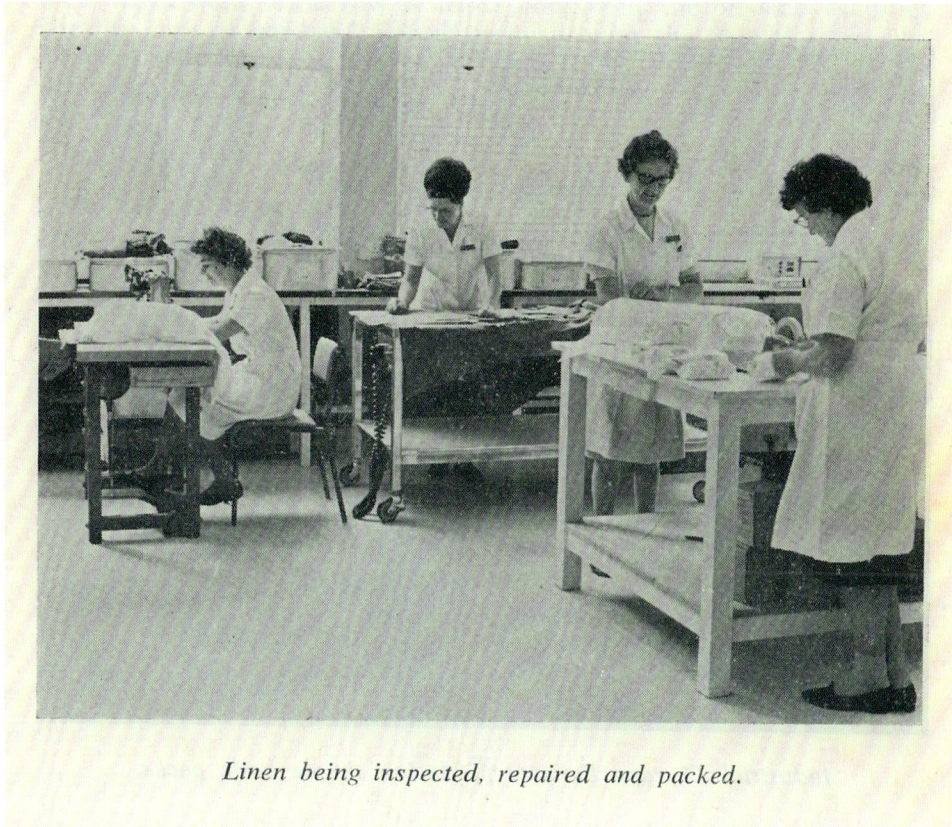

Linen being inspected, repaired and packed.

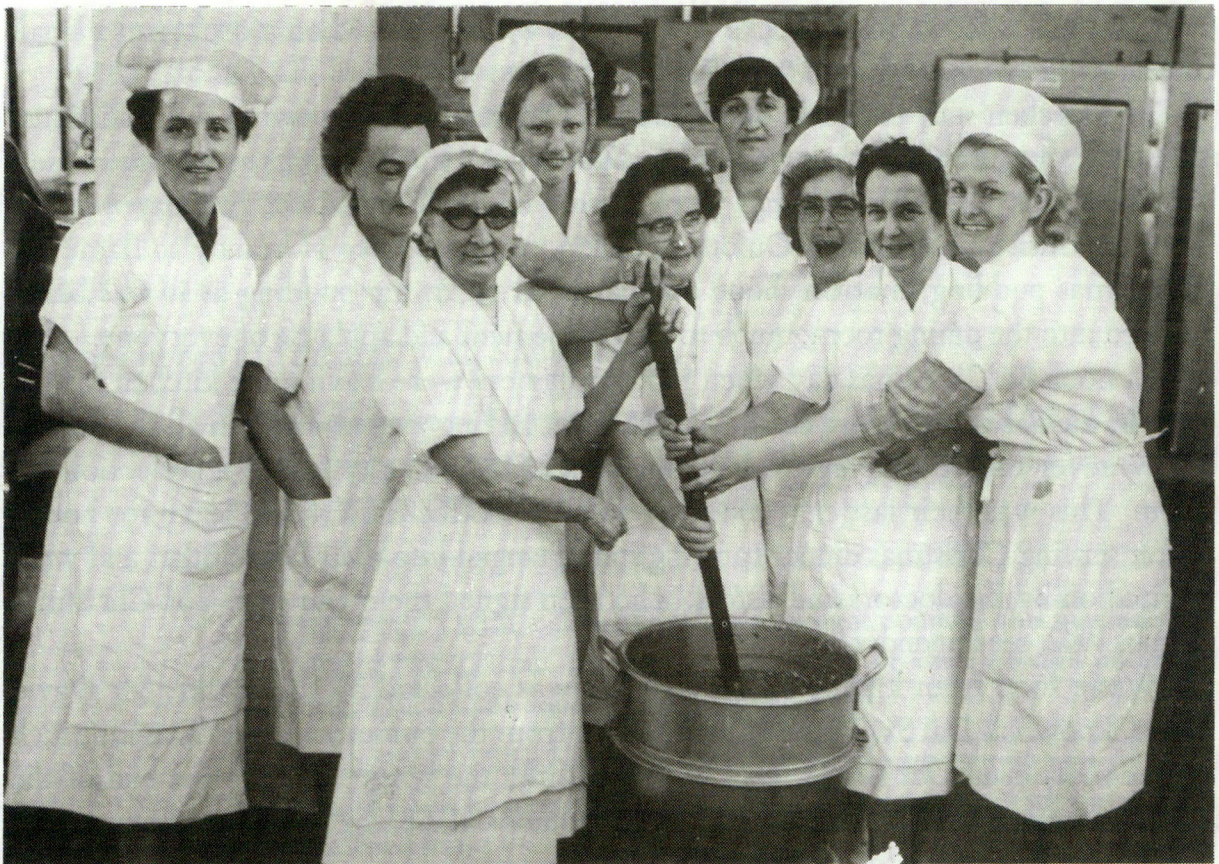

Catering Staff, 1955. Stirring the Christmas Pudding. Left to right: Margaret Charles, Kay Hopkins, Evelyn Pugh, Eira Parry, Cordelia Prosser, Doris Powell, Bessie Jones, Phyllis Heywood, Glenys Watkins
(Photograph courtesy of Mrs Margaret Charles)

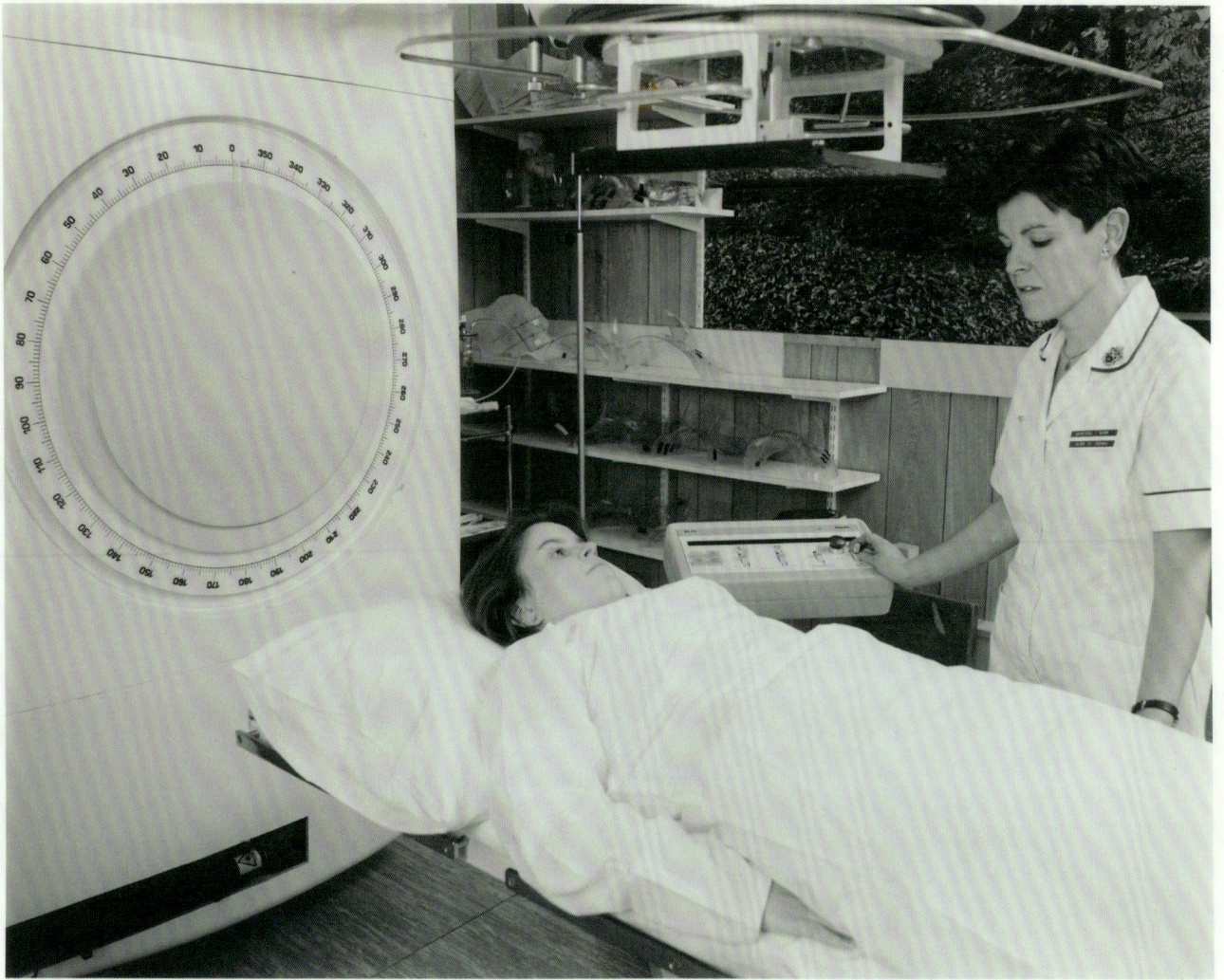

Radiotherapy in Singleton Hospital

Below: Singleton Hospital outpatients department cafe 1990s

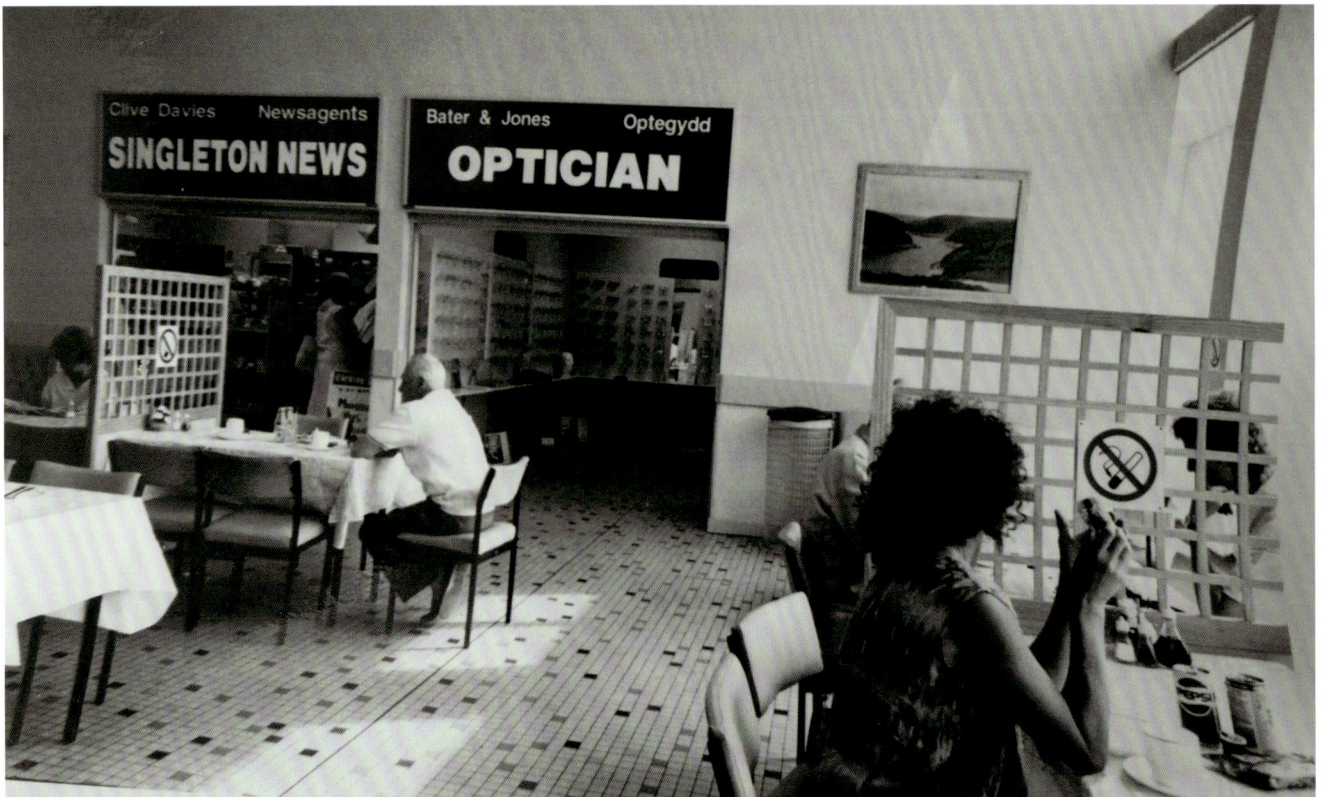

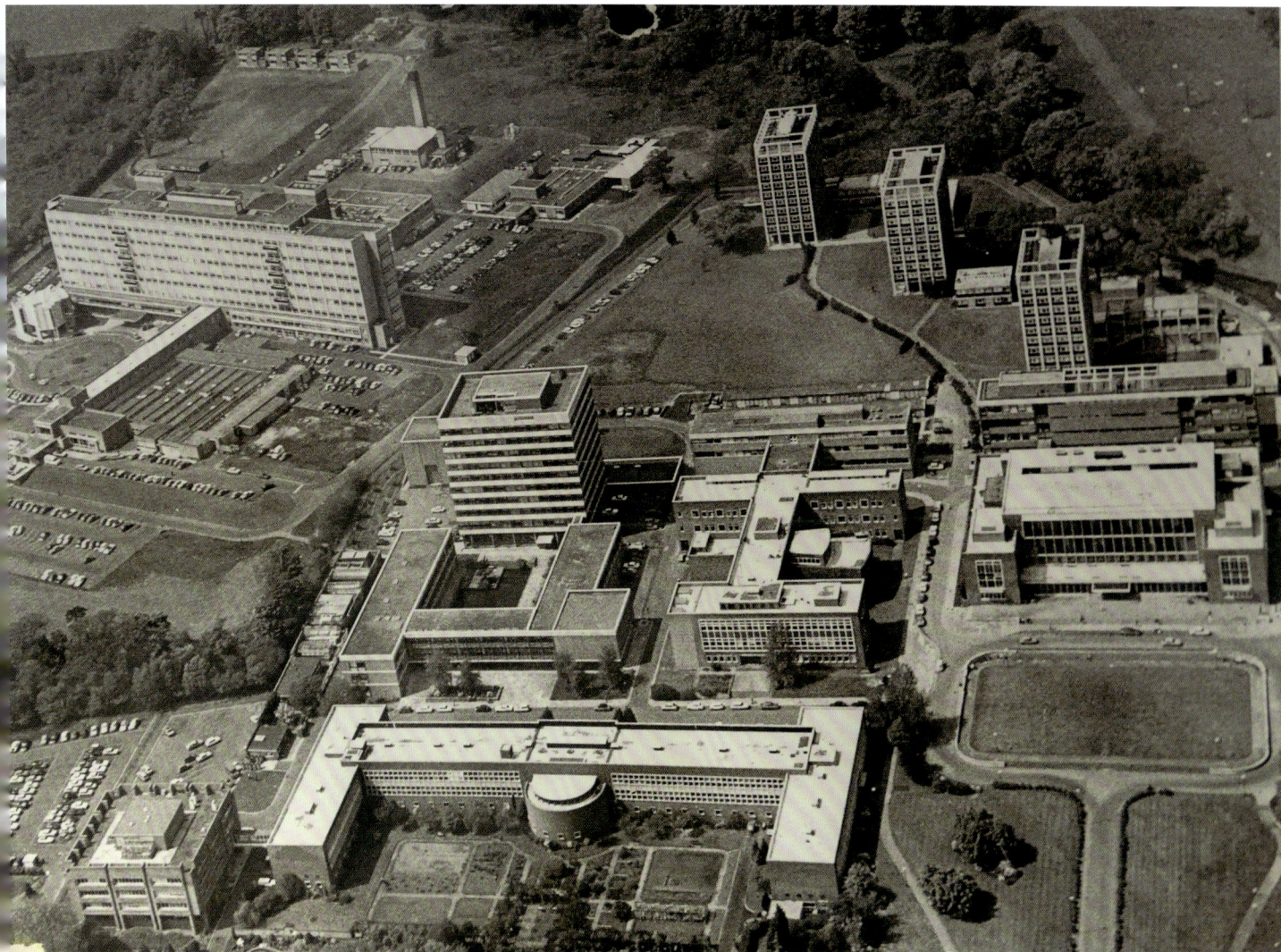

An archive photograph of Singleton Hospital and Swansea University

Below: Bridgend General Hospital shortly before demolition

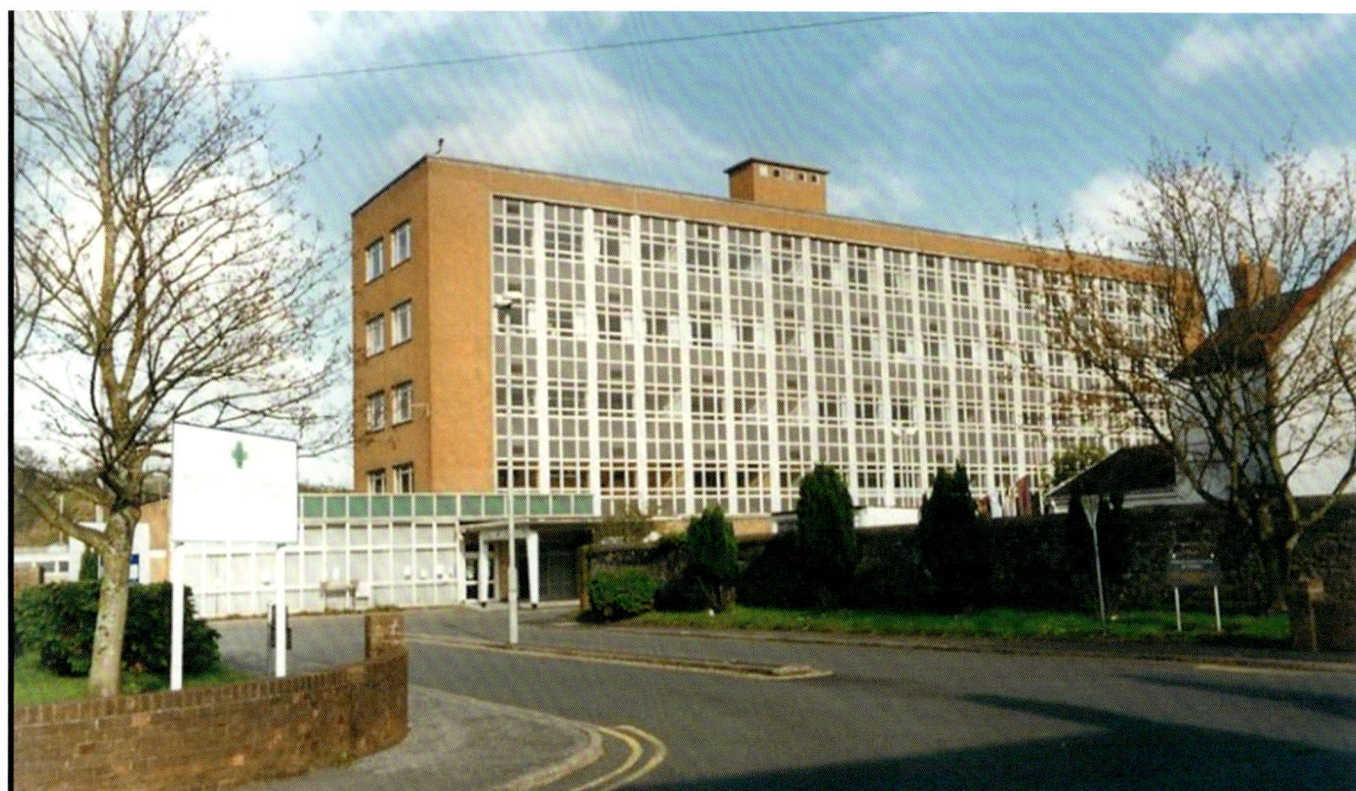

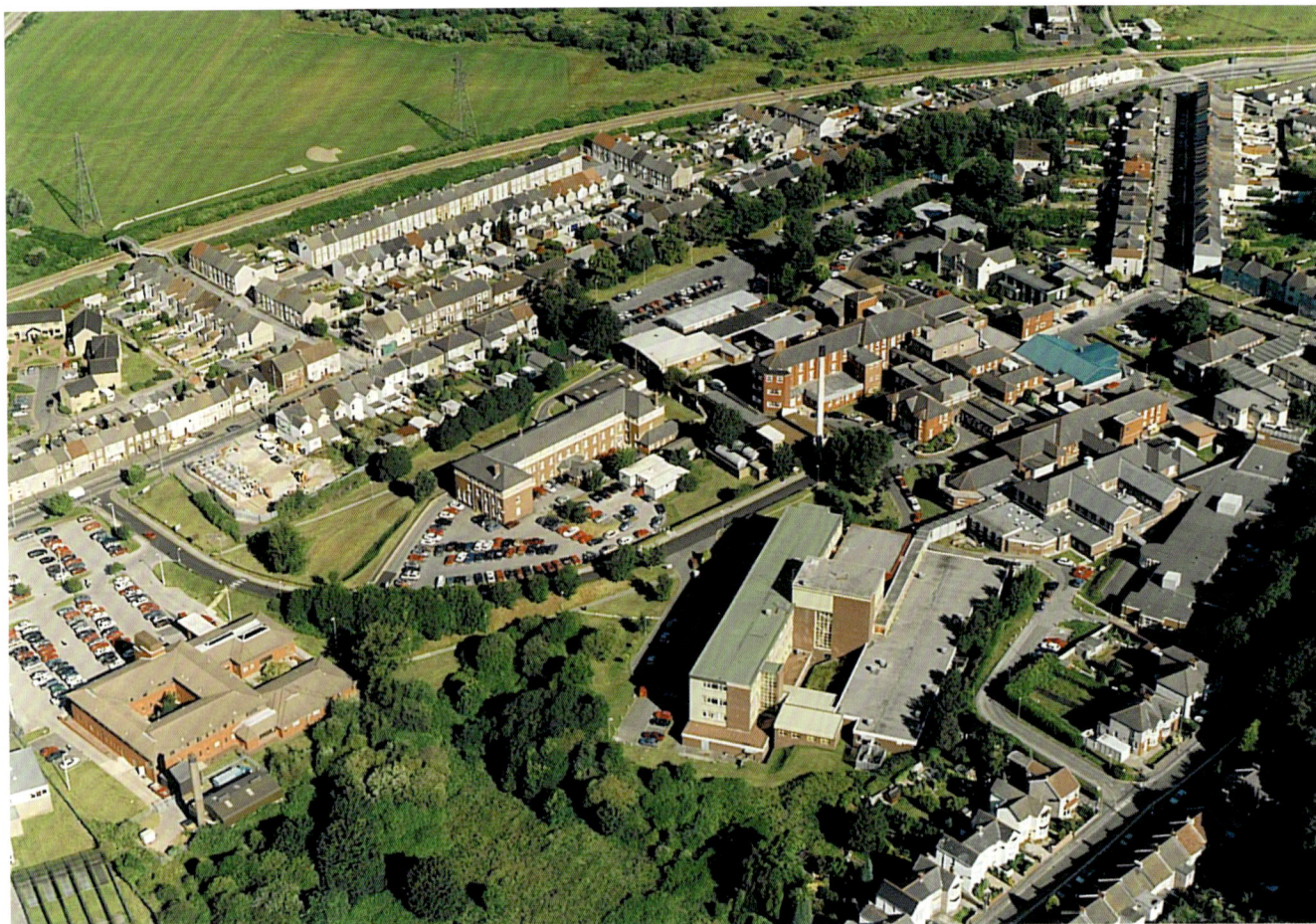

Above - Neath General Hospital. Below - Groeswen Hospital, Port Talbot. Both these sites, along with the old Port Talbot General Hospital, have since been turned into housing estates. Another hospital in the area, Cimla, is now the Cimla Health and Social Care Centre, which provides a range of seamlessly integrated community services, clinics, education programmes and more.

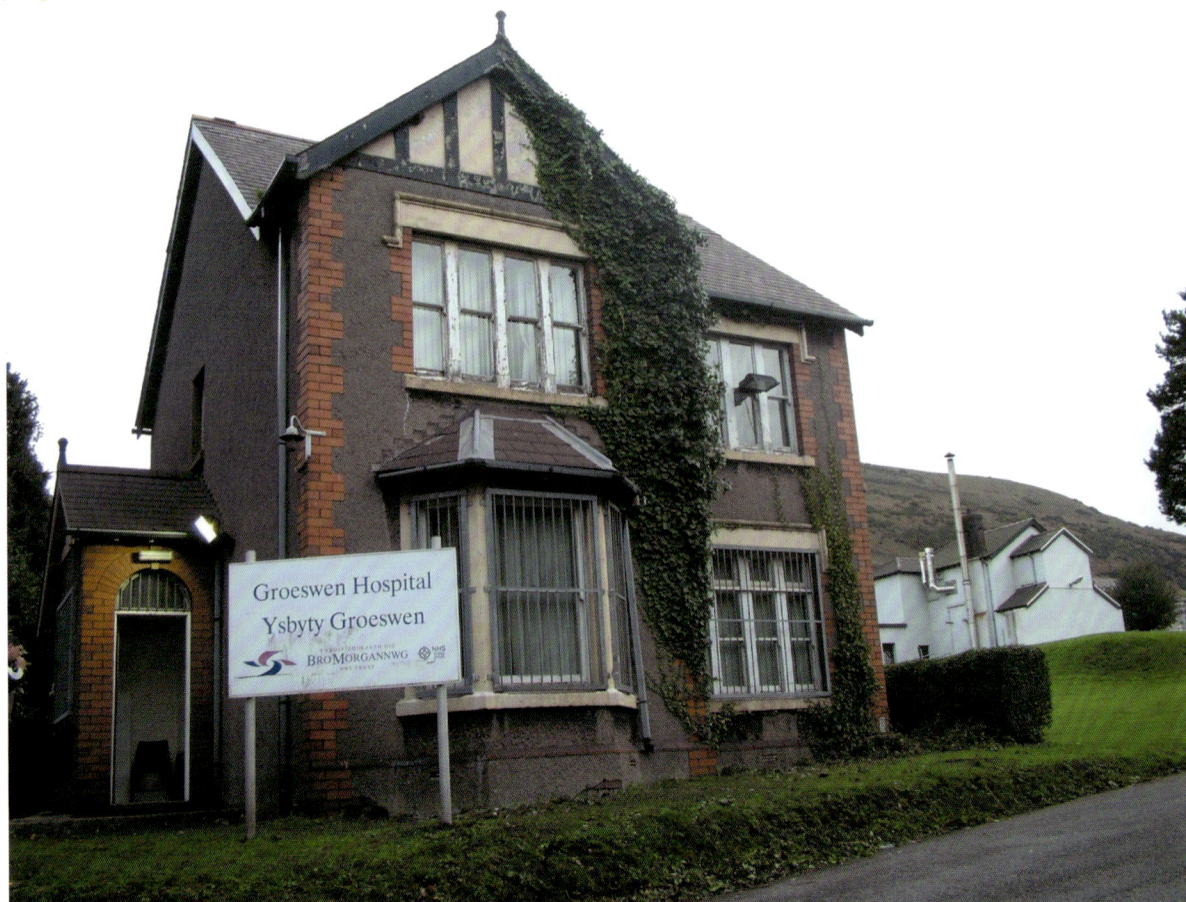

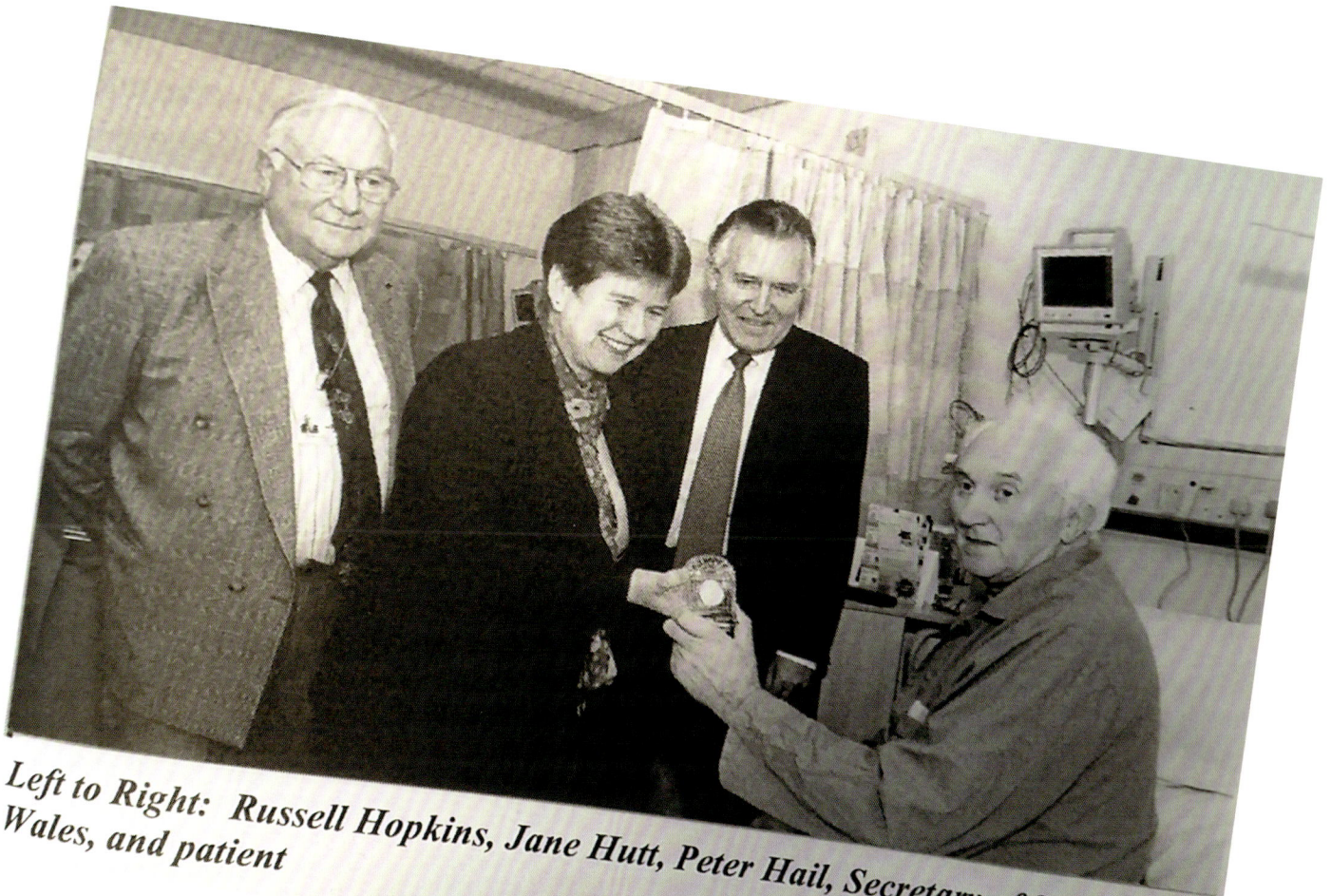

Left to Right: Russell Hopkins, Jane Hutt, Peter Hail, Secretary of State for Wales, and patient

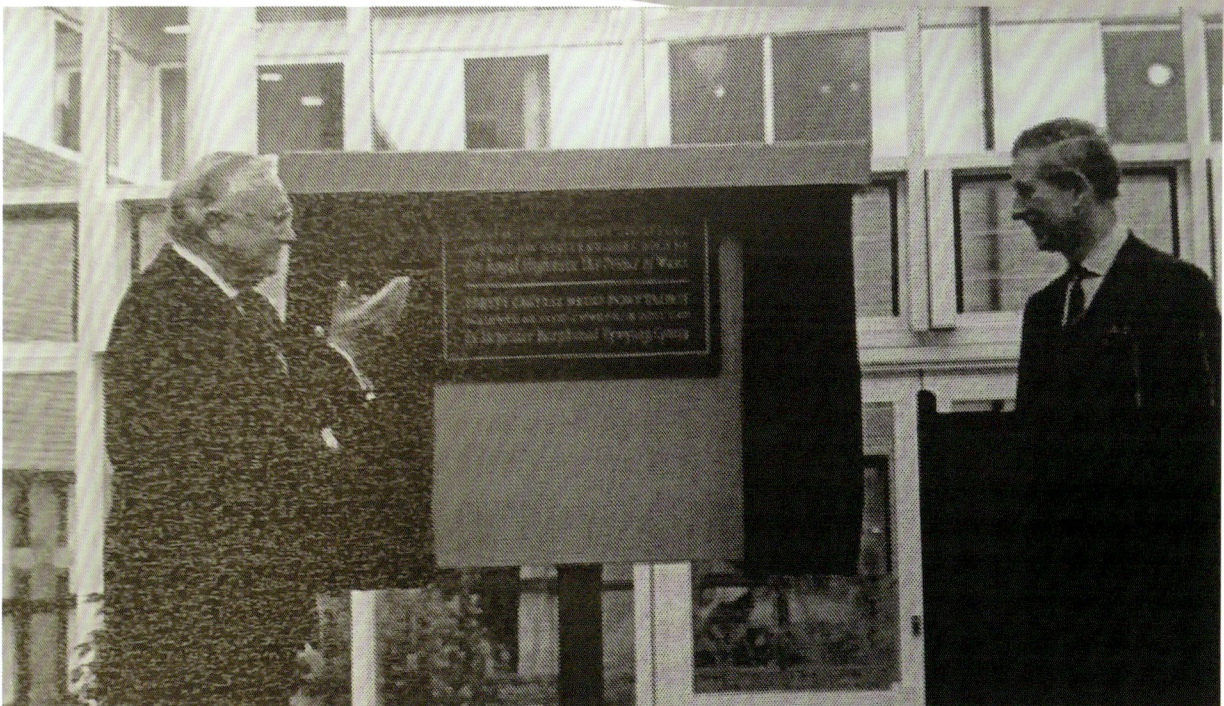

Top: The first patients arrived in Neath Port Talbot Hospital in November, 2002. The name of this patient is not recorded but with him are, from left, Bro Morgannwg NHS Trust Chairman Russell Hopkins, Welsh Health Minister Jane Hutt, and Welsh Secretary and Neath MP Peter Hain.

Below: The new hospital was officially opened by HRH The Prince of Wales in February 2003.

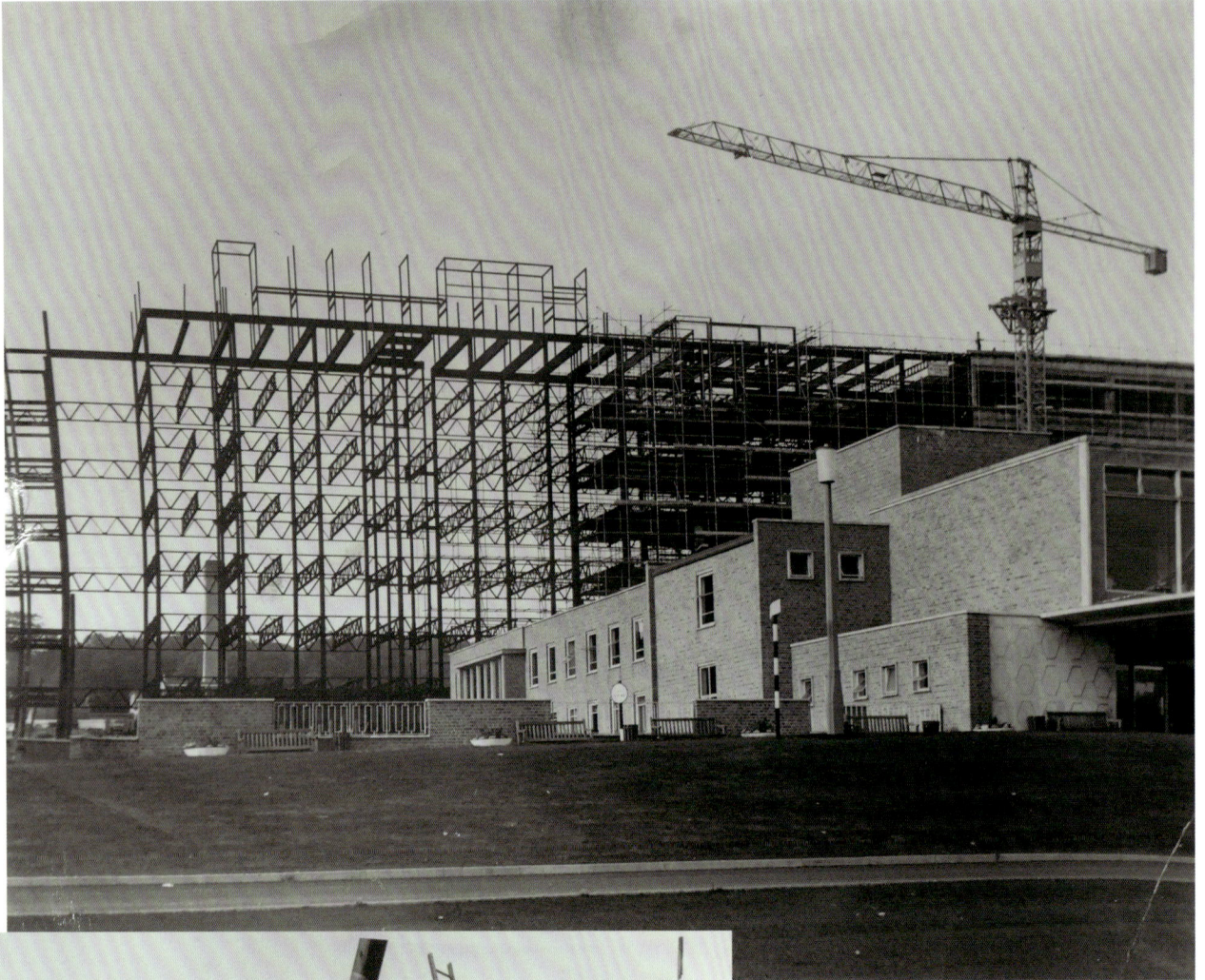

Singleton under construction over the decades

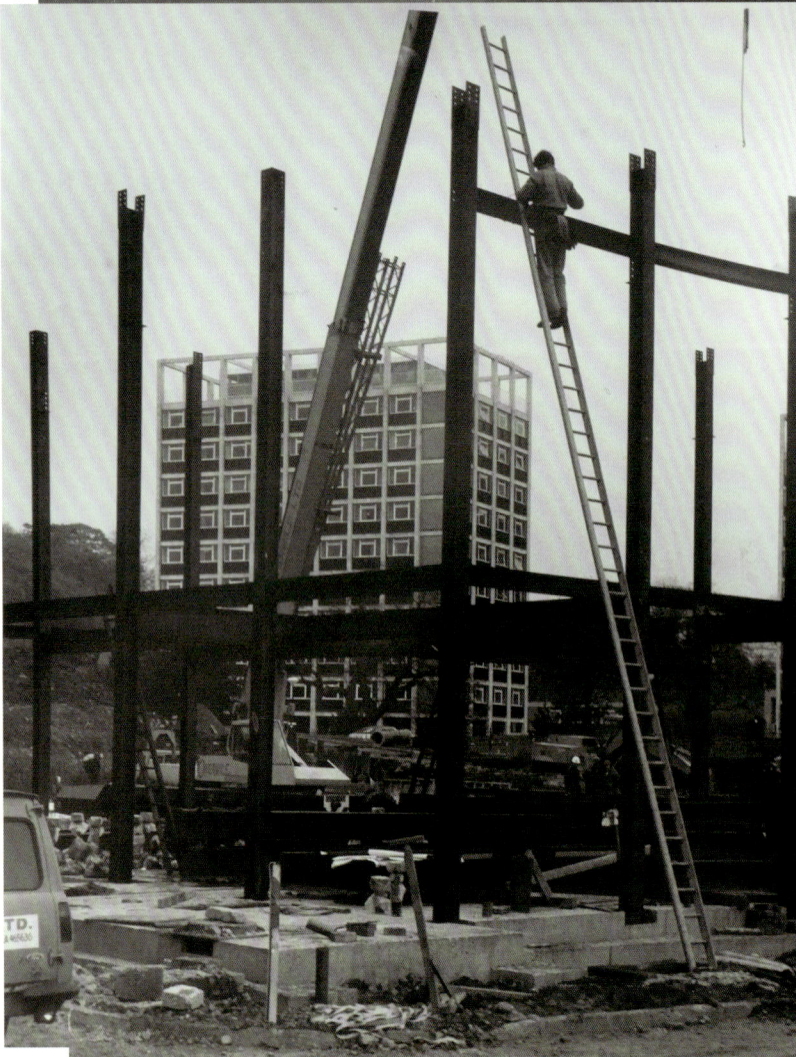

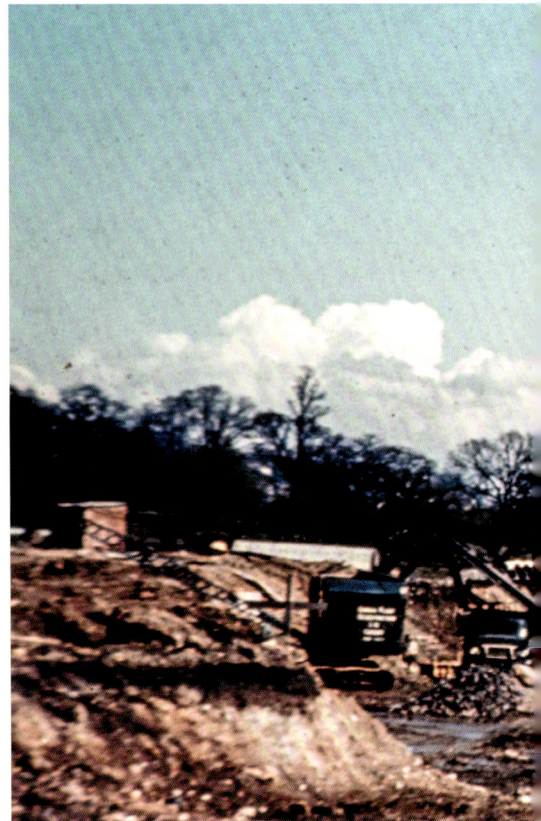

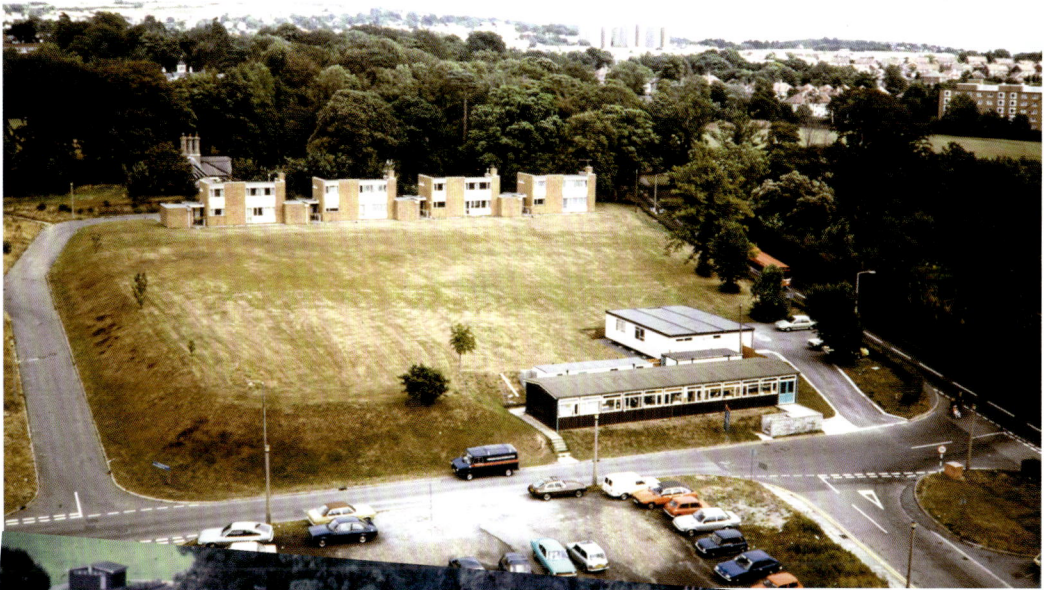

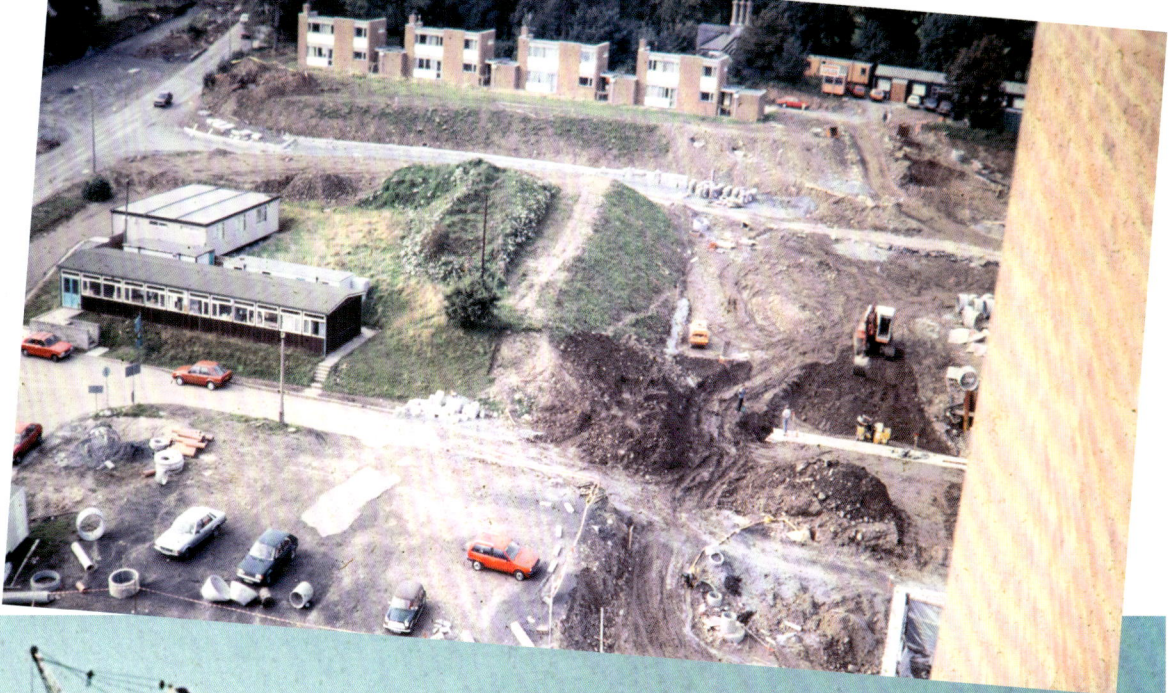

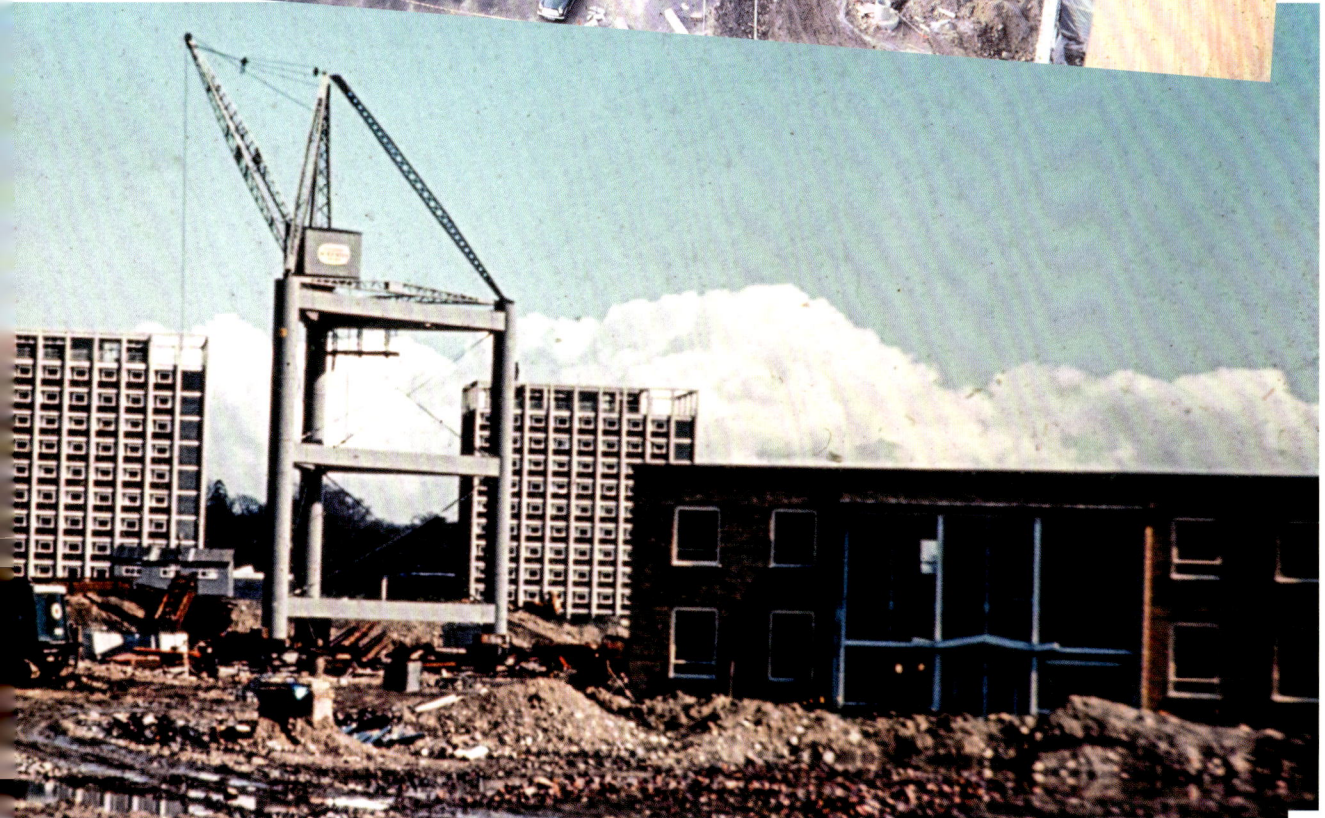

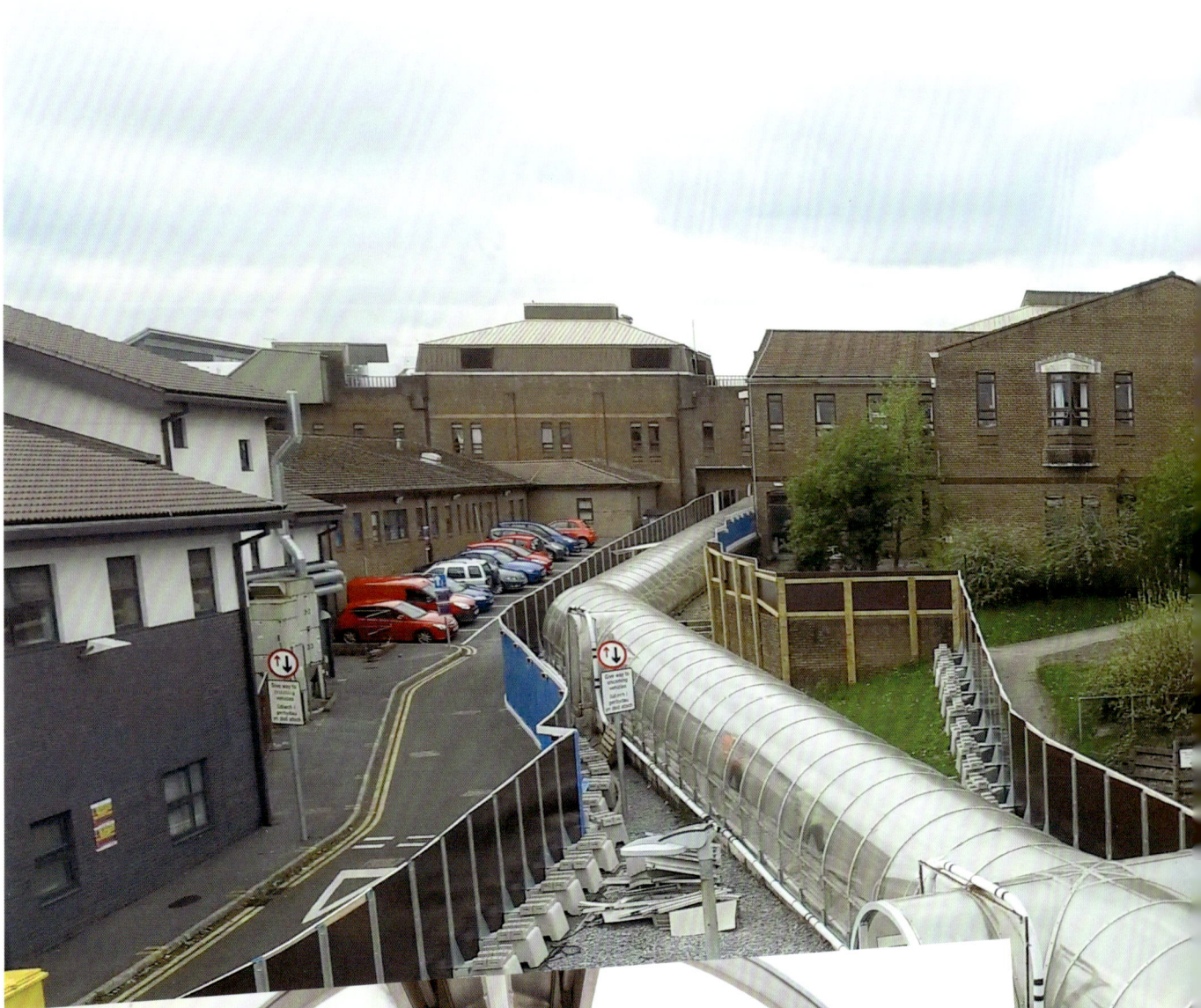

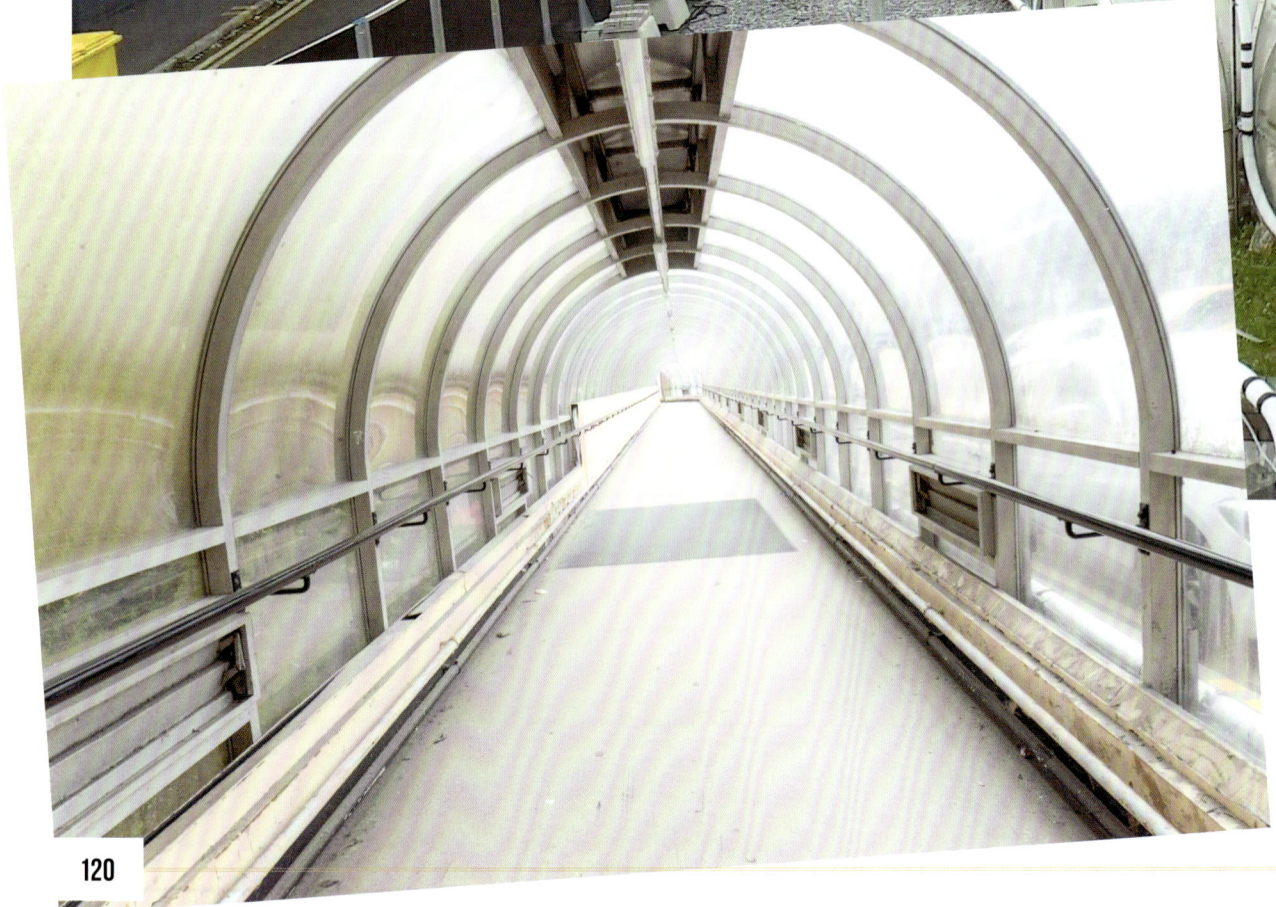

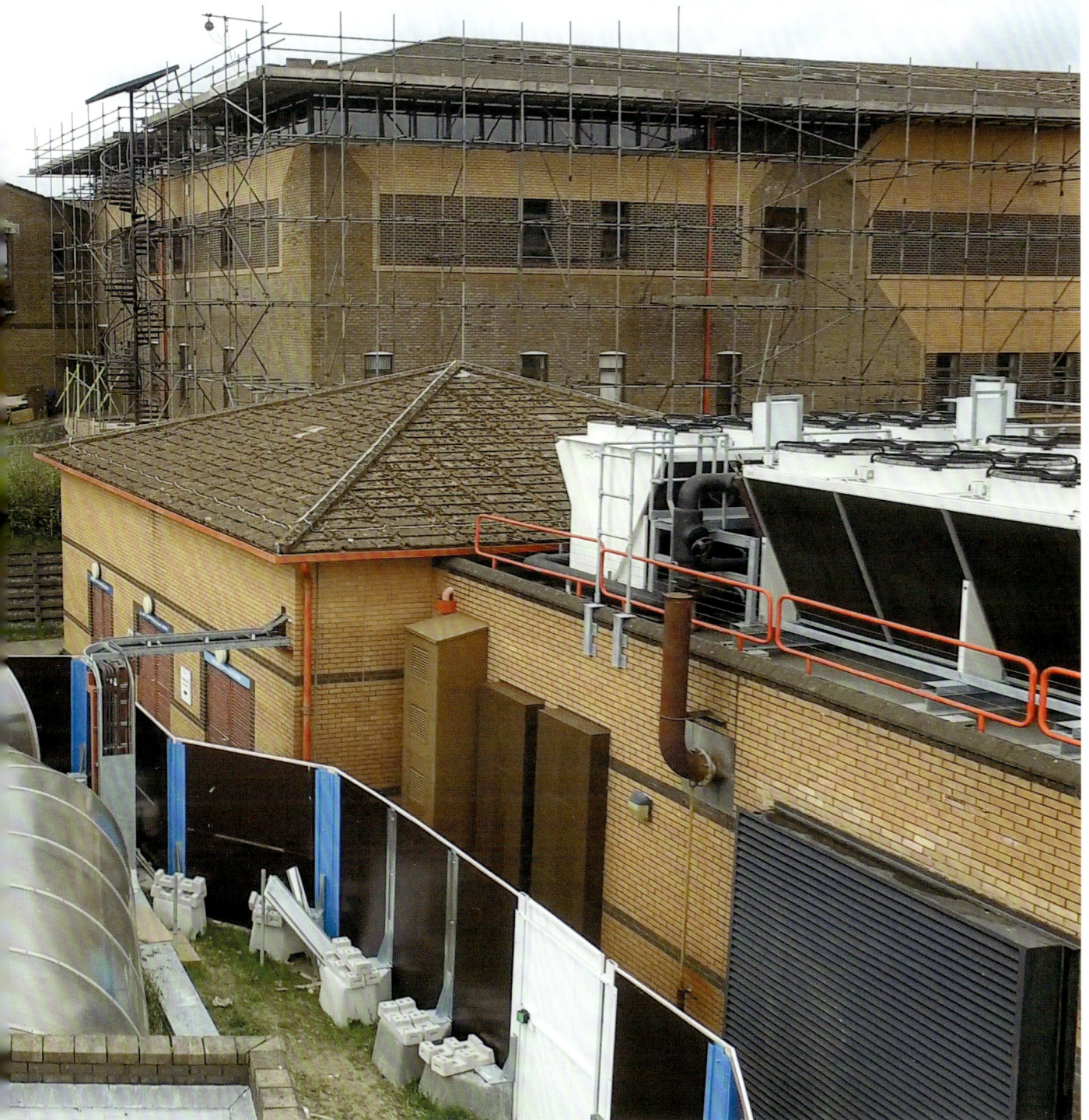

The famous "bubble tunnel" at Morriston Hospital which was demolished in 2017 as part of the ongoing redevelopment of the site.

Changing times

Not enough staff…not enough beds…not enough money. And not taken from today's headlines either!

They say there's nothing new under the sun. Turn back the clock 60 years and the pressures facing the 1950s NHS sound all too familiar today.

"This ninth year of the National Health Service has seen a continuance of many of the difficulties mentioned in previous reports – shortage of nursing staff and medical auxiliaries…a heavy demand for chronic sick beds, and a continued call for economy.

"In spite of financial restrictions which have prevented the fulfilment of many of the Committee's plans, there has been a continued development towards a more efficient service."

This was taken from the ninth annual report of the Glantawe Hospital Management Committee, covering 1956-57.

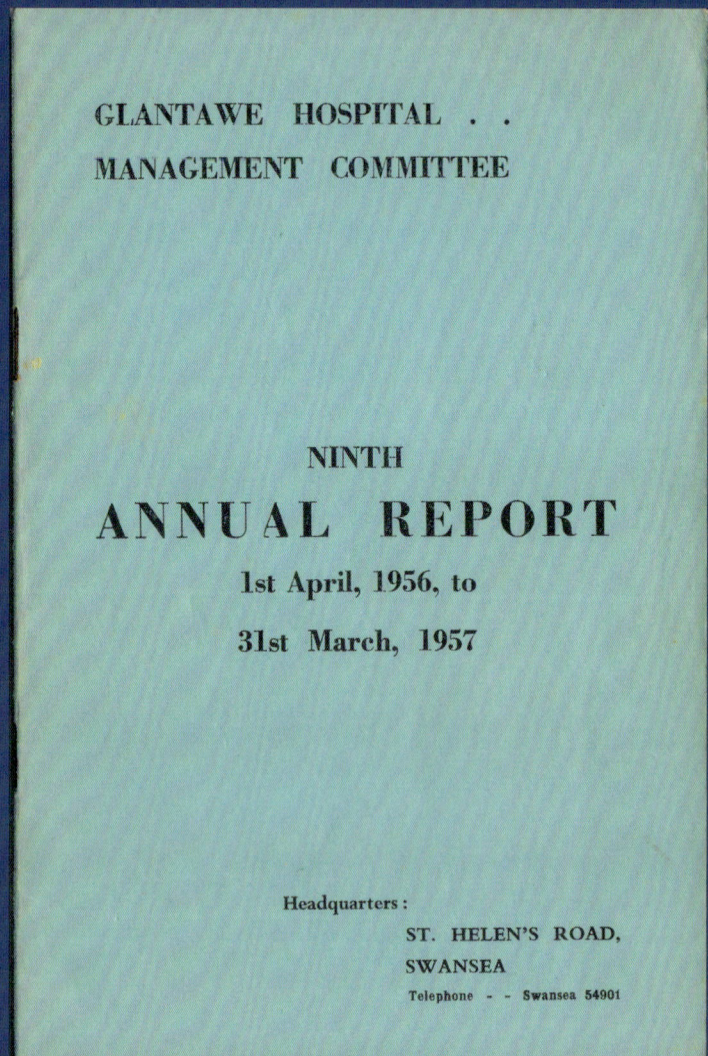

GLANTAWE HOSPITAL . .
MANAGEMENT COMMITTEE

NINTH

ANNUAL REPORT

1st April, 1956, to
31st March, 1957

Headquarters :
ST. HELEN'S ROAD,
SWANSEA
Telephone - - Swansea 54901

The committee was responsible for hospitals and clinics not just in Swansea but the Amman Valley and Llanelli areas too.

At the time of the annual report, it administered 16 hospitals as well as chest clinics and a "new outpatient department, Singleton Park".

Fast-forward to 1962 and the 15th annual report was "pleased to record an event of outstanding importance: the beginning of stage II of the new hospital in Singleton Park…it should be ready for use in 1966 if all goes well".

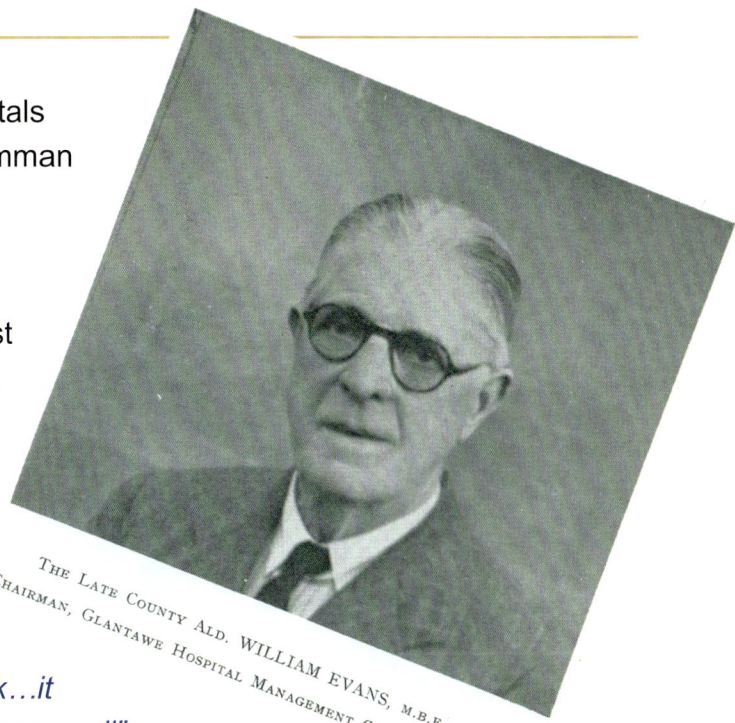

THE LATE COUNTY ALD. WILLIAM EVANS, M.B.E., J.P., (CHAIRMAN, GLANTAWE HOSPITAL MANAGEMENT COMMITTEE, 1948-57)

Things have changed dramatically since those days. Many of the sites referred to are now just memories, while Singleton is one of ABMU's major hospitals and home to the South West Wales Cancer Centre.

Another change is that services in Llanelli now come under Hywel Dda University Health Board.

But there is one constant across the decades – a determination to provide the best possible care despite those never-ending pressures on the NHS.

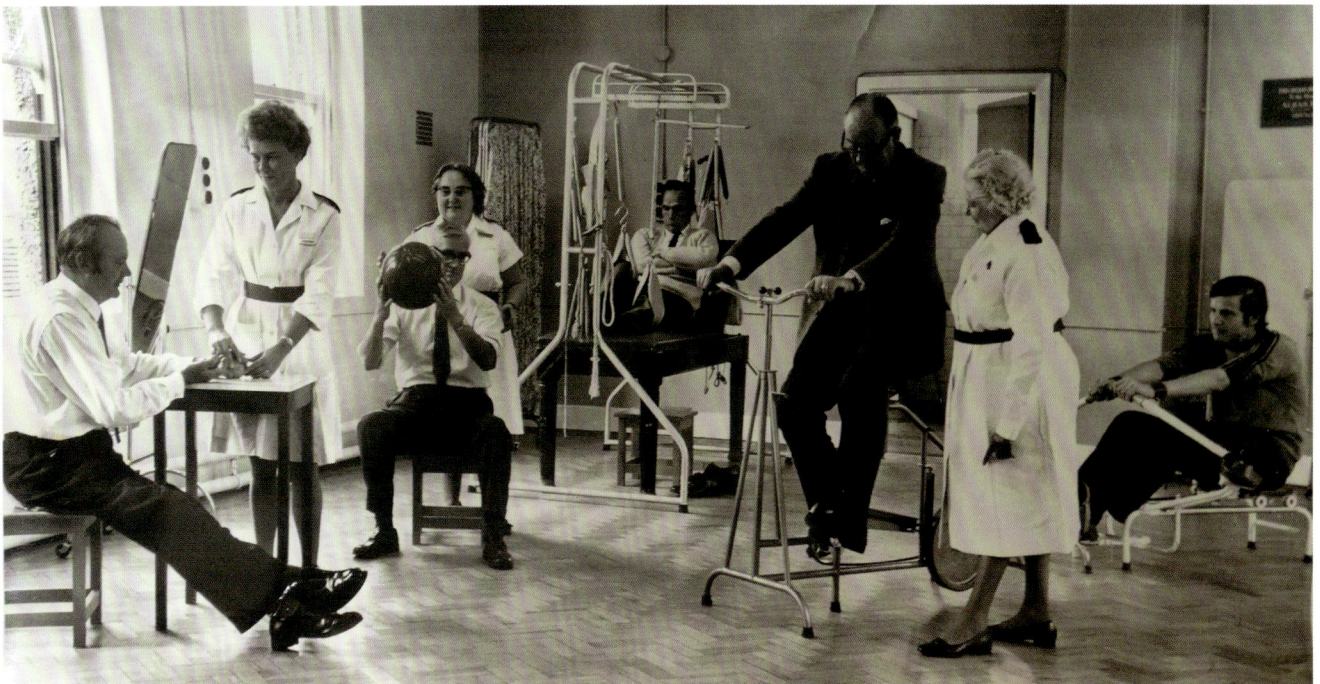

Phillips Parade circa 1970

Memories of the Workhouse…..

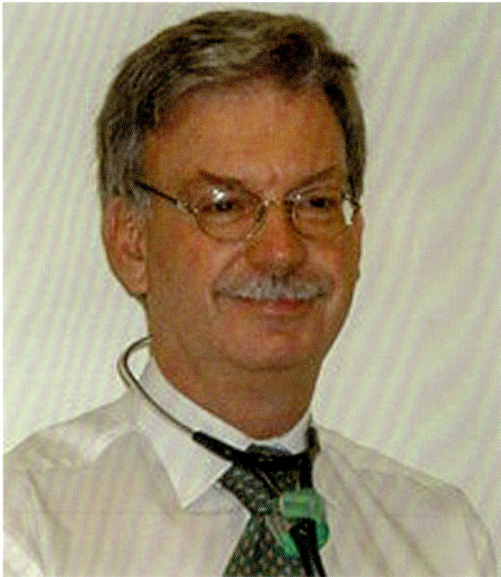

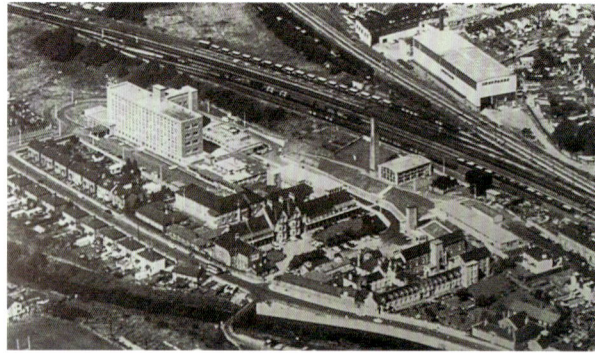

By Dr Ed Wilkins - Consultant Physician, Princess of Wales Hospital Bridgend

With the inception of the NHS in July 1948 the health services and associated infrastructures were taken over by the State.

These buildings reflected the endeavours of the local community to provide health care for its population and their origins date back to Poor Law Legislation at the end of the 18th century.

The Act originally referred to the care or containment of vagrants and those who were extremely poor and homeless. The Act was underpinned by a somewhat punitive 'let's accommodate them but make sure that they work'.

This led to the development of the workhouse providing accommodation for the homeless - males and females were kept separate whether married or not - and tramps were incarcerated in cells and made to carry out tasks before they were released and encouraged to move on. This was usually to the next workhouse - strategically placed within a day's walking distance - usually 25 miles.

As a consequence of the legislation, Workhouse Masters and Matrons took this part of the Act to heart and the institutions became cruel. Public outcry led to further legislation to provide care for the frail and infirm and there emerged the concept of the Workhouse infirmary.

In Bridgend, the workhouse became a key part of the NHS estate and remarkably played a key role in the provision of care until the mid 1980s - providing wards mainly for the elderly. Garw Ward was located in the female section of the workhouse with St David's and Glanogwr wards part of the original infirmary.

Administration was located in what were probably the Master's house and the men's section. The biochemical laboratory was originally located in the Tramp Ward cubicles!

Although much of Bridgend General including the newer section built later in the 19th Century is now gone - thanks to Cadw the workhouse building is visible with the Tramp Ward running along Quarella Road as you come off the Tesco Bridge. Likewise, the main body of the workhouse with its male and female entrance is clearly visible facing south.

I was appointed as consultant physician at the beginning of the 1980s. My specialty was care of the elderly and as such inherited the workhouse wards with an office in the upper section which was probably the mother with infant section.

There is a tendency for those advanced in their career to refer back to the 'good old days' but were they?

The standard of nursing care was very good but the accommodation was very poor and cramped - with the only advantage that hip fracture rate was low because inevitably any fallers fell on to the next patient's bed!

When I took up post there were 50 outlying patients - there was one physiotherapist shared with paediatrics – and over three times the number of care of the elderly beds there are at present.

Thus in addition to inheriting the workhouse building, the NHS of the day inherited and to an extent propagated the institutionalisation of older people, with service provision influenced inappropriately by the age of patients. Even during the early 1980s patients above the age of 65 were precluded admission to the Coronary Care Unit.

So, in the early 1980s and before - they were not really the good old days if you happened to survive into a reasonable old age and became ill.

However, during my subsequent professional career I have experienced astounding changes to patient care, coupled with associated remarkable changes in the demography of old age. Far greater numbers of people are living to a greater age and of equal importance the quality of life also greatly improved.

Thus from the days of the workhouse and its infirmary the NHS now provides a remarkable and continuously improving high quality of care irrespective of wealth creed or age.

Pathology

The service is often unseen by most of the patients who benefit from it, but pathology has long been a key part of hospital life.

One member of staff revealed that back in the early days of the NHS it used to take half an hour or do a test, now hundreds are done in the same time.

"Pathology used to be seen as a bit of a backroom service but, of course, doctors often can't make a decision until they get the results of pathology tests.

"When I started we used to do all the public health work, testing things like milk and water. If there had been an outbreak of food poisoning at a wedding, all the food would come to us for testing."

He said one of the biggest differences over the years were the incredible advances in the way tests are carried out. Today, for example a woman can tell if she is expecting a baby in minutes using a simple test from a supermarket.

Back in the 1950s however it was a different story.

"Pregnancy tests then involved four virgin white mice. We first needed to prepare over 24 hours a sample of urine from the lady to concentrate the hormones in it. Then we would inject the urine into the mice.

"We would wait five days and then check for changes in the mice to see whether or not the urine contained pregnancy hormones. Sometimes the changes were so small that we had to use a magnifying glass to see them."

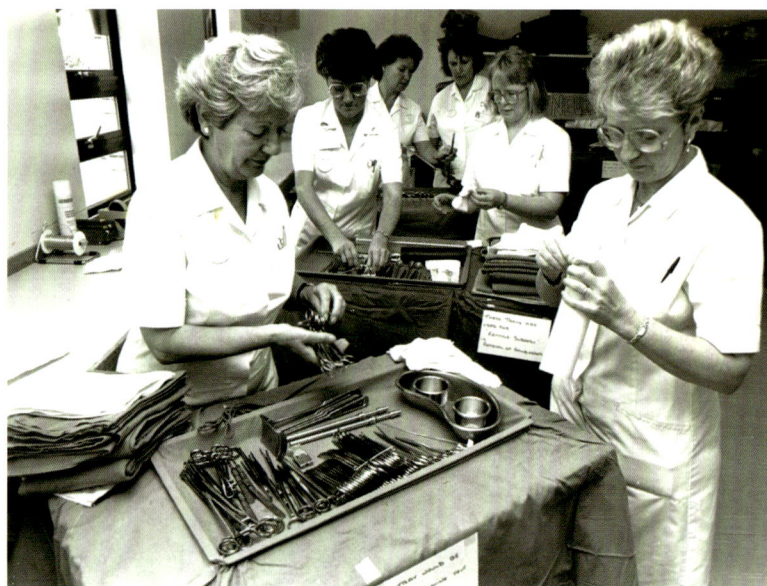

Children in hospital

It certainly is good to talk, but it was much more difficult to do if you were a child in hospital in the early days of the NHS.

The emotional problems of sick children in hospital were not fully understood on children's wards across the UK. It's well documented that staff might only allow parental visits for a limited time, and would discourage telephone enquiries.

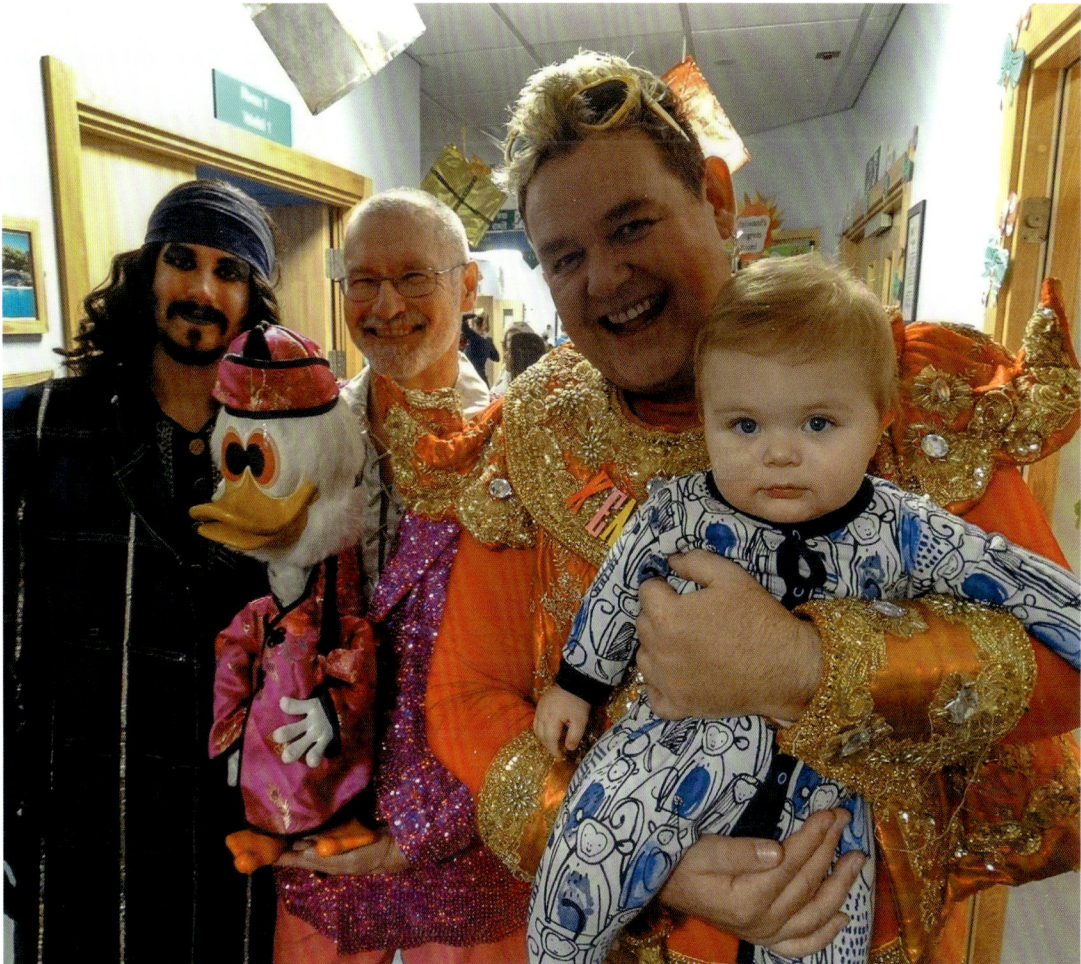

Some colourful characters help to heer up children in hospital

The great distress caused by the 'no visiting' policy would never be more evident than when the infant forgot the mother and clung to the nurse when the time for discharge came, to the distress of all three.

All a far cry from the games, toys, computers and even visits from entertainers and celebrities that are normal service today.

And to make a visit to hospital even less stressful for young patients there is even a warm welcome from other children available.

The children of hospital colleagues star as staff in a video tour of the children's wards at Morriston. In the video they wear miniature versions of adult uniforms and play doctors, nurses, play leaders and domestics.

The idea is children who need to go into hospital and their families can simply access the video on ABMU Health Board's website to find out more about what lies ahead of them.

Head of nursing for Neonatal & Children's Services Eirlys Thomas said:*"We wanted to look at how we could support children and young people who need to come into hospital and decided the best way was to use other children to do it."*

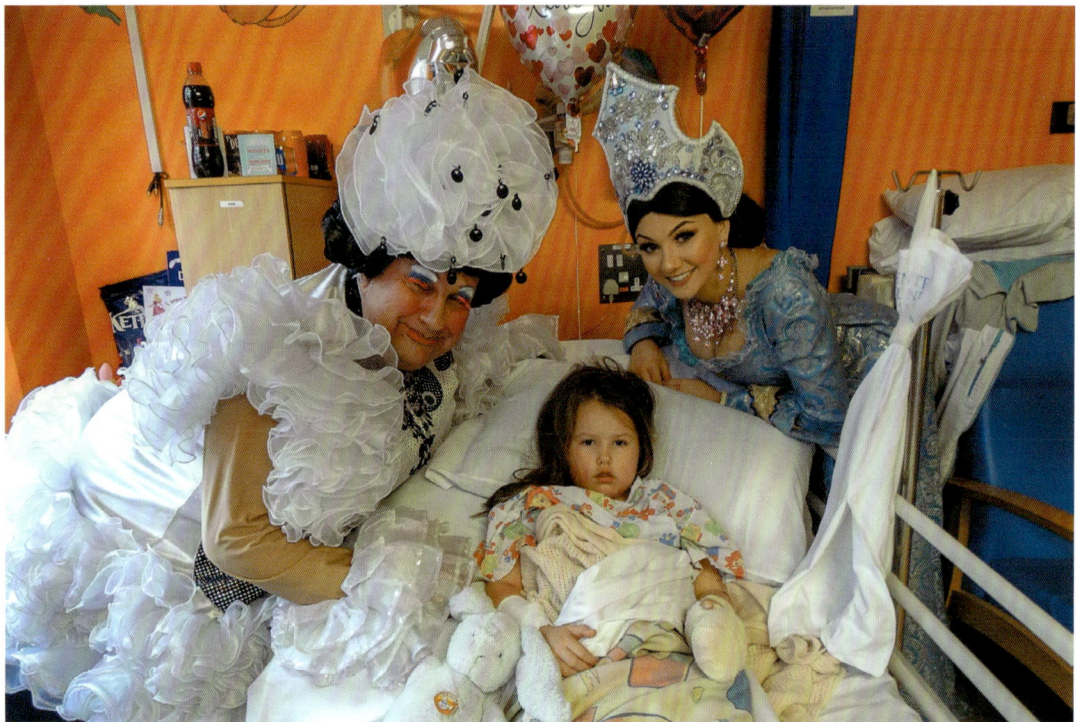

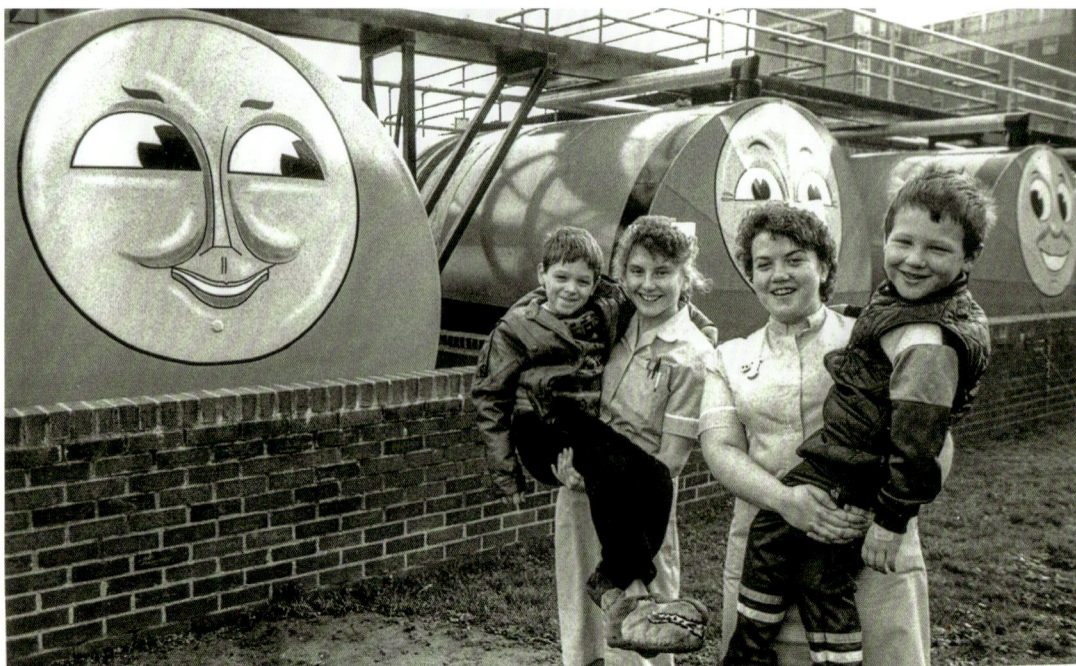

Martin Green

Pictured with his Preliminary Training School set at Frenchay Hospital in Bristol back in 1976 is Martin Green who is now bed site manager at Morriston Hospital.

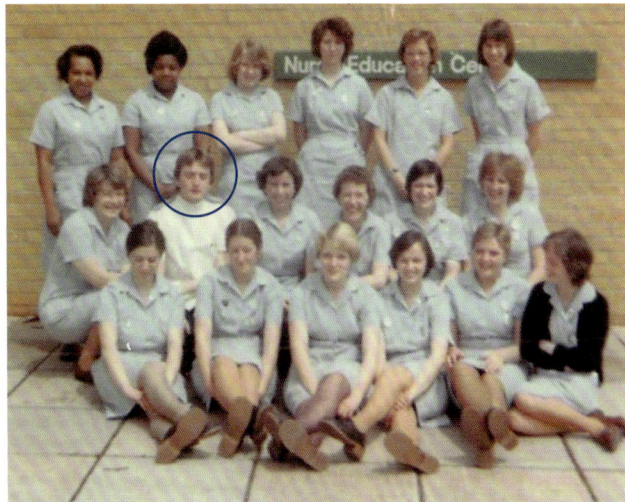

But his earliest memory of the hospital where he now works is the bench in the corridor alcove at Morriston *(below)*. He was waiting there for news while his mum gave birth to his baby brother.

Martin has gone on to have a 42 year nursing career - part of it spent as charge nurse in A&E when it was still in the same old corridor.

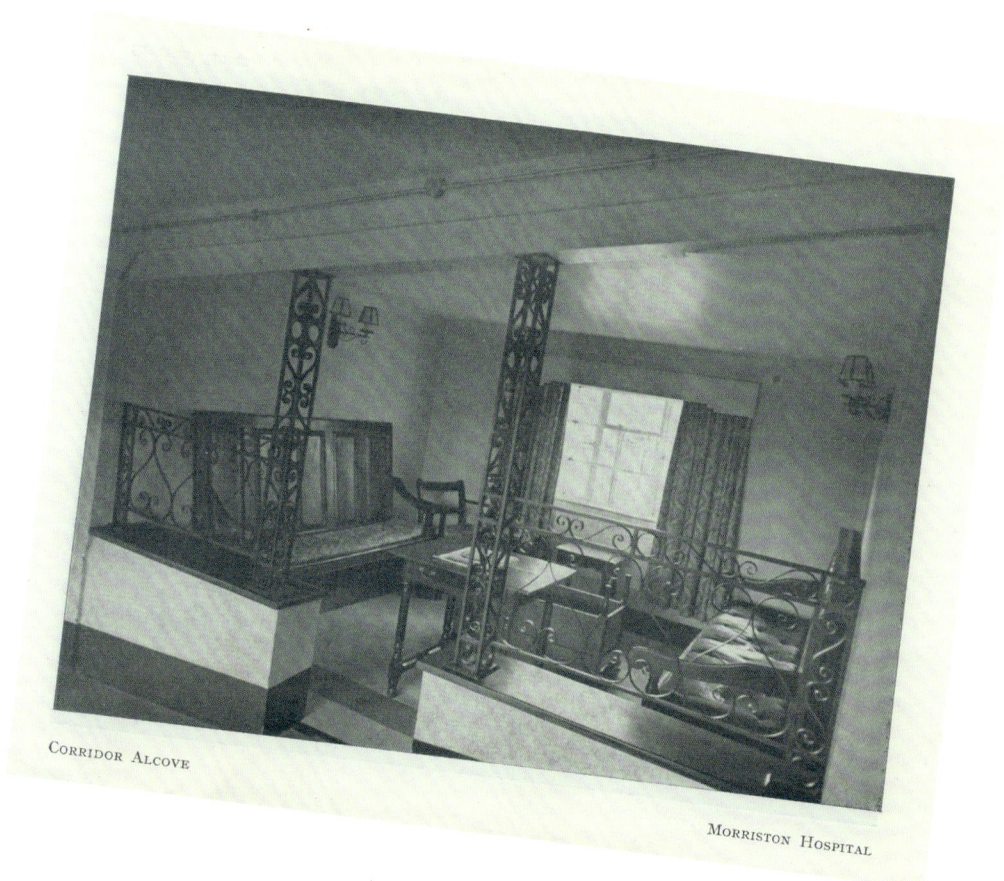

CORRIDOR ALCOVE

MORRISTON HOSPITAL

We couldn't do without you

Whether it is sitting in a bath of baked beans, pushing tea trolleys or hitting the high notes, the variety of support the community provides for our health services is quite remarkable.

Groups of fundraisers and volunteers have made a life-changing difference to care in our community throughout the past 70 years.

From the pioneering work done by our Leagues of Friends to raise funds for equipment and services to the friendly voices of presenters hosting hospital radio and providing a welcome distraction to patients in the days before wifi and mobile phones – what unites all their endeavours is a shared desire to help our staff and we remain very grateful!

South West Wales Cancer Centre

The depth of community support for health services in our area was clearly demonstrated by the £1 million raised locally in a very short period of time. This sparked the creation of the South West Wales Cancer Centre.

This determination of our community combined with the personal passion of a remarkable doctor led to the appeal's success and now – almost two decades later - the cancer centre at Singleton Hospital is thriving.

The centre is the realisation of a vision by consultant oncologist Salah El-Sharkawi which began back in 1996. When he became clinical director of cancer services he felt the necessity to develop facilities locally.

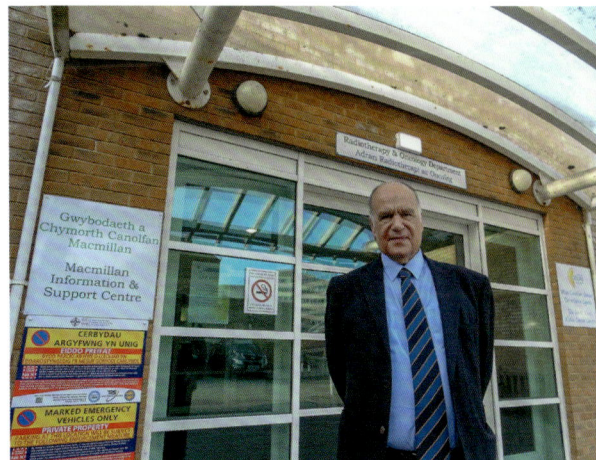

Dr Salah El-Sharkawi outside the radiotherapy department at Singleton Hospital.

"I sat down with Chief Executive of Swansea NHS Trust, David Williams and I told him about my vision for the future. He said 'You can rely on my full support as long as the financial aspects of the venture will not interfere with other services in the trust'. "

Dr El-Sharkawi outlined his proposals for future services, including the creation of a cancer centre, to hospital chiefs and began to think about how he could turn them into a reality.

"I knew the community would come to our aid, they would not let me down - and they didn't."

Fortuitously at the same time the *South Wales Evening Post* was looking to get behind a campaign to mark the millennium and Dr El-Sharkawi had the perfect suggestion for them.

"That is how the Evening Post Cancer Appeal began in 1998 – we set an ambitious target of raising £500,000 but we ended up making more than double that."

At the appeal's launch Dr El-Sharkawi decided to highlight one case, that of Sally Davies who had a very rare type of cancer which meant she couldn't be treated close to home and had to spend long periods in London.

"You can have the best cancer treatment in the world but if you have it away from your friends and your family, you lose a lot.

"Sally was being treated at one of the best centres but she just wanted to come home.

"I wanted to touch people's hearts and minds, to make the appeal vivid to the public. I used Sally's case so they would understand just why having a cancer centre here was so important.

"It struck a chord, it gave people the idea that all of us working together could make a difference."

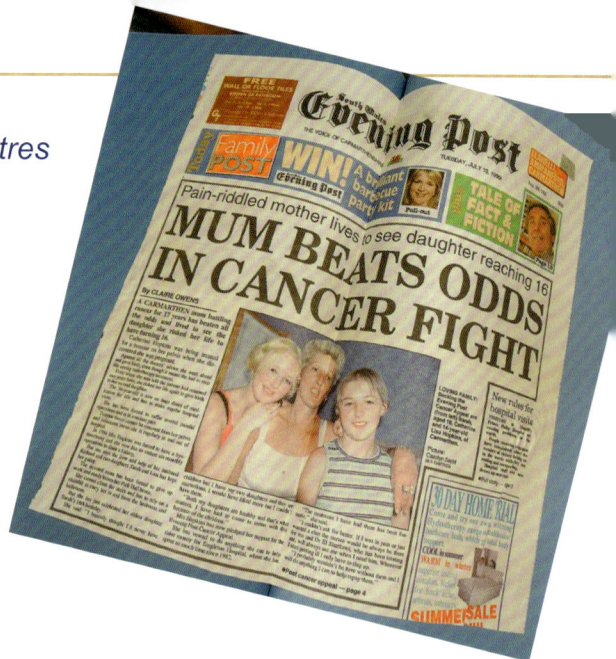

And it certainly did. Money poured in from clubs, sports teams, schools and individual donors with the total – recorded daily in the Evening Post – kept going up. And Dr El-Sharkawi was on hand to receive the cheques in person.

"We were out three or four times a week, I went to every school, to every pub and club. We wanted people to know it really was so appreciated."

He was often accompanied by his late wife Bana and as a result his three daughters grew up influenced by their parents' dedication to cancer patients – Dima is now a consultant haemato-oncologist in the Royal Marsden Hospital while Lamah is a GP partner and Reem is a pharmacist, both in the Bay GP Cluster in Swansea.

Reem said:

"We are all very proud of Dad's contribution, we didn't realise at the time just what he had done. But he would always tell us how overwhelmed he was by the support of the local community."

Dr El-Sharkawi said:

"When we got to £100,000 in just 80 days we thought we had done well, but it just kept going.

"I involved a lot of sporting personalities and we had money from all over West Wales. I also had support from the health authority and the Welsh Office."

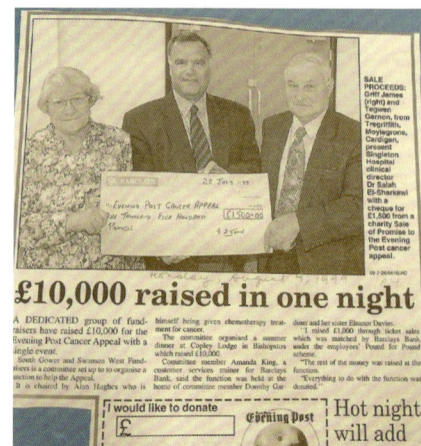

The donations kept flooding in, pushing the target up through the £1 million mark.

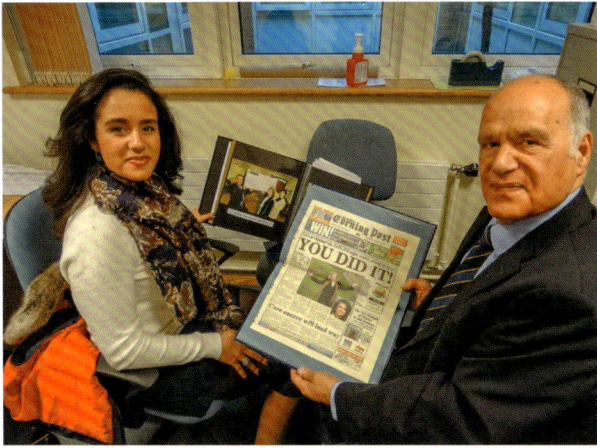

Dr Salah El-Sharkawi with his daughter Reem looking at some of his collection of cuttings and pictures from the successful cancer appeal.

Besides group donations the appeal was boosted with significant sums from larger donors – and one in particular played a key role.

"Evan Davies, known to everyone as JCB, raised £250,000 for the cancer unit over the years, he is remarkable and has done more for the cause than anyone else," he said.

A former patient of Dr El-Sharkawi, Mr Davies was one of the first to get involved and staged a string of major money-spinning events, including concerts attended by hundreds of supporters.

He was appointed MBE for his fundraising efforts, an honour which was also bestowed on Dr El-Sharkawi in 2010.

The appeal money was an incentive for the health authority and the Welsh office to invest £30million that went towards creating the centre which now provides 45,000 treatments a year to patients who come from Bridgend to Aberystwyth.

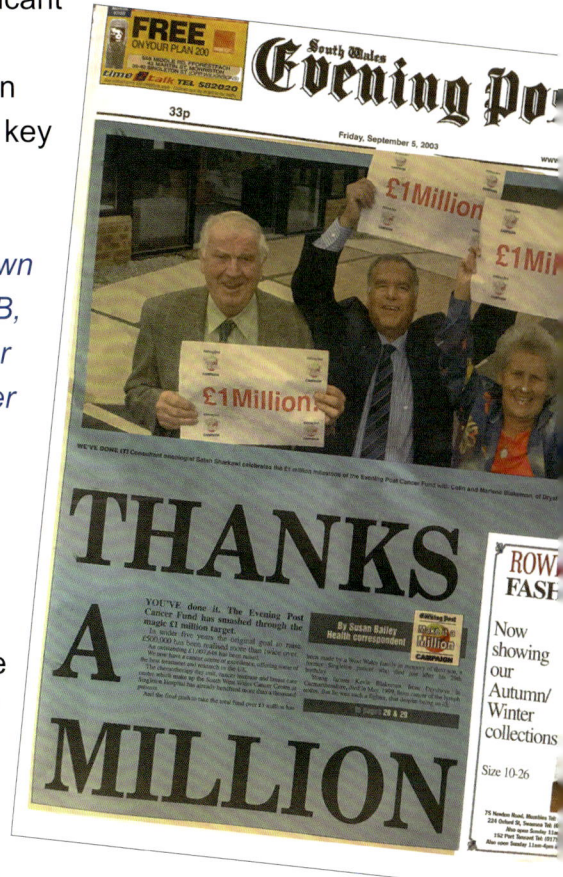

Besides the care offered at Singleton, which has a chemotherapy day unit breast care unit, bone marrow transplant unit and radiotherapy department, there are also clinics and wards at hospitals across the region.

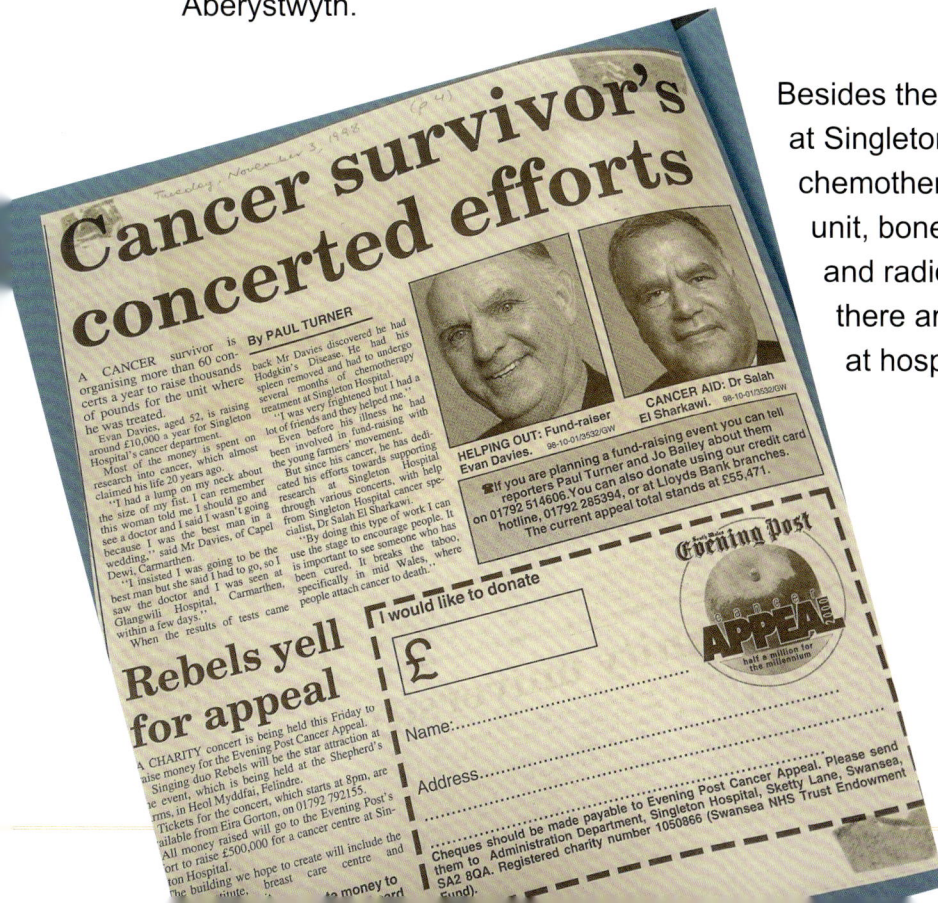

"Now every patient's case is reviewed by 15 or 20 people in a multi-disciplinary team, all of that wouldn't have happened before."

One legacy of the appeal is the creation of the Cancer Institute where vital research is carried out.

Dr El-Sharkawi added: "I wanted to improve academic aspects of the service. Now our staff contribute towards cancer research at the university and educating students at the medical school.

"The more your reputation grows, the easier it becomes to attract staff. When people ask 'where did the money I raised from that sponsored walk go?' this is what it has done."

One of the final projects Dr El-Sharkawi was involved with before retiring in 2007 was the creation of the Seaview Hostel on the top floor of the main hospital building. This is used by patients who need to stay overnight while undergoing radiotherapy treatment.

"We couldn't tell people who had come here for treatment from Aberystwyth that they would need to get a hotel to stay during the period of their treatment.

"This hostel makes things easier for everybody – staff can call them at any time and patients are near to their treatment centre without being hospitalised."

Dr El-Sharkawi's affection for the hospital endures. He is still involved with the Golau Cancer Foundation, ABMU's charity which supports the work of the cancer centre.

"This is something that was a mission for me for more than 25 years. I felt I had a moral duty to the public.

"I felt I must leave something behind. It would have been a lot easier to just do my job and go home but I felt if I don't do it, who is going to do it."

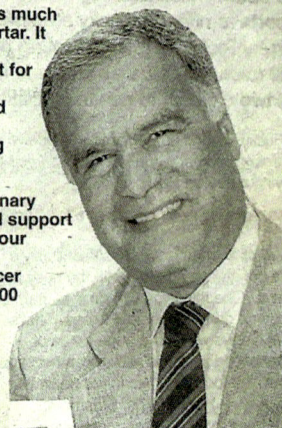

Why I am so proud of all your efforts

READERS of the Evening Post are well aware of the Evening Post Cancer Centre Appeal that was launched in September 1998. The appeal was designated to raise half a million pounds for the benefit of the Cancer Centre that would serve the people of South West Wales.

The efforts and the preparation for the cancer centre, however, go back far back as 1991 when I referred the late Sally Davies to London for specialised treatment that was not available locally at the time.

Soon afterwards Sally rang me with a plea to come home to be near her family and friends. Sally's plea and the pleas of other patients have sparked a chain of events which led to the establishment of South West Wales Cancer Centre, and the Evening Post Cancer Centre Appeal to fund three of its main components — a chemotherapy Unit, a cancer institute and a cancer breast unit.

But the cancer centre is much more than bricks and mortar. It is about providing a cutting-edge environment for promoting excellence in cancer care, research and education.

It is also about building upon the track record of quality medical care and leading with multidisciplinary programs to respond and support the specialised needs of our cancer patients.

The Evening Post Cancer Centre Appeal set £500,000 as a target.

The people of South West Wales, with their boundless generosity and their innovations in fund-raising, managed to raise £1million — double the amount set as target for the appeal. It was truly an impressive achievement to which I remain eternally grateful.

Staff at the Evening Post also played an important role in the planning, management and co-ordination of the appeal. They all deserve credit for their encouragement, creative minds and for the shouldering a disproportionate share of burden in making this appeal a success.

For this, I thank them all.

If anyone, around 1990, had predicted the changes that would take place in cancer services in South West Wales in the next 10 or 15 years, he would have been dismissed as hopelessly optimistic.

But this vision of transforming cancer services, education, and research has been turned into reality with the creati of the Cancer Centre whic will continue to serve ma generations to come.

The Evening Post Canc Centre Appeal has, in effe offered every member of community, whether they contributed £1 or £1,000, opportunity to help shape the future of cancer servi in South West Wales.

Dr Salah Sharka
Clinical director of can
servic
Singleton Hosp

Evening Post

Make it a Million

CAMPAIGN

The end result saw the establishment of the cancer centre with all its components – the South West Wales radiotherapy centre, chemotherapy unit, breast care unit, cancer institute, bone marrow transplant unit, the IT unit and Sea View Hostel.

In addition, the appeal contributed greatly towards setting up the Teenage Cancer Trust unit in Cardiff to serve our younger population.

He added:

"In short with the help of the generosity of our local population, the Evening Post and its staff, West Glamorgan Health Authority and the support of the Welsh Office we have managed to set up a nationally renowned cancer centre."

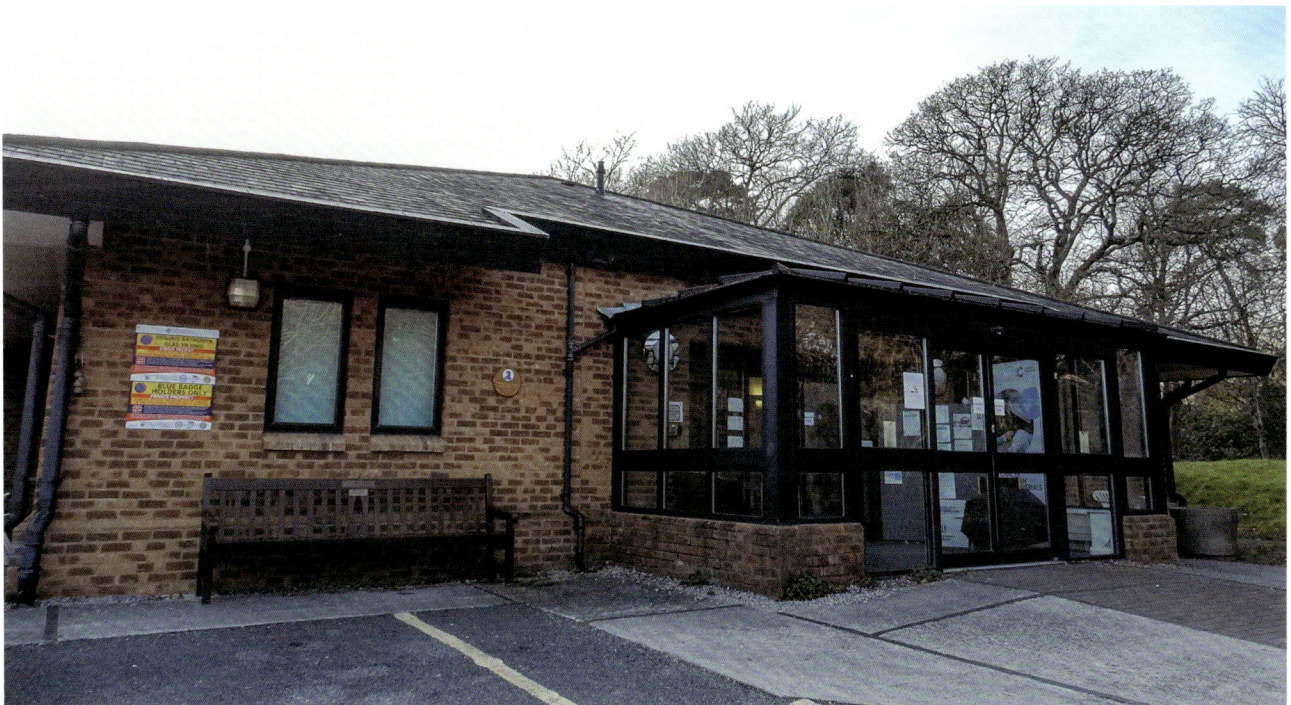

Part of the South West Wales Cancer Centre at Singleton Hospital

Hospital radio.

In the days before smartphones and tablets provided instant access to news and entertainment, patients had one vital way of breaking the monotony - hospital radio.

Beds came with their own headsets, linking patients up to the latest hits and dedicated programmes keeping them informed about hospital life.

The importance of entertainment for hospital patients has long-been recognised – one of the earliest contributions made by Morriston Hospital's League of Friends was wireless headphones paid for by the proceeds of a darts league.

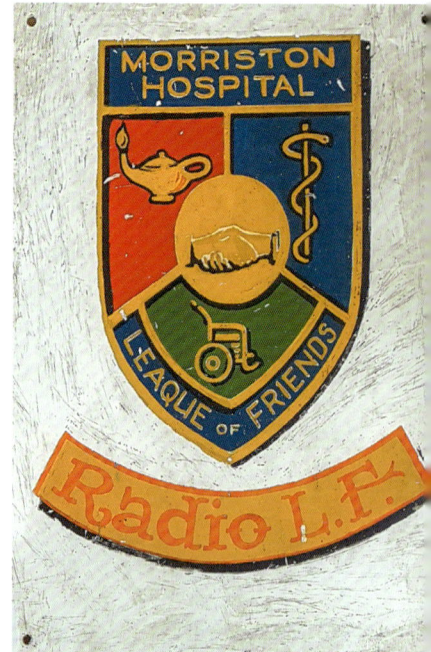

In 2017 six friends who helped found one of the first hospital radio services in the UK when they were still schoolboys reunited to mark its 50th anniversary.

The Swansea Hospitals Radio Service was created by Dynevor School pupils Clive Thomas, Rob Rees, and David Vaughan and operated out of a small studio at Morriston Hospital before opening a year later at Singleton.

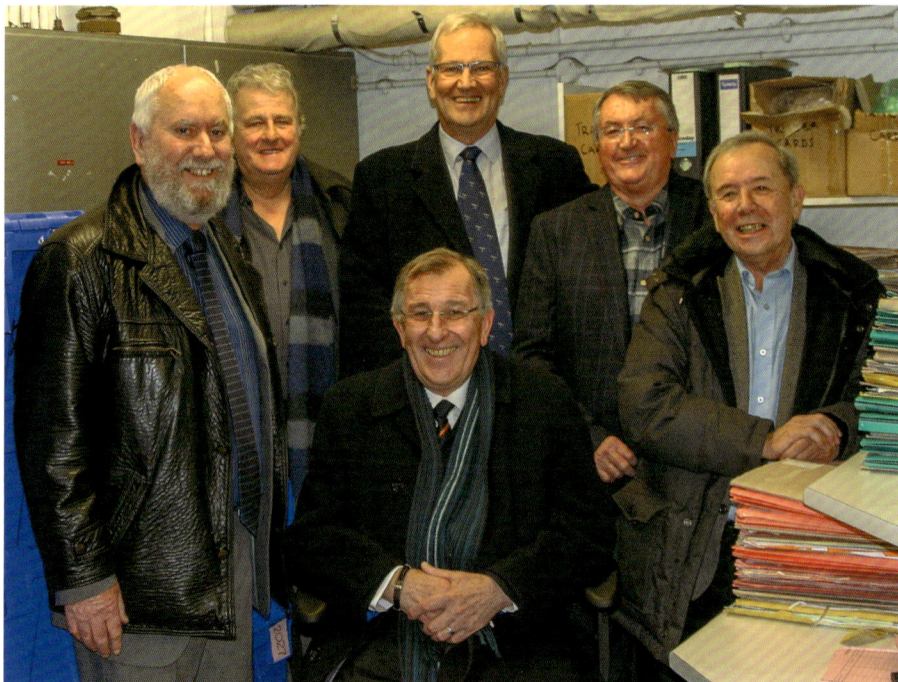

Fifty years on they returned to the site of their very first studio at Singleton *(pictured above)* . The group included Swansea barrister Ieuan Rees, law lecturer and Private Eye journalist Tim Richards, as well as retired teachers Roger Brown and Jeff Lewis, and music entrepreneur Mike Evans.

Also involved at the early stages was former hospital chaplain and retired bishop of Swansea and Brecon, Tony Pierce, and the reunion was organised by GP turned international sports broadcaster Dr Robert Treharne Jones.

"We've lost many founder members and lost touch with so many more, but it was a very special day to get this group back together to celebrate such a significant anniversary," said Dr Treharne Jones.

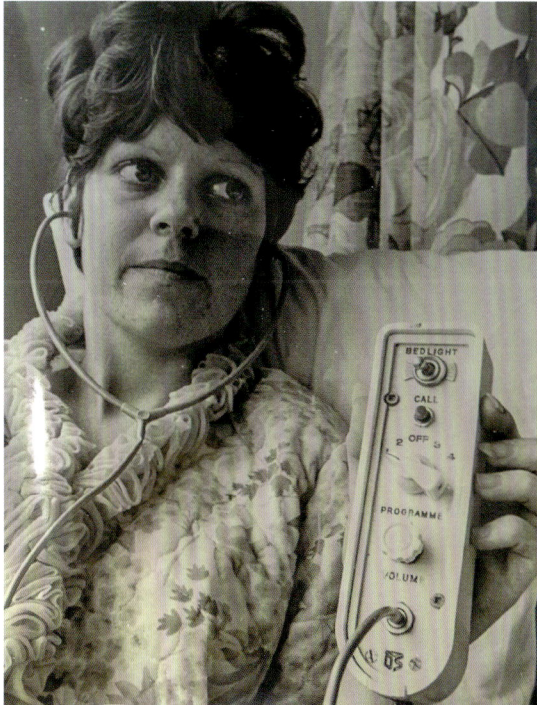

"In retrospect it was very forward thinking of the hospital management to allow a group of young people to put on this service without any particular degree of supervision. We were all just 16 or 17, but we'd like to think we took a responsible attitude to the whole project and that really paid off.

"Not only did we have the chance to go on air for the very first time, but also a chance to go around the wards and speak to the patients and gather record requests – I'm not sure that would necessarily be allowed these days."

Writing in the Swansea History Journal Tim Richards explains that their earliest equipment was just a record player, a microphone and a tape recorder which they used to record music at their homes before playing it back at Morriston using landlines round the hospital.

"We were delighted when we moved into the 'studio' in the basement at Morriston. You will have noticed the quotation marks as this was as basic as you could get, set up on a table on a bare floor with water-pipes above and as dusty at you might expect."

The boys broadcast at the weekends and would go round the wards to get requests from patients and made every effort to cater for all musical tastes.

"Our enthusiasm was for all music and being a DJ like our pop pirate heroes. My own three-hour slot on a Saturday morning was named the Tatty Tim Fiaso which gave me enormous licence and the programmes were at times totally anarchic which suited me perfectly as you could get away with loads of rubbish."

But one day the boys certainly got something right – and managed to beat the rest of the media to break the story that Swansea was to become a city.

"It was at the time of Prince Charles' investiture in 1969 and he was finding out all about his new Principality and it was when he got to Swansea that I got early news of the announcement by chance."

Tim's father was the BBC's West Wales representative at the time and when Tim took an urgent message for his dad from the Town Clerk he got wind that something was up.

His father knew the Prince was going to make an important announcement when he visited Swansea's Guildhall later that day and a curious Tim was determined to find out what it was and when he did, from his father's colleague, he made sure he shared the story.

"I borrowed my Dad's car and set off to Singleton Hospital to break the news. Ironically I was delayed by a traffic jam caused by the Prince while he passed through Sketty, finally got down to the studio where Chris Harper was doing his show and there and then around the same time as the Prince was making the announcement Radio City broke the story, beating the BBC to it by an hour and all the newspapers by a day."

When an attempt was made to centralise the broadcasts at Singleton Hospital patients and staff at Morriston opposed the studio closure. The League of Friends installed a new service and Radio League of Friends was born, complete with a badge specially designed by the Friends' general secretary William Randall Hughes. Radio City 1366AM, as the station is now called, is still on the air broadcasting from Singleton and offering a schedule featuring a wide variety of music as well as live commentary of sporting fixtures.

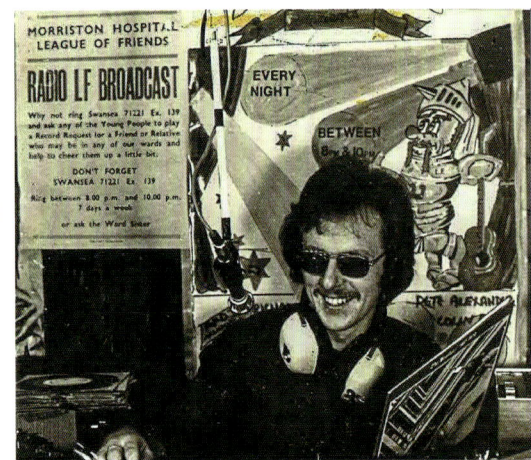

It is eager to sign up new volunteers who would follow in the headphones of established broadcasters including Jason Mohammad and Radio Wales's Mark Buckley and Simon Davies.

Also still thriving are Bridgend's Hospital Radio – formally known as Bridgend League of Friends Hospital Radio (BLFR) which has provided a service at Princess of Wales Hospital since the vinyl days of 1982.

Radio Phoenix was established in 1986 and broadcasts to Neath Port Talbot Hospital.

Meet our fantastic volunteers

Did you know that more than 450 people regularly volunteer throughout the health board? By giving their time, volunteers aged from 17 to 90 plus make a unique and valued contribution to our services, enhance the experience of our patients and families as well as providing added support to staff teams.

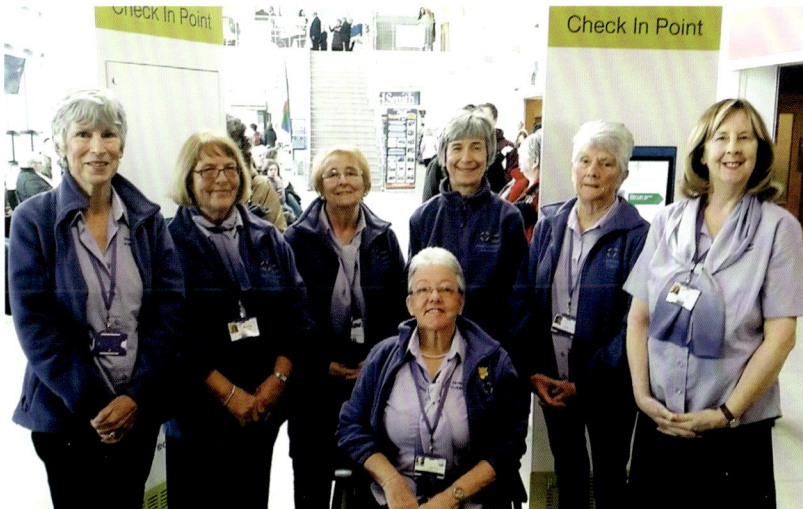

Volunteers do not replace paid staff, but provide an invaluable service in improving care by doing things like providing companionship for patients, helping at mealtimes, running errands or helping with feedback surveys.

Every year they are invited to a festive celebration event to say thanks for their hard work. ABMU's Director of Therapies and Health Science Christine Morrell described the volunteers' work as *"putting the icing and hundreds and thousands on top of our cake"*.

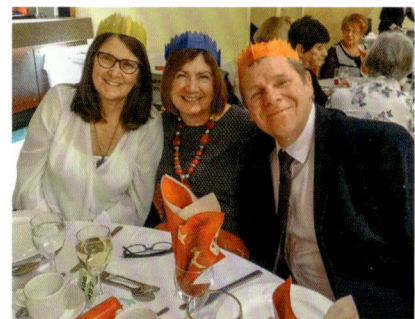

She told them: *"You do the things that we can't do. The rich diversity of volunteers also helps us to develop our services. Your contribution is a hugely valuable and ABMU is better for your input."*

Feeling part of a team is one of the things that makes Wendy Jones value her days helping at the Regional Cardiology Unit at the Princess of Wales Hospital.

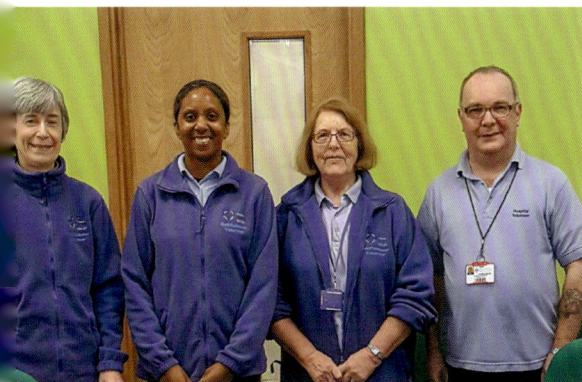

"The staff are wonderful, I feel included and trusted. I welcome patients, show them where they need to go, fetch them drinks, basically anything that helps the staff.

"I needed something to do after my husband died, I didn't want to just vegetate, now I feel I am useful and I have met so many interesting people. I love it."

League of Friends

Morriston

The NHS is not the only institution celebrating this year - Morriston Hospital's own League of Friends is also marking its 75th anniversary.

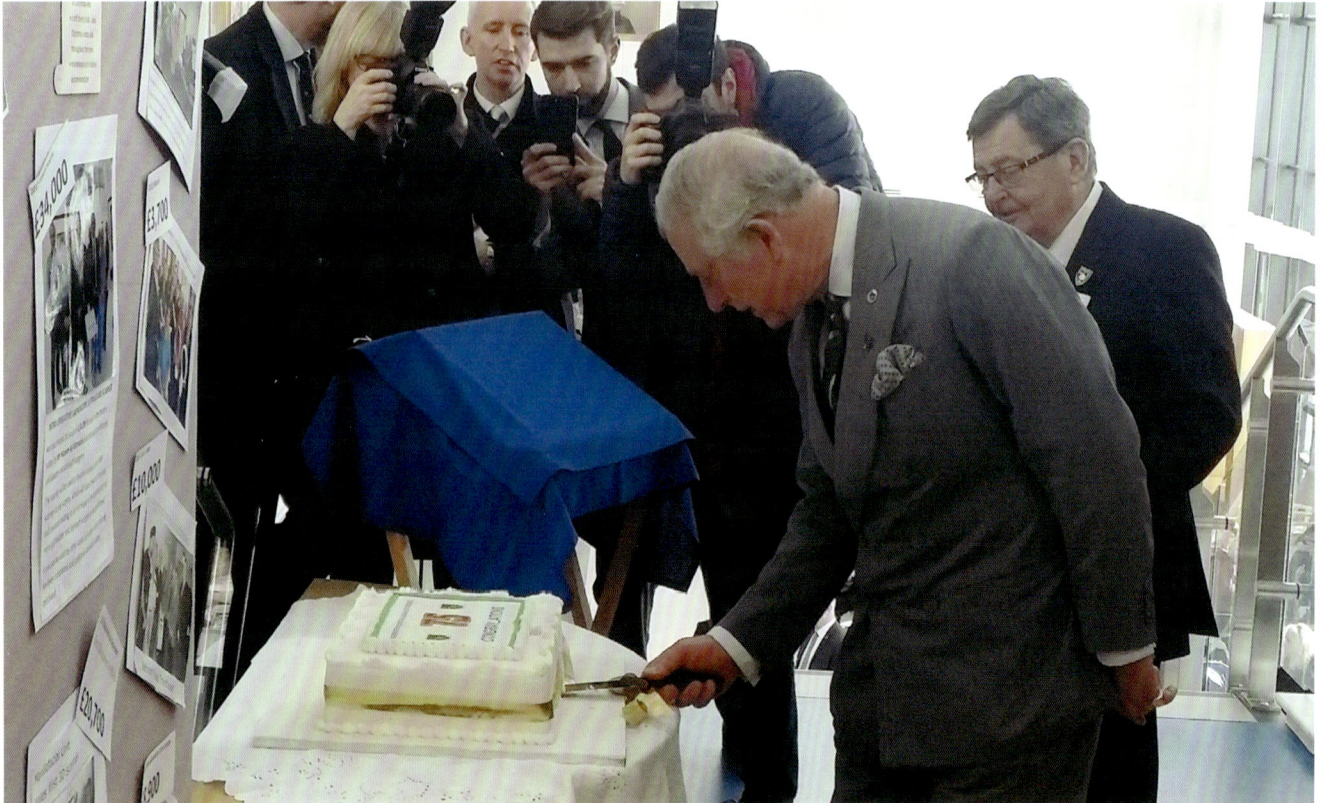

The group received the royal seal of approval earlier this year when Prince Charles paid a special visit to the hospital to meet the team and get a close-up look at some of the equipment and services their hard work has paid for.

Now the oldest hospital league in the UK, over the years the group has been responsible for raising a remarkable £2,100,000 which has gone directly into supporting patient care.

Among those welcoming the Prince was League chairman John Hughes, whose father William Randall Hughes was one of its founder members back in 1943.

Pre-dating the NHS, it was established to provide film shows and concerts for wounded servicemen and the very first pieces of equipment it bought were headphones for each hospital bed.

Mr Hughes said: *"My mother Gladys was also a member and I was brought up to be a part of it. I remember being a 12-year-old boy helping to show films on the wards and it has just gone from there."*

The League's current secretary is John's wife Trish whose own mother and father were also involved. In fact the League of Friends is a real family affair for several of its seven-strong committee who are continuing the proud tradition of fundraising their own relatives started.

Over the years the group's fundraising has paid for a variety of support including cutting edge equipment such as the hospital's first 3D scanner as well as its chapel and its organ which opened in 1964 at a cost of nearly £10,000. Now the hospital's multi-faith room, League members still help bring patients to worship there regularly.

"We are now only a small group but we are very proud of everything that the League has been able to achieve over the decades. Our aim has always been to do whatever we can to help the patients."

Many staff and patients have fond memories of the annual carnival which was a popular fundraising event run by the league for many years.

"One year we had 51 lorries taking part, it took hours before the final one reached the hospital at the end of the parade from Morriston town centre.

"We would have major celebrities of the day coming to open it – people like Clive Dunn from Dad's Army, Blue Peter's John Noakes, stars of Coronation Street."

Mr Hughes and his fellow committee members are particularly proud of the League's ongoing support for patients' families. Originally it provided furnishings for alcoves along main corridor where relatives could wait.

Over the years the League was able to pay for dedicated accommodation, known as The Bungalow which officially opened in 1976. Now the hospital is a regional treatment centre many patients' loved ones have to travel a long way to see them, making family accommodation on site even more vital.

In 2010 the Bungalow was replaced by the new League of Friends accommodation *(right)* and Mr Hughes says plans are now in the pipeline to extend it further.

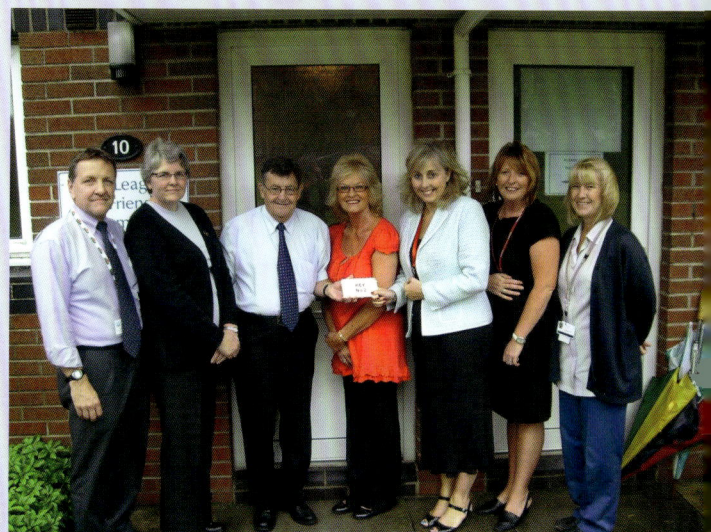

"It is occupied all the time at the moment, there is always a demand and we know what a difference it can make to patients if their families can stay close to them."

Singleton

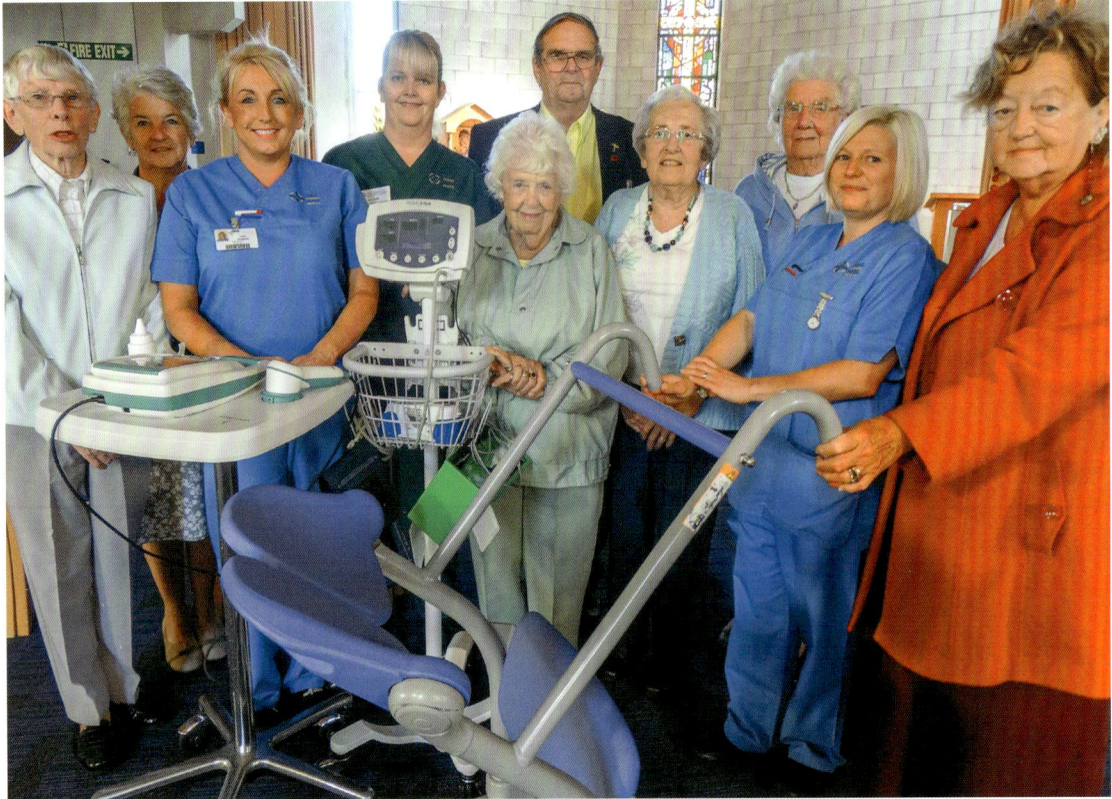

The Friends of Singleton Hospital have been raising hundreds of thousands of pounds to support patients since 1970.

Members of the group are a familiar sight as they man their fundraising stand in the hospital's foyer and the donations they receive, along with the proceeds of raffle ticket sales, go towards continuing that support.

Over the years they have been able to provide a variety of equipment for different departments around the site.

More recent donations have paid for high-tech equipment to support cancer patients having radiotherapy, blood pressure monitors used constantly across the wards and new toys for the hospital's Hafan y Mor children's centre.

Unit service director for Singleton Jan Worthing said: *"They are a dedicated group of people who do so much to improve the experience of our patients.*

"I am truly amazed and extremely grateful for what they achieve. As well as purchasing equipment, they do other things such as buying a small gift for patients who unfortunately have to remain in hospital over Christmas. For many patients it will be the only gift that they receive."

The group is eager to continue its good work and so is looking to enlist new recruits to help support its ongoing fundraising.

Neath

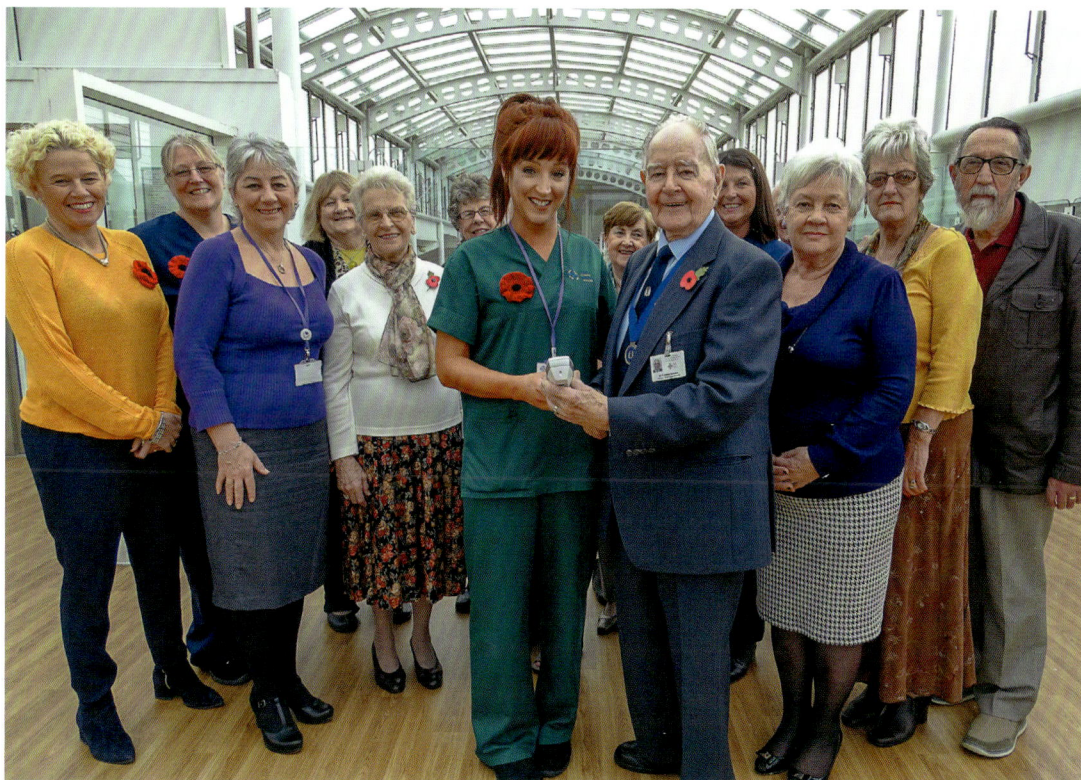

Neath Hospitals League of Friends have been supporting patients in the area for more than half a century.

Chairman Arthur Bowden first got involved with the group in 1969 – six years after it was formed.

Mr Bowden said: *"We must have made close on £2 million in that time.*

"We usually put in around £25,000-£30,000 a year but for the last two years, thanks to a large donation we received, we have been able to put in £50,000 a year."

The group has committees in Neath town centre, Skewen, Bryncoch, Glynneath, Cadoxton and Crynant which hold regular fundraising events.

Volunteers also have regular collections in Neath Port Talbot Hospital.

Mr Bowden said *"Neath Port Talbot received the lion's share of the money but the group also supported Tonna Hospital."*

The most recent large contribution was to support Tonna's Forget Me Not garden, where day patients can sit and enjoy the outdoors.

Mr Bowden said: *"We also buy a parcel of items for every patient who is in Tonna at Christmas."*

Port Talbot

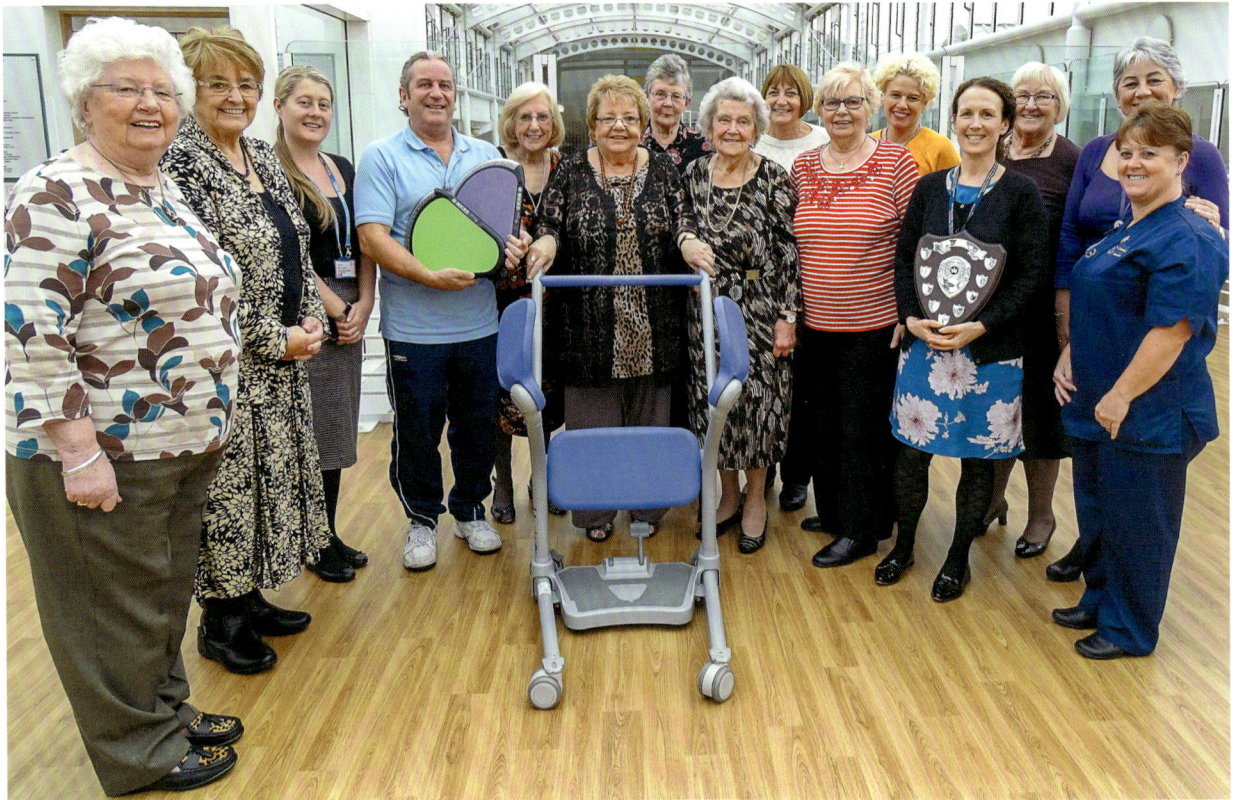

Tireless fundraisers with Port Talbot League of Friends are still going strong more than 60 years after the organisation was founded.

The biggest event in their calendar is the annual fete which has taken place in the grounds of Neath Port Talbot Hospital for 15 years – and in the old Port Talbot General Hospital before it closed - every year since 1969.

The 2017 fete was the most successful yet, generating a record-breaking £23,915. That took the group's fundraising efforts to £573,164 since 2002 after Neath Port Talbot Hospital opened.

Vicky Weekes, who chairs the group which her father Roy Hamer founded in 1953, said:

"The fete is the big event but we do fashion shows, raffles, collections and lots more. We have around 20 people who do all the work and without them it wouldn't be possible."We always have fantastic support from the people of the town and we hope that will continue in these difficult times."

In 2011 ABMU bid a sad farewell to the **Bridgend League of Friends.**

The volunteer group, which looked after the Bridgend based hospitals for 40 years and raised over three quarters of a million pounds, decided to disband after its membership declined and no new younger members came forward.

Neath Port Talbot Cancer Challenge

Run entirely by volunteers, the Neath Port Talbot Cancer Challenge aims to help with the prevention, early diagnosis and treatment of all types of cancer.

The charity was formed in 1997 and was followed two years later by the launch of the Neath Port Talbot Cancer Challenge Singers, *(pictured below)* a mixed choir which is still going strong today.

Over the last 21 years, the Cancer Challenge has raised around £800,000 to buy equipment for hospitals in Neath Port Talbot and Swansea.

In 2006 Neath Port Talbot Cancer Challenge was presented with the Queens Award, the highest award given to local volunteer groups across the UK, to recognise outstanding work done in their own communities.

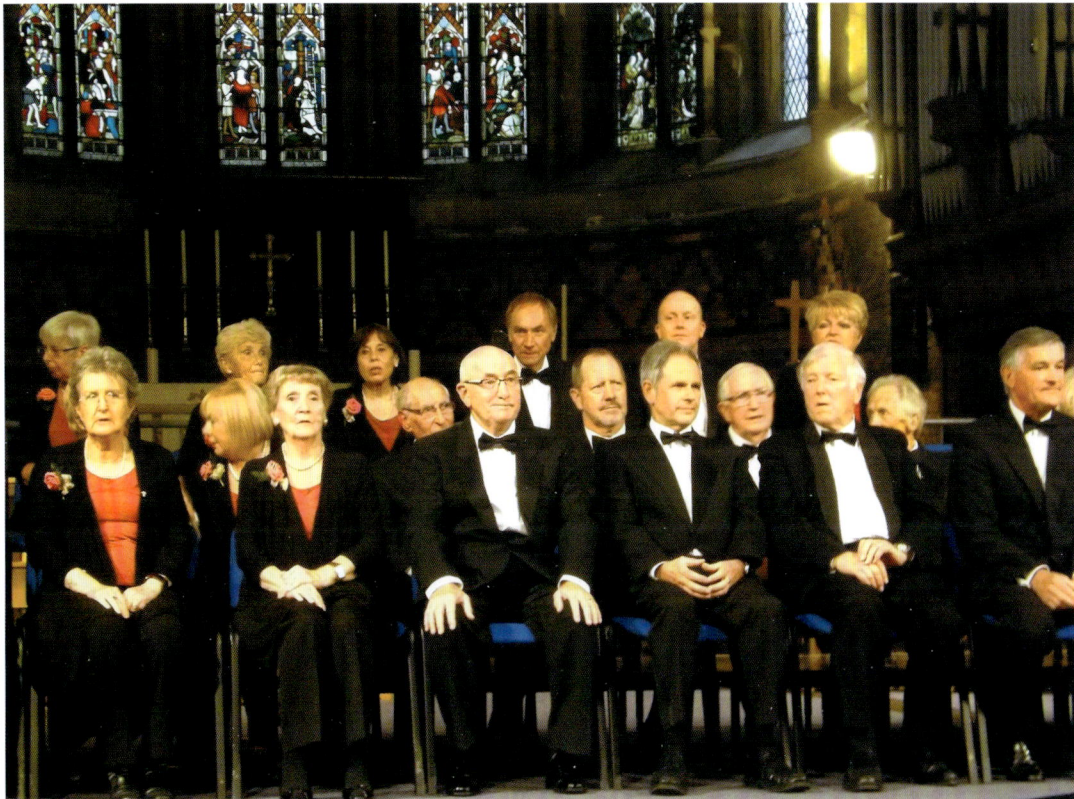

Royal seal of approval

Earlier this year another important anniversary saw Morriston Hospital welcoming Prince Charles – the latest in a long line of occasions when our staff played host to royalty.

The Prince joined celebrations to mark the 75th anniversary of the League of Friends and met staff and members of the fundraising group.

League Chairman John Hughes said: *"We are so honoured and very grateful that His Royal Highness found time to come and find out more about our work here at Morriston."*

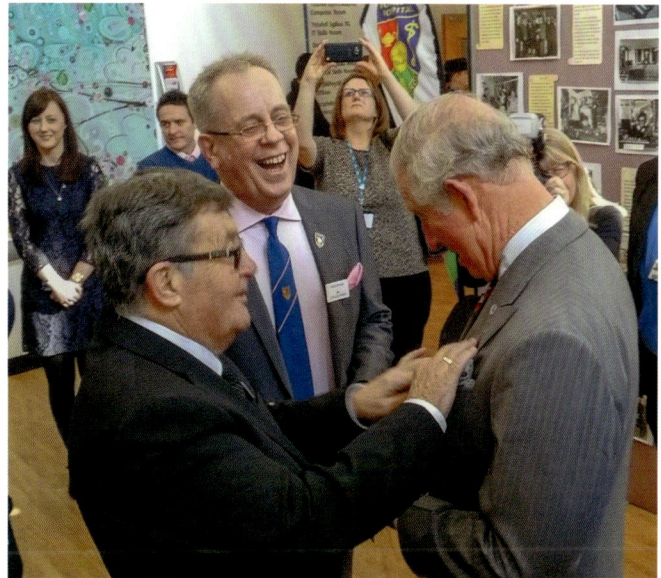

Prince Charles also met outpatient volunteers including Brenda Broad, *(below)* the hospital's longest-serving volunteer.

"He asked me how long I had been a volunteer here and I told him 28 years."

Caroline Kirk was an auxiliary nurse when the brand new Princess of Wales Hospital in Bridgend opened in 1985 and was there on a very special day eight months later.

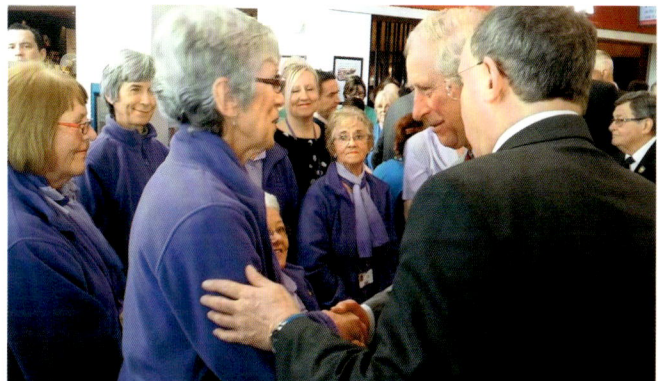

"I was on duty when Princess Diana came to open the hospital. She visited the ward I was working on, she was so friendly and spoke to everyone."

The Princess returned to the hospital in 1990 accompanied by Viscount Tonypandy to open the George Thomas Scanner Suit.

Prince Charles was the special guest when he opened Phase 2 of the hospital's development, which houses services from areas of what remained of Bridgend General Hospital.

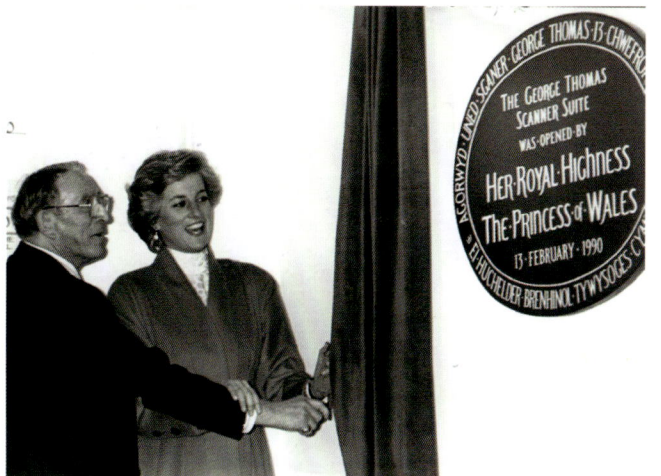

The Duchess of Kent returned to Wales to perform the opening of the Bridgend Diabetes Centre at the hospital.

She had previously met health staff when she carried out the formal opening of Singleton Hospital in Swansea in June 1968.

The Duchess was also the guest of honour when Ty Olwen, offering inpatient specialist palliative care, opened officially in May 1982.

It was a day paediatric diabetic clinical nurse specialist Geraldine Phillips remembers well.

Back then she was working as a nurse on the hospital's children's ward and she and a colleague were part of the crowd of staff and visitors lined up to greet her.

"We had a patient, a four-month old baby with ostegenis imperfect – or brittle bone disease on the ward, a long-term patient, so we took her out with us to see the Duchess arriving.

"As she walked past the Duchess spotted the baby and stopped to talk to us and ask about her. She was very interested," said Geraldine.

The unit had soon outgrown its original space and the Duchess returned in 1991 to open a much-needed £750,000 extension. Funded through a public appeal the extension houses a purpose-built day centre and kitchen, chapel, physiotherapy room, therapy areas, library, lecture rooms and a larger office for the Home Care teams.

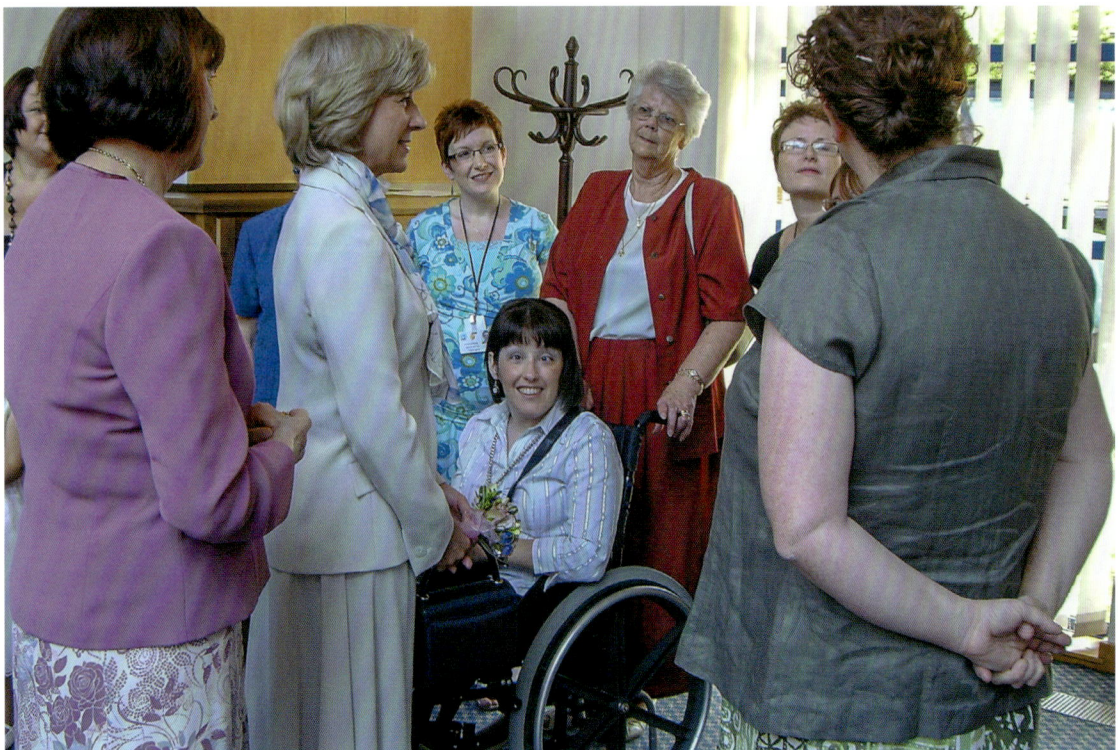

A further £1.2 million renovation at the hospice saw the Duchess of Gloucester come to visit in 2007. *(pictured above)*

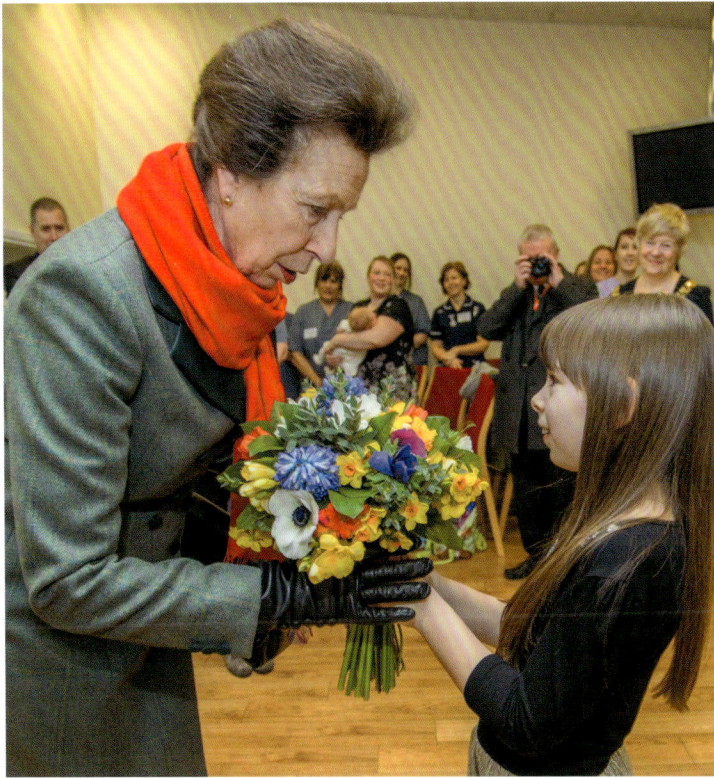

She met and chatted to staff, patients, volunteers and trustees, and was given a tour of the refurbished facilities, which include a new light and airy lounge built in the former quadrangle area.

Sophie Countess of Wessex officially opened Ysbryd y Coed at Cefn Coed Hospital in September 2015. She met ABMU officials, staff and patients and was given a guided tour of the new facility, a 60-bed inpatient unit with assessment and treatment facility for older people with dementia.

In February 2016, the Princess Royal visited the Birth Centre at Neath Port Talbot Hospital in her capacity as patron of the Royal College of Midwives.

After a private tour, she attended a reception during which she met staff, mums and children and received flowers from eight-year-old Elizabeth Rawle who was born at the centre. *(see picture above)*

Back in 1962 her predecessor Mary, Princess Royal, visited Swansea to present the certificates and prizes at the annual prize day at Swansea Hospital's Nurse Training School. The event was held at the outpatients' department at Singleton Park – where work on phase two of the hospital's development was progressing ahead of a planned completion date of 1965.

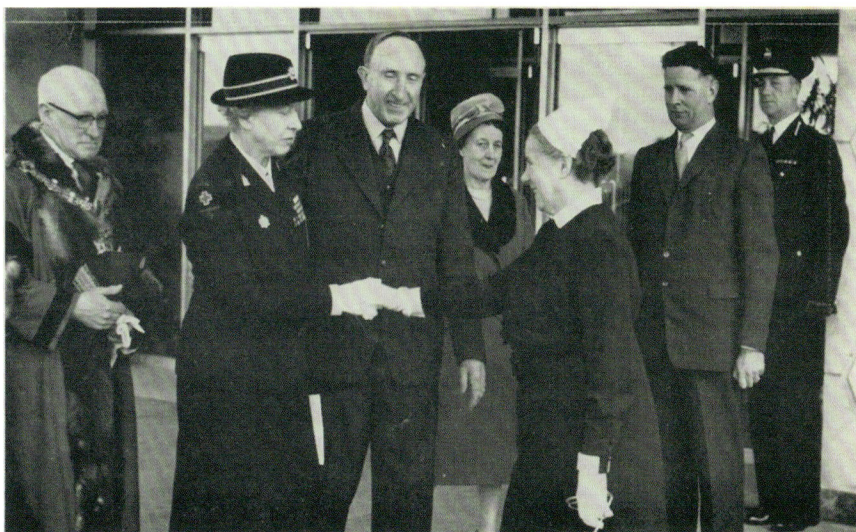

Visit of Her Royal Highness The Princess Royal to the new Out-Patient Department, Singleton Park, Swansea - 16th May, 1962.

At the cutting edge

Our hospitals are not just about providing care. They are leading the way in finding new and better ways of looking after people too.

The way services are delivered has changed dramatically over the years, thanks to advances in medicine and science.

This section highlights just a few examples of how such advances have transformed healthcare in a way no-one could have imagined only a few decades ago, let alone in 1948.

It's down to the expertise and commitment of our staff, and he health boards commitment to cutting-edge research and development. This is not just good for patients but helps attract the best people to deliver services too.

The health board works in partnership with Swansea University and other academic institutions across the UK and beyond, developing research collaborations involving a whole range of fields.

Patients often get the opportunity to take part in clinical trials which gives them access to new medicines or devices.

Research and Development is also an important strand of the ARCH (A Regional Collaboration for Health) project involving ABMU and Hywel Dda health boards and Swansea University.

All this pioneering work often results in headline news not just here in Wales but sometimes nationally and even worldwide. What was science fiction in Nye Bevan's day is now science fact.

And who knows what else the future might bring...

Morriston Cardiac Centre

Life-saving procedures now used routinely when people have heart attacks were unheard of when Morriston became Wales's second cardiac centre in October 1997.

In fact anyone needing any kind of cardiac intervention would have needed to go to Cardiff.

The Morriston centre now provides a regional service covering South West Wales, carrying out 750 heart operations a year along with thousands of other procedures.

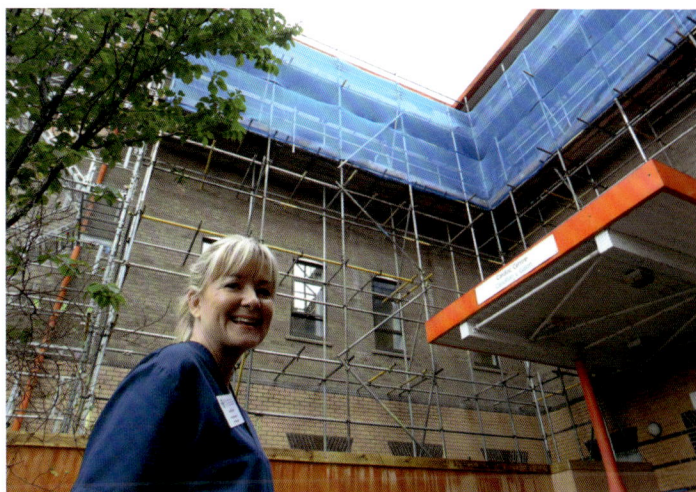

The Cardiac Centre underwent a £6.6 million upgrade in 2016. Centre manager Julie Barnes is pictured as work starts.

Some of the centre's staff have been there since it opened. Among them is consultant cardiologist Mark Anderson.

Dr Anderson said: *"I can remember arriving here in September 1997 and it was just an empty building – all the beds were there but no people.*

"It has been fascinating watching it develop since then. It has progressed and changed almost out of all recognition in many respects and the treatments have evolved greatly during that time.

"For example, the way heart attacks are treated has changed radically since 20 years ago. If you had a heart attack in Aberystwyth then, you would have been taken to Bronglais Hospital and given clot-busting drugs.

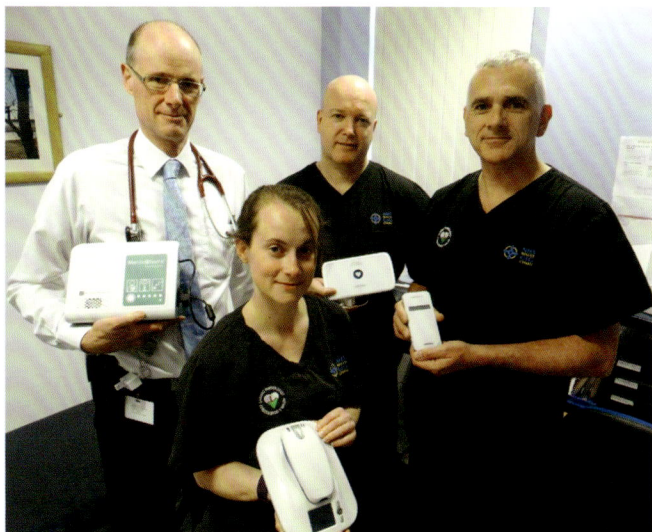

Dr Anderson with some of his team

"Now, you will be brought straight here, and have an angioplasty instead of clot-busting drugs, which greatly improves your chances of surviving. We do around 500-600 of these procedures every year now, something not even considered back in 1997."

A heart attack is a blockage by blood clot in one of the arteries, damaging that area of heart muscle.

It's treated through an angioplasty, which uses balloons and stents to open the blocked artery and restore blood flow to the heart muscle as quickly as possible. Morriston has carried out some 18,000 of them, along with 13,700 cardiac surgery procedures, and 9,800 pacemaker and defibrillator procedures.

From the initial small teams of three cardiologists and cardiac surgeons it now has a team of 12 cardiologists and five cardiac surgeons.

The Cardiac Centre also provides thoracic services and undertakes urgent operations for patients with lung cancer – 4,400 of them since 1997.

Its performance has also been consistently high. In 2015 Morriston was ranked sixth out 39 in the UK for survival rates. This is despite the fact that these operations are particularly complex because this area has more severe levels of heart disease and other serious illnesses.

Morriston's cardiac surgeons were also deemed excellent.

In 2009, Morriston became the first hospital in Wales to undertake a procedure called a transcatheter aortic valve implementation (TAVI). This is a minimally invasive procedure for people with aortic valve disease but cannot have the valve replaced through conventional open heart surgery.

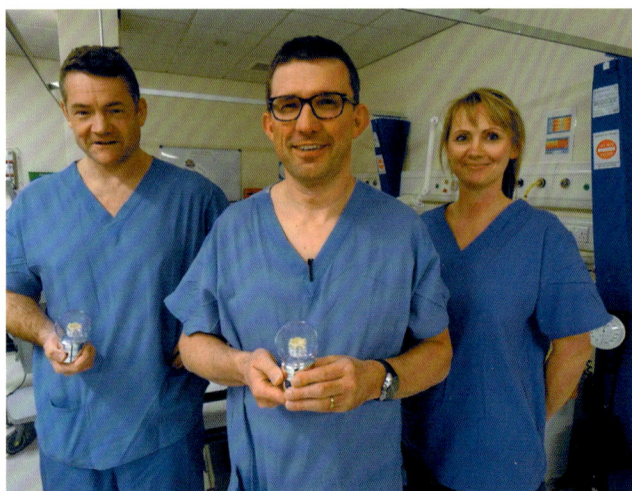

The TAVI team: consultant cardiologists Alex Chase and Dave Smith with catheter labs manager Anwen Jenkins

The cardiac centre has two dedicated surgical theatres along with two catheter labs – recently upgraded with a £2.43 million investment – where procedures such as angioplasties and TAVIs are carried out.

A third lab specialises in pacemakers, while other facilities include an expanded cardiac intensive therapy unit, which opened last year following a £6.6 million investment, along with wards and outpatient services. Morriston also provides a full range of cardiac diagnostic services.

A series of events took place in 2017 to mark the cardiac centre's 20th anniversary, including a celebratory gathering of almost 300 staff at Swansea's National Waterfront Museum.

The South Wales Cochlear Implant Programme

A service available in Bridgend since the early 1990s has transformed the lives of people with profound hearing difficulties.

The South Wales Cochlear Implant Programme has offered cochlear implants to suitable patients since autumn 1993.

The Bridgend team has been based in Princess of Wales Hospital since 1997.

Working together with the cochlear implant team based in Cardiff, the two programmes provide a regional service, with the Bridgend-based service accepting referrals from South and West Wales.

A cochlear implant is an electronic hearing device under the scalp, with stimulating electrodes inserted into the inner ear 'hearing computer' (cochlear).

The implant works by electrically stimulating directly the nerves of hearing in the cochlear, bypassing the outer and middle ear structures of ear drum and bones of hearing (ossicles).

When worn with an external sound processor that attaches magnetically and sits outside the scalp, it provides a sensation of sound to people with severe-profound hearing loss and unable to benefit from traditional hearing aids.

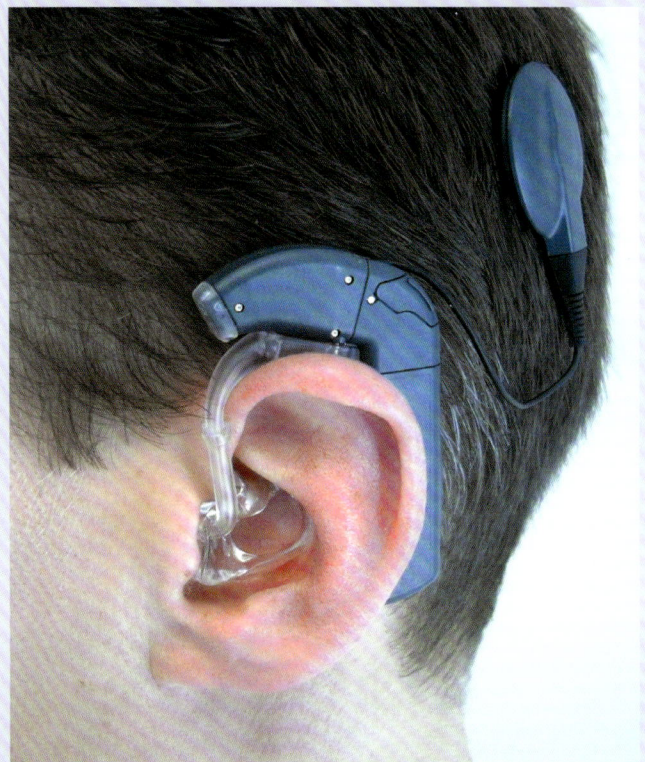

The POWH-based cochlear implant team comprises an audiological scientist, audiologist, consultant clinical psychologist, secretarial administrator, ENT consultant surgeon and a speech and language therapist to undertake assessment, surgery and rehabilitation of appropriate patients.

Additionally, for adults, the team also includes a hearing therapist, and for children, a teacher of the deaf and specialist community paediatrician.

A truly multidisciplinary team-delivered service!

3D printing

Not long ago 3D printing was the stuff of science fiction – but today it's making a real difference to patients and surgeons at Morriston Hospital.

Specialist staff there have pioneered the use of digital technology to 3D design and print implants and cutting guides.

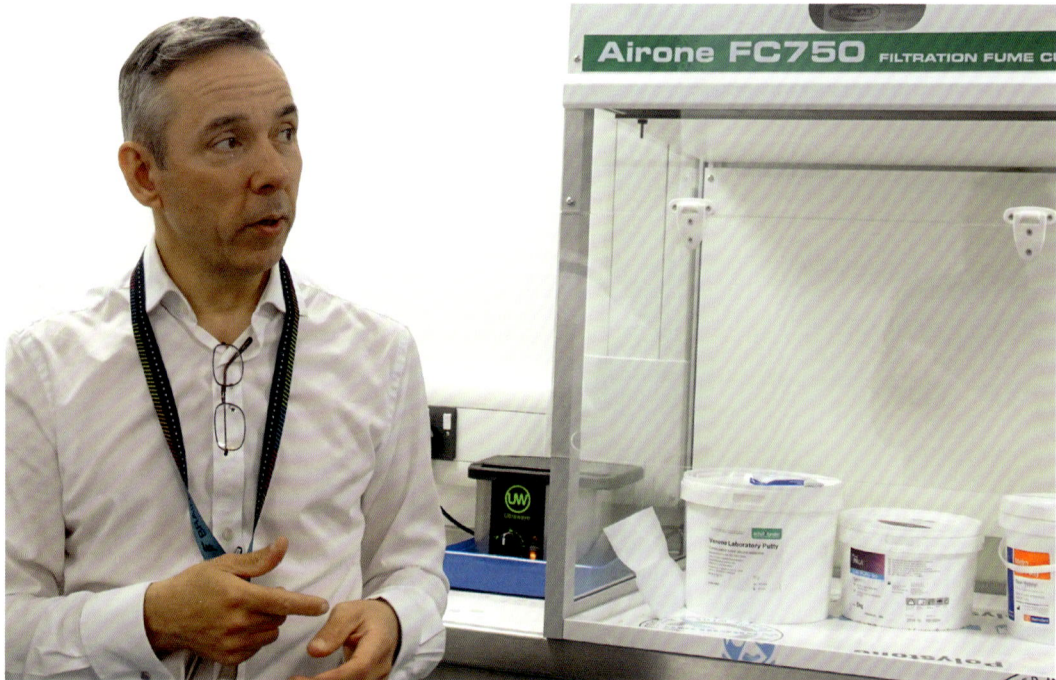

These are created using the patient's own CT images, meaning they are as anatomically accurate as possible.

This ensures a better outcome for patients and saves time for surgeons who previously had to bend implants by eye to the correct fit.

Maxillofacial Laboratory Services manager Peter Llewelyn Evans *(above)* said: *"In the past, a lot of what we do now would have been done by hand.*

"If we were making a facial prosthesis, for example, we would have hand-carved it. "Which is fine. We're trained to do that. But it takes a degree of artistic skill and takes quite a bit of time to do."

Now Mr Evans and his team, working with the surgeons, use the patient's own CT scans to design implants and cutting guides.

These can then be created using 3D printers. Morriston has a range of cost-effective printers of its own which it can use for just about anything other than titanium implants – these are printed off-site.

The results have been remarkable and have led to the hospital making headlines nationally – and sometimes internationally.

In March 2014, patient Stephen Power, who had been badly injured in a motorbike accident, had his face rebuilt at Morriston using 3D technology.

The hospital was in the news again in 2017, with a world-first procedure that combined a traditional bone graft with 3D printing to reconstruct patient Debbie Hawkins's jaw after it developed a tumour.

This involved removing the area of jawbone with the tumour and replacing it with bone cut from Debbie's leg. A 3D printed titanium implant held the bone in place, with perfect results.

Earlier this year, Abergavenny grandad Peter Maggs became the first person in Wales to have his chest wall rebuilt with a 3D printed prosthesis following the removal of a large tumour.

The implant *(pictured below)* replaced three ribs and half of Mr Maggs' breastbone, which had to be removed along with the tennis ball-sized tumour.

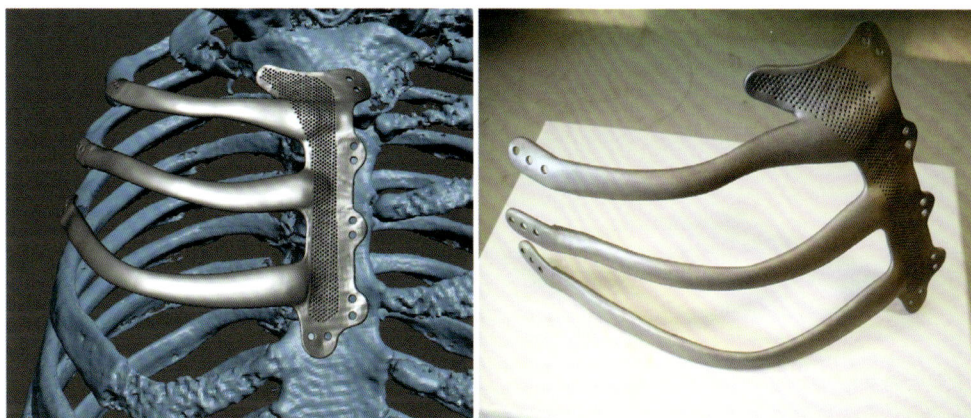

And if what once seemed like science fiction is now science fact, the technology may yet be taken to another exciting level.

Plastic surgeons at Morriston's Welsh Centre for Burns and Plastic Surgery have been working with engineers and scientists to develop 3D printed tissue made from human cells for the first time.

Led by Professor Ian Whittaker, the team hopes that, before long, patients who have lost all or part of an ear or nose could have reconstruction using new tissue grown from their own cells.

Mr Evans said: *"We have probably reached the ceiling of creativity because there isn't anything we can't design or make in metal now. But bio-printing, the work that Professor Whittaker and his team are doing, that is going to be the next big jump. It's probably some years off yet, but it is getting there."*

Supporting people with dementia

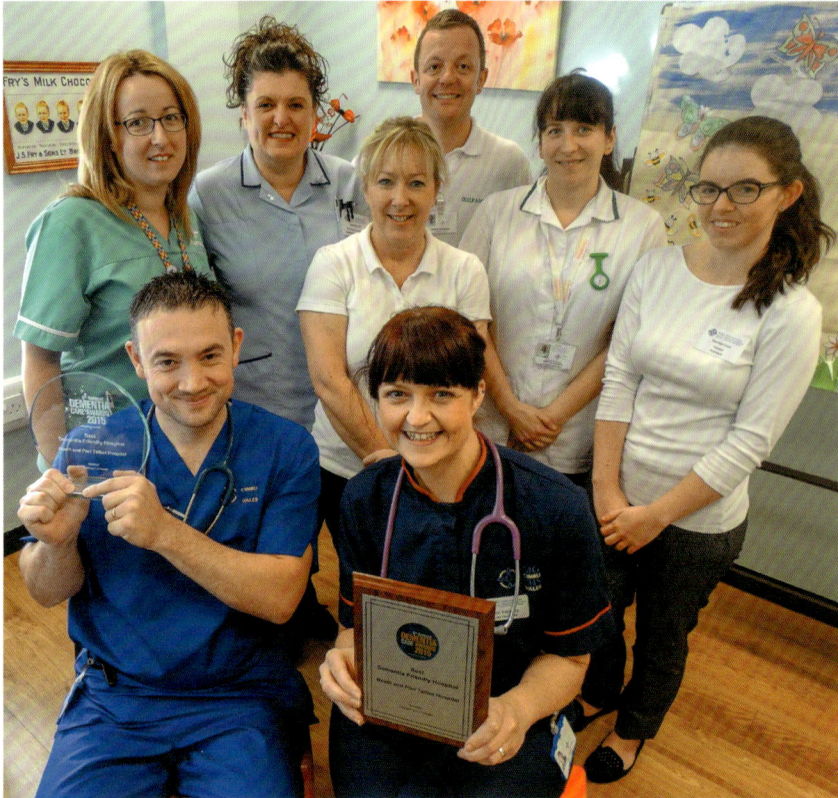

Recognising the ongoing challenge posed by an aging population has seen some radical steps taken to support those with dementia.

More than 7,200 people living in Swansea, Bridgend and Neath Port Talbot are known to have dementia and there are many more yet to still be diagnosed.

And as the risk of dementia increases with age and more people are living longer, that number will grow. So ABMU introduced an ambitious training programme to ensure all staff – not just frontline clinical colleagues - are more knowledgeable about dementia.

This led to the health board becoming the first in Wales to be honoured by the Alzheimer's Society's for its efforts to become dementia friendly.

In 2015 Neath Port Talbot Hospital was named the best dementia friendly hospital in the whole of the UK at the National Dementia Care Awards *(pictured above)*. The judges were impressed the collaborative approach of staff which sees clinical teams - nurses, doctors, occupational therapists, physiotherapists and pharmacists - working together to improve care.

In addition several wards offer a variety of activities aimed to keep patients with dementia stimulated - Ward 18 at Princess of Wales Hospital has decorated its main corridor with pictures of movie stars and the royal family to trigger memories and conversations while Angelton Clinic even has a games room with mock bar and sporting memorabilia to help engage patients.

Emergency Medical Retrieval and Transfer Service (EMRTS).

Medical care isn't just provided by staff at hospitals and health centres these days – since 2015 ABMU has hosted the Emergency Medical Retrieval and Transfer Service (EMRTS).

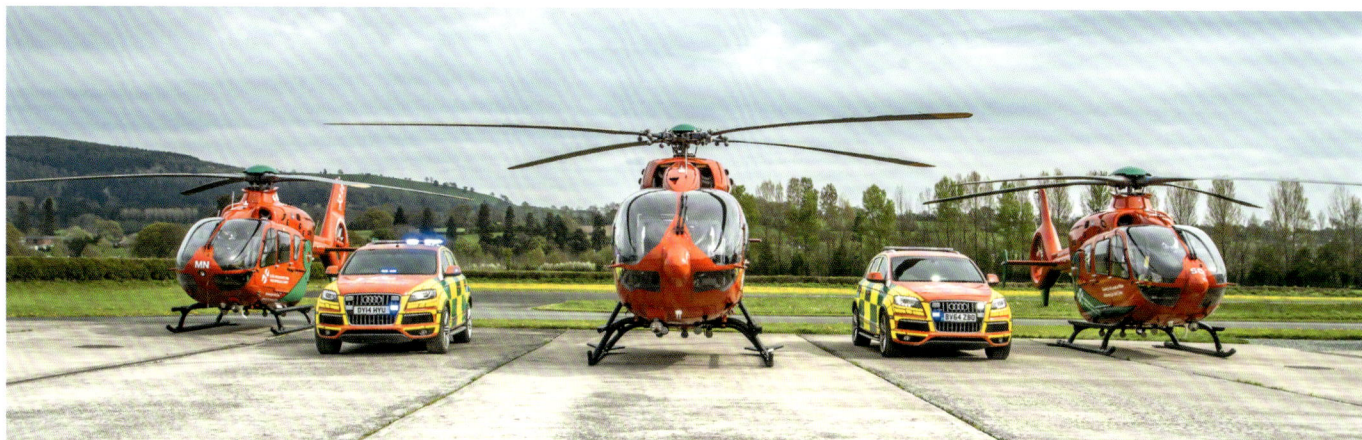

The flying doctors service provides innovative pre-hospital critical care across Wales, by air and by road in partnership with Wales Air Ambulance, the charitable trust that relies entirely on public generosity to fund the helicopter operation.

In 2017, EMRTS medics received 2,554 calls, attending 71 per cent of incidents by air and 29 per cent by road. A total of 53 per cent of patients had received a trauma while 43 per cent had experienced a medical episode. During that period, medics carried out 50 blood product transfusions and 161 emergency anaesthetics.

The service has attracted international interest and has influenced the design of other Helimed services across the world. It has received two Air Ambulance Association Special Incident Awards (2016/2017) for cases that produced 'unexpected survivors'.

Dr Ami Jones, EMRTS interim National Director said: "I am proud to be part of an NHS team that provides platinum-level medical care to Wales' sickest patients, wherever they may be and when they need it the most."

Renal services

Morriston Hospital is home to a renal service which cares for thousands of people from across South, Mid and West Wales.

The services covers an area from Fishguard to Bridgend in the south and from Tywyn to Llanidloes in the north.

It receives referrals from GPs throughout this area as well as from clinicians based in seven district hospitals.

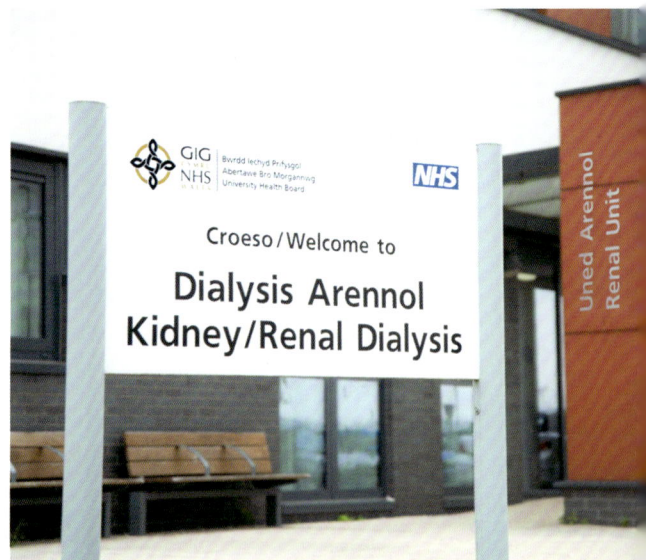

Morriston has its own haemodialysis units but is also clinically responsible for others in hospitals in Carmarthen, Haverfordwest and Aberystwyth – between them providing dialysis for hundreds of people.

There is also a community support service working out of Morriston and extending throughout the wider area.

Outreach clinics are held in other hospitals, while Morriston itself has clinics where patients with renal transplants and potential kidney donors are seen.

Developments within the renal service include establishing a nocturnal dialysis programme in 2011. It involves training patients to dialyse themselves at home overnight, greatly improving their quality of life.

More recently, the specialist Renal Medicines Service has pioneered the use of digital technology to electronically prescribe and manage medicines used by patients across the region.

Earlier this year, work was completed on a £5.8 million upgrade of Morriston's main renal unit.

It saw improvements to the local and regional renal dialysis units, renal outpatient department and renal day case and self-care service.

The refurbishment, funded by the Welsh Government, includes direct access from the wards into the dialysis units. There are also more cubicles, more bed space and more outpatient consulting rooms, plus a new main entrance.

It followed the opening of the new renal annex within Morriston Hospital's £60 million main entrance and outpatients department in late 2015. The annex provides additional dialysis machines and other services.

Mental health services

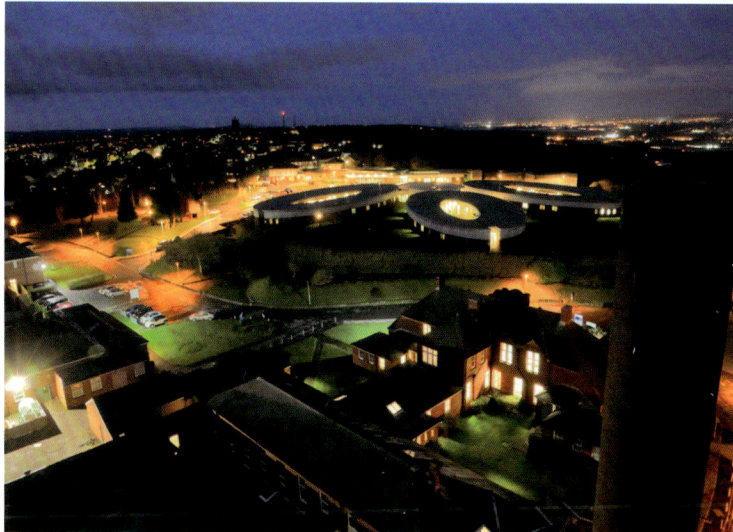

The view from the top of Cefn Coed Hospital tower pictured by Jono Atkinson

Seventy years ago at the dawn of the NHS over half its hospital beds were designated for mental health services, with thousands of psychiatric patients often living in huge institutions for years or even decades on end.

At one time Cefn Coed Hospital alone looked after 700 patients and there were three huge mental health institutions in the Bridgend area alone: Penyfai; Parc and Glanrhyd. As recently as 1979, the three Bridgend psychiatric hospitals still had over 1,400 beds between them.

But the service has undergone major modernisation. Those old buildings are no longer fit purpose and have been replaced with specially designed facilities as part of a rolling £100 million programme for mental health projects.

These have included the opening of Cefn yr Afon residential unit and Angelton Clinic in Bridgend, along with Ty Einon, Gwelfor and Ysbryd y Coed in the grounds of Cefn Coed Hospital. Ysbryd y Coed, for dementia patients, has three oval shaped wards so patients can find their way easily, and the loop provides a continuous path to walk with cushioned seats along the route.

Taith Newydd low secure unit at Glanrhyd Hospital supports patients with more complex needs and means people who had previously needed to travel to England for treatment can stay closer to home, somewhere with better living facilities, garden areas and therapeutic space.

Nurse Director for Mental Health and Learning Disability Hazel Powell said: *"Mental health is one area where the NHS has taken massive strides during its 70 years. "We now put much greater emphasis on providing care in a community setting. We have a better understanding of mental health and the range of treatments and approaches that can support people."*

The Welsh Centre for Burns and Plastic Surgery

Welsh mythology took centre stage when the health board hosted its first event to mark the 70th anniversary of the NHS.

This was the unveiling of a visually stunning sculpture in a courtyard at Morriston Hospital's Welsh Centre for Burns and Plastic Surgery.

The rusting steel sculpture, the Lady of Llyn y Fan Fach, *(pictured right)* uses the themes of regeneration and healing.

It was inspired by the Lady of the Lake from Welsh mythology and embodies the close relationship between the centre and Port Talbot's steelworks.

The sculpture, created by West Wales-based artist Sarah Tombs, was paid for by Community, the principal trade union at Port Talbot steelworks, using materials donated by Tata Steel.

In 2014, the Welsh Centre for Burns and Plastic Surgery celebrated its own landmark anniversary – 20 years since the service moved from St Lawrence Hospital in Chepstow to a purpose-built site in Morriston.

Consultant burns and plastic surgeon Bill Dickson, who retired in 2015, was one of the original members of staff who transferred from Chepstow.

Mr Dickson, *(right)* among the guests at the sculpture unveiling, recalled: *"The reason the service moved was because St Lawrence was a single-specialty hospital. It had plastic surgeons and maxillofacial surgeons. If you wanted a medical opinion you had to seek it from other hospitals.*

   "Linking the service to a large district general hospital with a whole number of other medical, surgical and paediatric disciplines has certainly been hugely beneficial in terms of patient care."

The centre started with six consultants in 1994. Today it has 17, along with an array of specialist clinicians including anaesthetists, nurses, physiotherapists, occupational therapists, psychologists and support staff.

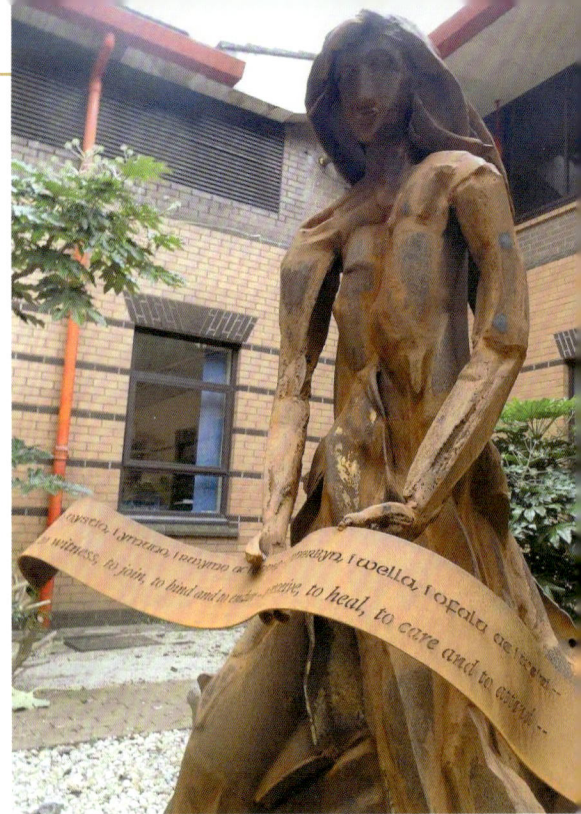

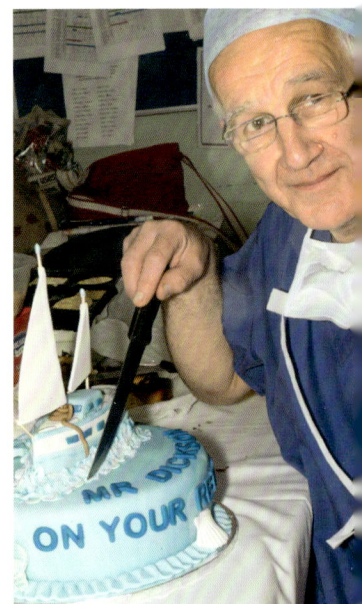

It provides a service for the people of South, Mid and West Wales – and beyond.

In 2010 it was designated the adult burn centre for the South West UK Burns Network, responsible for a population of 10 million as far afield as Aberystwyth, Portsmouth and Oxford.

Although the team treats children with quite severe burns, those with more extensive injuries are transferred to a specialist facility in Bristol.

The Welsh centre's director, consultant burns and plastics surgeon Peter Drew, said the number of serious burns – particularly those involving children – and major industrial accidents had decreased.

"There are fewer patients but we can do more for them. They are surviving with very extensive burns – we recently treated a patient with 90 per cent burns who is doing very well.

"Compared to Chepstow we have much more advanced intensive care input, which I think is what has made the difference. We also have access to donor skin, which is a huge benefit for patients.

"Medicine and science have moved on, and our understanding of wound infection and microbiology now is much better. The outcome for patients with serious burns has vastly improved."

Although the centre has links with industries across the region, providing advice and information, and treating any injuries, it has a particularly close relationship with the Port Talbot steelworks.

The sculpture launch featured music, a poem by William Ayot, which was developed with contributions from Port Talbot steelworkers, and a tale from storyteller David Ambrose.

ABMU Chairman Andrew Davies came up with the original idea for the sculpture some years ago, and was supported by then-Aberavon MP Hywel Francis in making it a reality.

Professor Davies said: *"The sculpture is a reminder of the origins of the NHS but also that injuries and death in industry, while reduced, are something we still have to deal with.*

"That is why the Welsh Centre for Burns and Plastic Surgery is crucial. It is a global centre of excellence that has put Morriston on the map for world-class, cutting-edge treatment and research."

Looking to the future

Developing healthcare services

Hamish Laing, *ABMU's Medical Director, and Chief Information Officer, provides his view on how healthcare is likely to develop for the future, particularly through technological advancement*s.

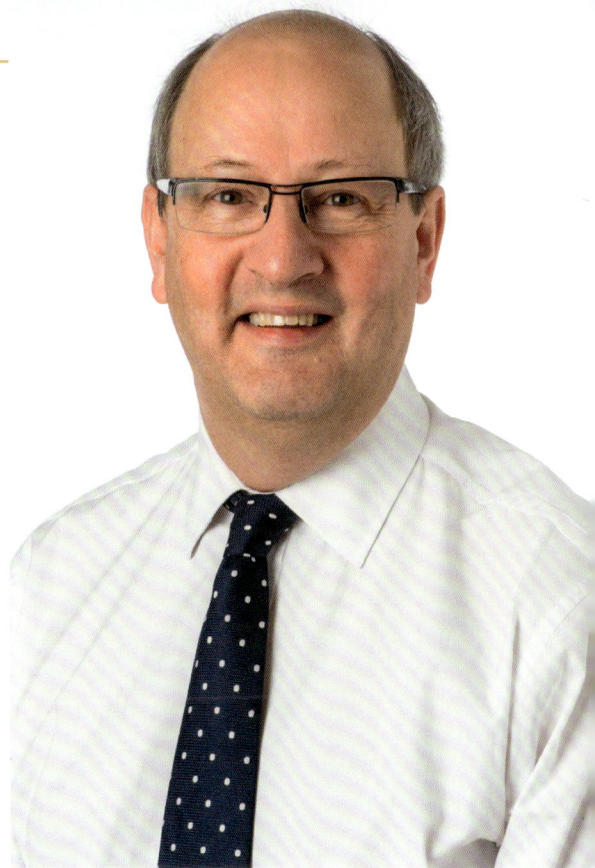

"Things have changed hugely over the 70 years since the NHS was established.

My mother was born in the Afan Valley where her father was the local GP. Her childhood memory was if someone was poorly you came to see her dad, if you were very poorly you went to hospital in Cimla and if you were really, really poorly you went to hospital in Swansea – and you never came back!

How things have changed. Now we have amazing treatments and cancer, for example, has moved from being something you were either cured of or died from to a chronic condition, something patients can live with for years.

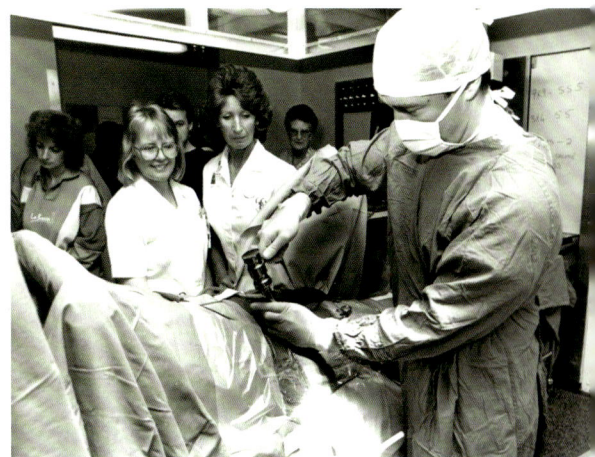

As a young surgical registrar I did a lot of operations to remove gall bladders. Patients would be left with a big scar, they would be in hospital for 10 days and would feel really rotten. Now it is almost down to being a day case procedure done by keyhole surgery, it leaves a couple of small scars and the recovery is so much better.

In every aspect of healthcare we've seen advances which have made a huge difference to patients with better outcomes and better use of resources.

But as a result we are living longer and have many more people living with not just one but several long-term chronic conditions.

Individually heart disease, lung disease, diabetes, cancer or mental health issues could all have been life-shortening, now we have people with five or six conditions alive in their 80s or 90s.

This has made healthcare much more complicated and means we have more frail people to care for. Our challenge for the future is how do we look after them well and how do we meet their needs in a more personalised way?

You can't put frailty off for ever, it will still be the case that most of the expenditure on people's health will occur in their last year of life. What we are doing at the moment is moving that last year later and later.

Dying is still going to happen, but we need to get better at helping people manage the "glide path" towards the end of life. We want to try to keep people in their own homes, in their own communities so that hospital is somewhere you only go for a short time, for something specific.

The challenge is to get healthcare and social care working together more effectively, to simplify the system and make it more efficient.

One small part of doing that involves technology. There are fantastic new technologies developing but some more straightforward advances already exist that we need to make better use of.

People are used to being able to do things online – whether it is shopping or booking tickets but healthcare isn't like that yet. We expect people to engage with us in a very old fashioned way and that makes services quite hard to access.

If you look at an NHS website you can see who the members of the board are, but probably can't get an answer to a simple question about your health. What matters to most people is 'how do I get the phone number for this?' or 'Should I call a doctor about this?'

Our approach needs to be about empowering people to care for themselves, giving them the advances they need and making it easier to find out how they can get the right help.

Patients will be able to use the Patients Know Best app to access their own information blood results and, in due course, letters appointments and discharge summaries as well as uploading data that they collect themselves. This will put them in charge of their healthcare and transform how we can help them with their condition in future.

The technology involved was just one side of it; the greatest thing has been the cultural and philosophical change surrounding the sharing of medical information with the patient.

But if you let patients know about their conditions they will be able to look after themselves better and feel in control of their lives.

In addition I am proud to say we were the first health board in Wales to provide free Wifi at our hospitals and this has been such a success.

I had a conversation with a patient on the renal dialysis unit at Morriston Hospital who was running a small business but had to spend four hours three times a week in the basement receiving his treatment. He couldn't get a phone signal, let alone internet access, and as a result was struggling to run his business. *'For about half of every week, I cannot work,'* and said he needed a phone signal. I asked: *'How about if we got you Wifi instead?'*

Now we have rolled out free Wifi at all our hospitals and can have over 10,000 concurrent users. It's allowed patients to stay connected to their businesses, their families and friends. It also allowed us to completely transform our model of mobile working for the staff and has released bandwidth on our NHS network.

For a small investment it's made a massive difference, to our efficiency but most importantly to the lives of our patients.

Technology is going to help us for the future. For example technology connected to adaptive living can provide devices which help people with cognitive impairment stay in their homes for longer.

We have devices to monitor people's conditions, implantable defibrillators that upload data across the internet to tell us that the device is working well, sensors which monitor diabetes and blood pressure, all sorts of conditions.

There have also been major advances in artificial or augmented intelligence which is developing devices that will help clinicians to do their job. Then there is personalised medicine - medication tailored to an individual patient – and gene therapy. We are very excited in ABMU to be part of the first gene therapy centre in Wales and the potential of this is huge.

Technology everywhere will help clinicians do their jobs and help patients live better, healthier lives. **"**

Modernising primary care

Dr Alastair Roeves, *ABMU's Medical Director for Primary Care and Community Services, looks at how health services on your doorstep are transforming and adapting to cope with 21st century demands*

" Becoming a doctor fulfilled my childhood ambition. Ever since I was seven and the family doctor diagnosed me with measles on a home visit, I knew that was what I wanted to do and it's a decision I have never regretted.

After qualifying in 1991 I stayed on in London where I trained, working as a GP in some of the most deprived inner city areas before swapping the capital for general practice in Newport, and venturing into management with Aneurin Bevan HB.

Now I combine my role at ABMU with time as a GP in the Afan Valley and stints in our out-of-hours service and at Swansea Prison – it's a varied career but one I still love and remain passionate about.

Every day is different and presents a new challenge and I am able to enjoy continuity of care and the chance to build relationships with my patients.

The days when patients visited the doctor's own home for consultations have certainly long gone. I recall being deeply moved as a medical student by A.J. Cronin's The Citadel, in which the main character, a GP in a pre-NHS South Wales valley, was so over worked that he would see 3 or 4 patients at a time in his consulting room as the only way to deal with the huge number of miners with chest problems.

Now we face very different challenges to those NHS pioneers – we have an aging population, living longer with a variety of chronic conditions putting more demand on our GP services but in different ways.

In addition, across the UK we are finding it more difficult to recruit new GPs to continue those hard-pressed services.

This all means we have no choice - we have to think differently to previous generations and provide our care in new ways.

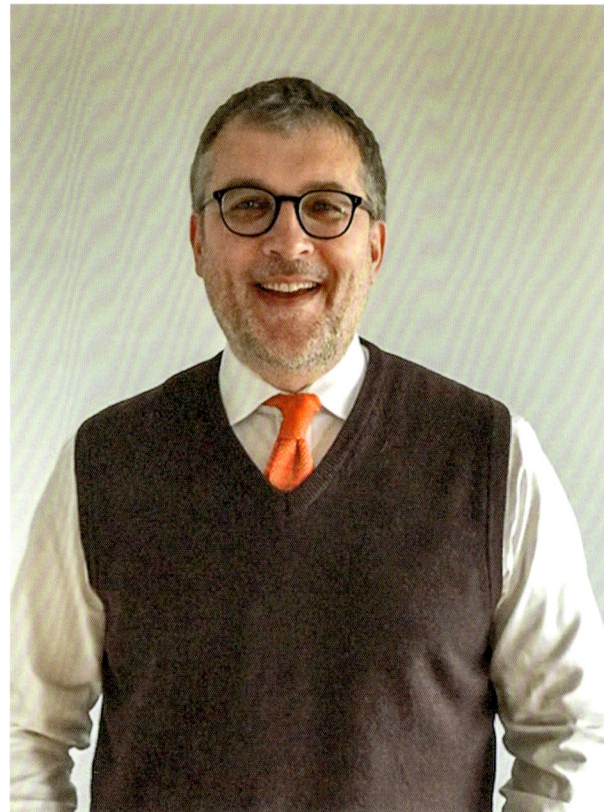

It is certainly challenging but also exciting as it opens up colleagues to different ways of working and new collaborations.

Most practices are now based in purpose-built health centres with multidisciplinary teams – allowing them to offer a one-stop shop which can mean patients no longer having to go to hospital for some appointments. Some of the beautiful new buildings that house GP teams also host social services, district nurses and specialist nurses, physiotherapists, children's centres, pharmacies, mental health and third sector.

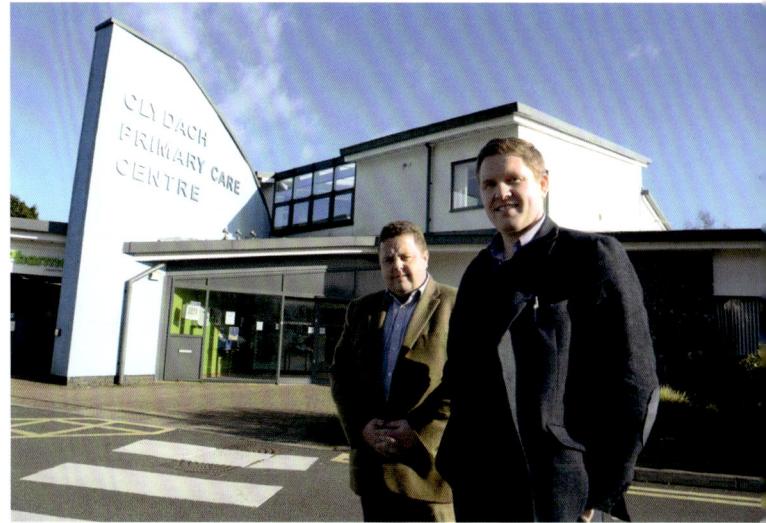

Dr Richard Tristham and Dr Iestyn Davies of Clydach Primary Care Centre

Innovative ways of working have been introduced, with many practices encouraging patients to speak on the telephone first, saving a visit to the surgery. In the early seventies, when I had measles, homes visits formed over 30 per cent of all GP consultations, now less than 5 per cent. Patients often get text reminders for appointments and practices have websites.

GP practices have also formed local clusters of practices, community nurses, therapists, local authority social services and third sector, so they can deliver sustainable services and better access. Practices are generally much larger, and some smaller practices have formed formal federations to help them deliver a wider range of services for patients to reduce the need to travel to hospital and make their own practices more sustainable.

The way people access GP services when their own surgery has closed overnight, at weekends and on bank holidays has also evolved.

We provide a GP out-of-hours service across Bridgend, Neath-Port Talbot and Swansea. This is very different from when I started; I had to cover my own practice patients at night and at weekends, and still work the next day.

If I needed to admit a patient to hospital from their home and the patient had no landline, I would have to knock on the doors of neighbours and ask to use their phone.

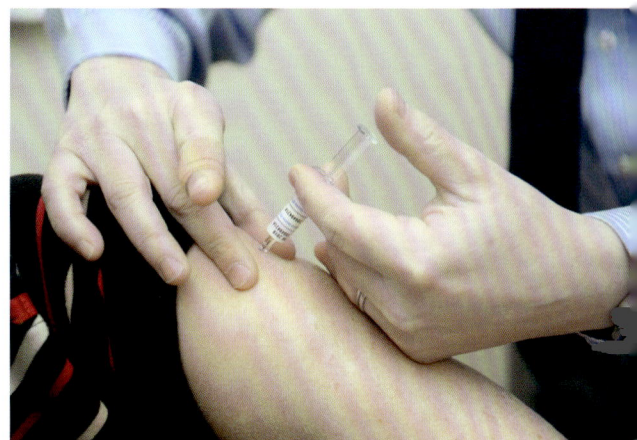

A patient receives their flu jab from a pharmacist

In 2016, this service was brought together with NHS Direct Wales, which provides urgent healthcare support and advice. Instead of having to call separate numbers to access each, anyone registered with a GP practice in the ABMU area can simply dial 111.

Before coming to ABMU I was Primary Care Clinical Director with Aneurin Bevan HB, the organisation that bears the name of the architect of the NHS. It was a daily reminder of the NHS's heritage and its ambition.

Being a GP is a privilege – to share our patients' lives, helping them through highs and lows is just as satisfying now as it was in 1948.

And while our surroundings, the equipment we use and medicine we prescribe may be very different today, the priority remains the same after 70 years – doing the best we can for our patients. *"*

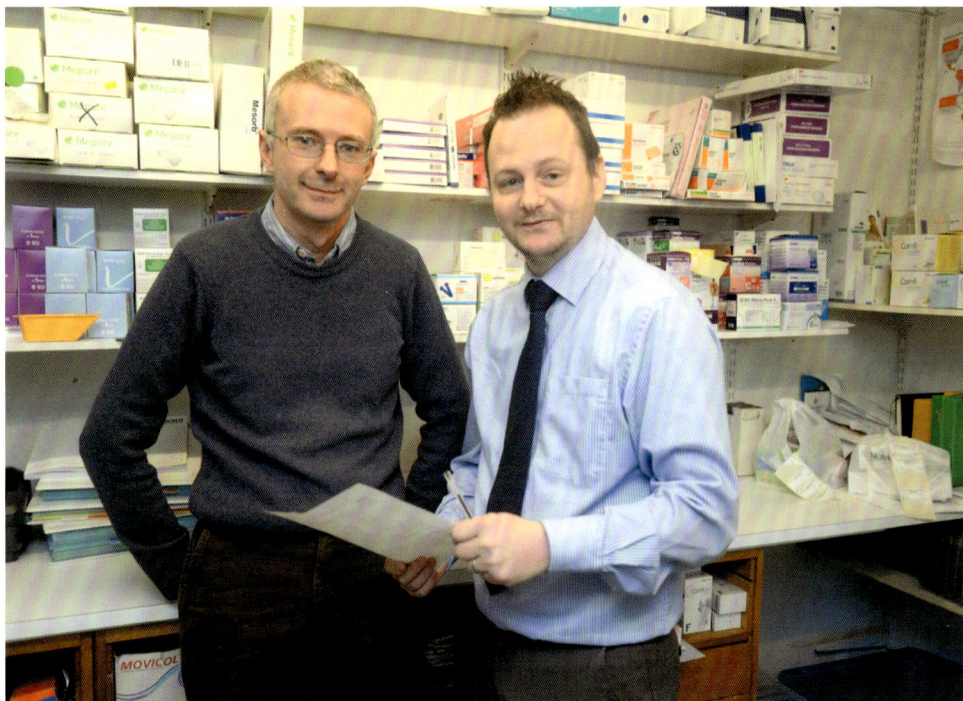

Dr Steve Harrowing (left) of the Vale of Neath GP practice with pharmacist Niki Watts of Dr Cecil Jones pharmacy, Glyneath

Advances in cardiac surgery

'It's a privilege to hold a person's heart in your hand . . .'

Consultant cardiothoracic surgeon **Professor Farah Bhatti** not only treats patients at Morriston Hospital's Cardiac Centre, she also teaches at Swansea University Medical School and is dedicated to encouraging and raising the profile of women in surgery.

During her distinguished career she has witnessed many life-changing developments and feels we owe a huge debt of gratitude to the NHS that has made them possible.

"It is hard for us to imagine that prior to 1948, if you could not afford medical treatment, you were simply left to suffer (and possibly die) from treatable conditions; we have much to be grateful for in the NHS.

"It is also remarkable how many technological and medical advances have occurred over the last 70 years. In my field, stopping and operating on the heart was simply inconceivable at the dawn of the NHS, the heart-lung machine not having been invented until the 1950s."

Prof Bhatti says that coronary artery surgery and heart valve replacements pioneered in the 1960s are now routine - though complex - procedures which can give people with angina and breathlessness a new lease of life.

"Advances in cardiac surgery include transplantation, minimal access surgery and robotic surgery, to name but a few. The development of artificial hearts is also being pursued right here at Swansea University by CalonCardio. The outlook for our future patients is bright!"

It was her passion for helping people in a practical way that made her determined to become a cardiac surgeon.

"The thought of helping patients with heart disease, and as importantly for me, to keep families intact, was the driving factor in my choice of career. "When I embarked on my medical training at Oxford University and then Cambridge, I knew surgery would not be an easy career to pursue, but I had no doubt that that is exactly what I would do.

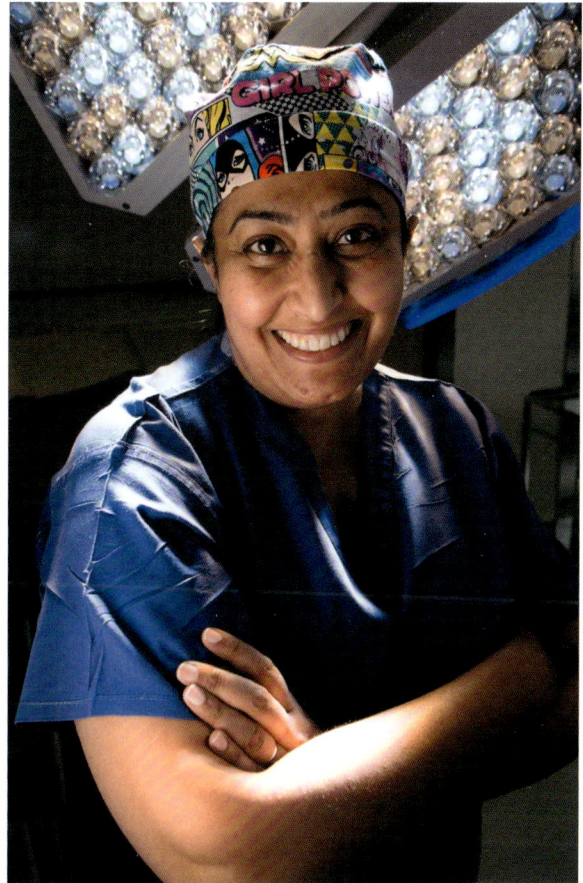

"I also had no idea that there were so very few women consultant surgeons in the UK (and none in cardiothoracic surgery) although again, it would not have deterred me had I known!"

Her training saw her going to the world famous Texas Heart Institute, as well as spending time at The Royal Brompton, Harefield and Papworth hospitals.

When she moved to Swansea in 2007 she was the first woman consultant cardiothoracic surgeon to be appointed in Wales and only the fourth in the UK.

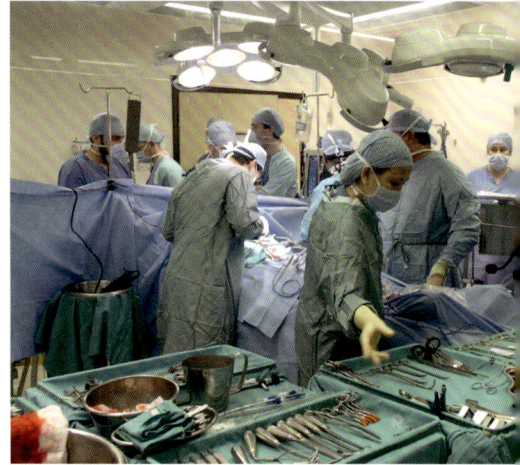

"Ten years on I'm proud to have served my patients from right across South West Wales, as well as help to educate the next generation of doctors at Swansea University Medical School.

"Of course, you are only as good as the team around you, and the staff I work with are some of the most dedicated and hard-working people I know."

Prof Bhatti's role as Director of Equality and Diversity for Graduate Entry Medicine at the medical school means she is particularly passionate about encouraging students to further their education, whatever their background.

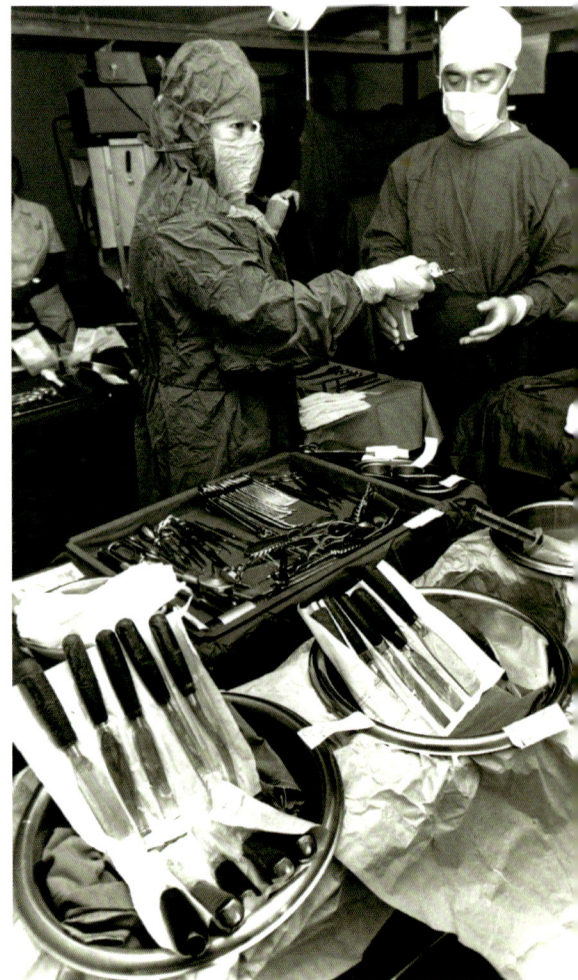

"I'm pleased to report that over the past two decades, the percentage of consultant surgeons in the UK who are women has increased from a tiny 3 per cent in 1991 to 12 per cent in 2016.

"As Chair of the Women in Surgery forum at the Royal College of Surgeons of England, I work towards encouraging and inspiring people from different backgrounds to consider a surgical career.

"I would like to say that it is a privilege to hold a person's heart in your hand and be able to 'fix it' - so thanks to my family for getting me here and to my patients for allowing me do what is one of the most rewarding jobs in the world! Diolch."

ABMyouth

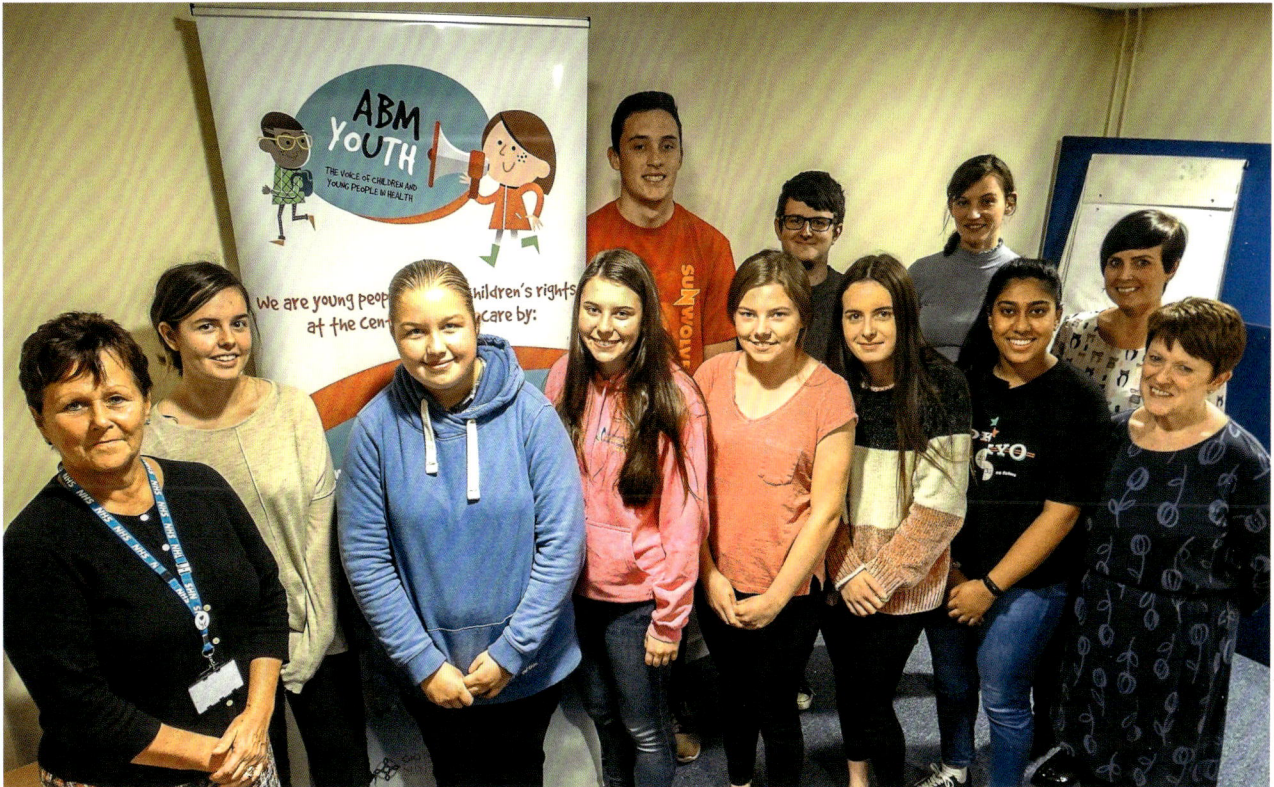

Members of ABMyouth with (left) paediatric patient experience nurse Janette Williams, project coordinator for the Children's Rights Unit Jannine Smith (second right) and head of nursing, women and child health Eirlys Thomas.

One of the innovations Aneurin Bevan could never have imagined is a dedicated group of young people speaking up for youngsters and their health care needs.

ABMyouth is the first youth health advisory panel in Wales and its members, aged between 13 and 23, are all passionate about shaping services for children and young people.

The groundbreaking group dedicated to improving health care for youngsters across South Wales is hard at work helping to make a difference

Supported by ABMU Health Board and Neath Port Talbot Children's Rights Unit, the 20-strong panel was set up to give young people a voice about things that affect them

Chair Sophie Millar, a 23-year-old medical student, said: *"We love being part of an evolving NHS that listens to children and young people and respects their human rights"*

"At ABMyouth we project children and young people's thoughts on the health issues that matter most and make sure they are heard by the professionals who can make a difference"

171

"We are incredibly proud to play a part in shaping health services in Wales for future generations."

The panel aims to highlight different issues and provide valuable feedback to health leaders from a young persons' perspective.

ABMyouth was originally launched in March 2017 at the same time as the health board's pioneering Children's Rights Charter which sets out the basic rights children and young people can expect when they use health services.

Since then it has gone on to win the Health, Social Care and Wellbeing Category at this year's Third Sector Awards Cymru.

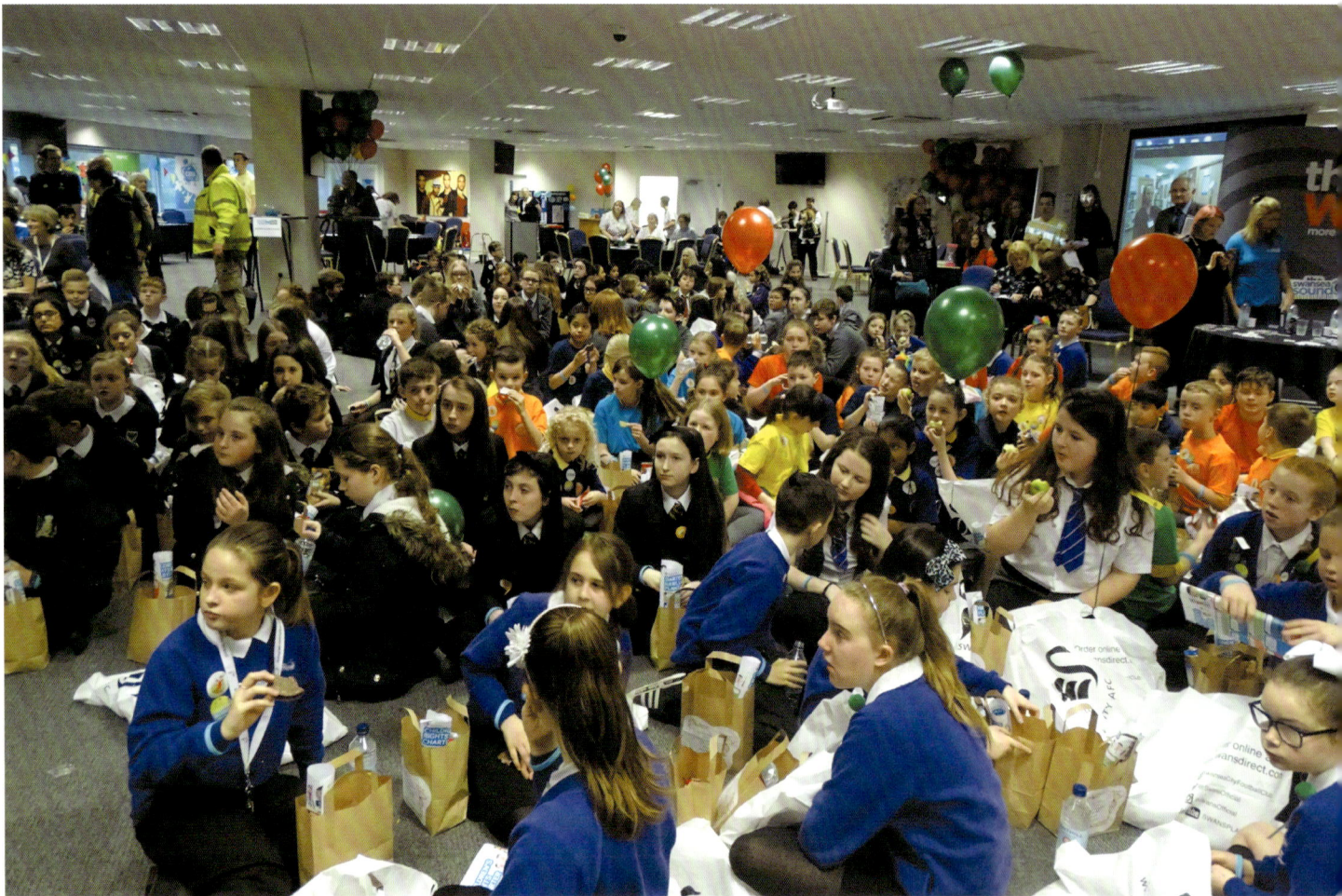

Hundreds of youngsters from local schools attended the launch of the Children's Rights Charter in Swansea

Promoting the rights of older people

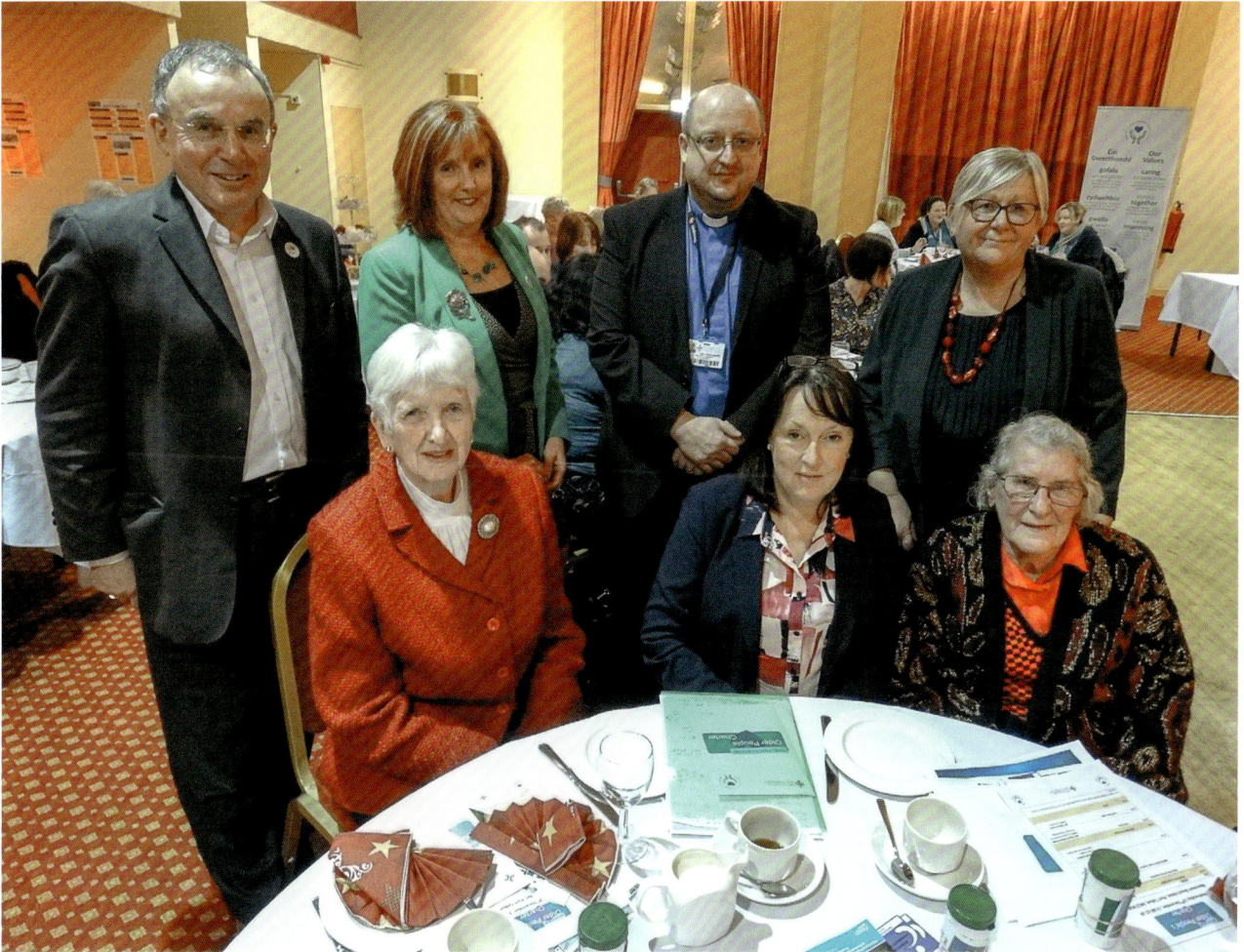

Chairman Prof Andrew Davies, Assistant Director of Strategy Joanne Abbott-Davies, Head of Chaplaincy and Spiritual Care the Rev Lance Sharpe and Director of Therapies and Health Science Christine Morrell with (front) Catherine Coombs, of Swansea Over-50s Forum, Older People's Commissioner for Wales Sarah Rochira and guest Kay Coleman.

ABMU is the first health board in Wales to introduce an initiative to promote and protect the rights of older people across South West Wales.

It has created its own Older People's Charter, developed following close consultation with people living in Swansea, Neath Port Talbot and Bridgend.

The health board's Director of Therapies and Health Science Christine Morrell said: *"We want to transform our perception of older people and shine a spotlight on the importance of their wellbeing as well as their health.*

"Older people are the largest users of our services so it is very important for us to develop this charter. It is something we're very proud of, especially as we have been guided by the public and what they want."

A series of engagement events were held last year giving third sector groups, carers and the public a say what was important to them – and nearly 600 older people and those who work with them took the opportunity. This was then further developed through discussions with staff.

Christine added: *"All older people possess the same lifelong rights as any other adult in Wales. We sometimes need to be reminded of these rights and that is the purpose of both the Declaration and our Older Persons Charter."*

ABMU Chairman Andrew Davies said: *"We know the average age of our patients is increasing and we are caring for more frail and elderly people. That is why we need to focus on older people's needs as reflected in our new Charter. "*

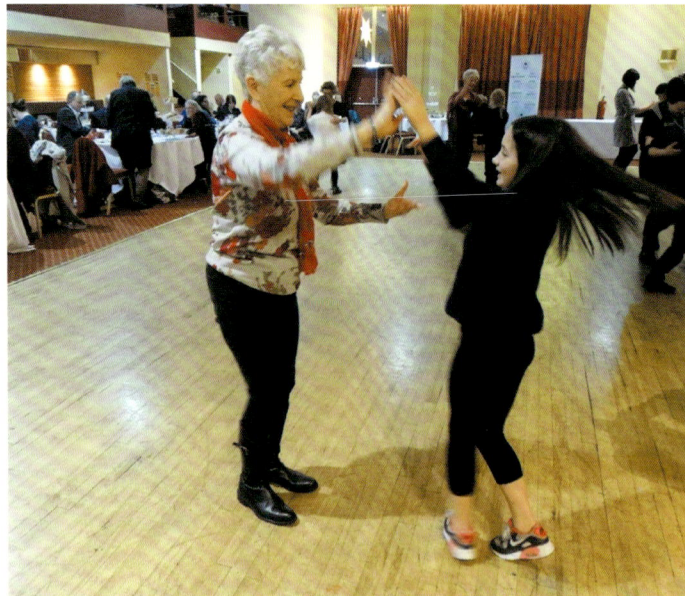

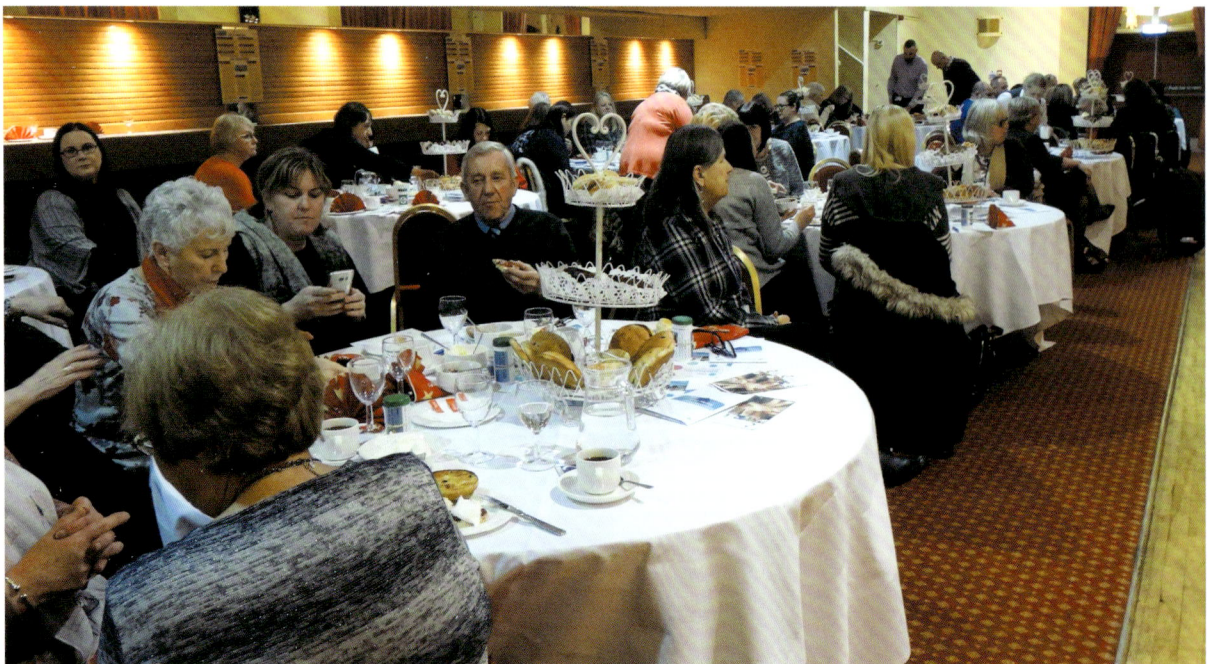

A tea dance brought the generations together following the formal Charter launch (top); and some of the guests at the launch event.

Celebrating health staff diversity

One area which has seen great strides over recent years is the celebration of diversity among health staff.

Calon, ABMU's LGBT+ & Allies *(right)* staff network, was established in 2016 and since then has gone from strength to strength promoting inclusion and diversity within the health board.

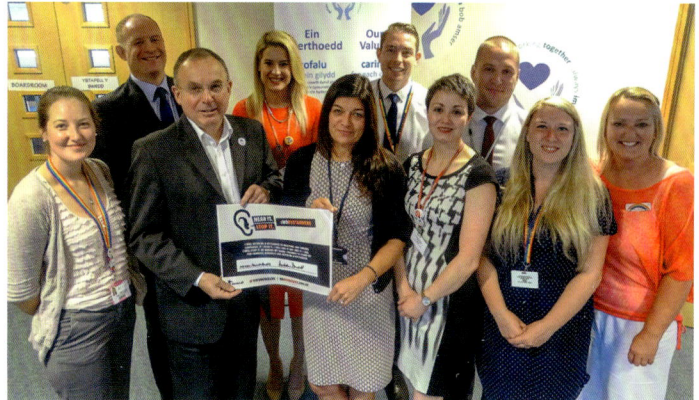

The health board is now a member of Stonewall's Diversity Champion programme and is moving steadily up the campaigning group's Workplace Equality Index.

Calon members, joined by friends and supporters also march at Pride Cymru, one of Wales's largest celebrations of diversity also hold regular events around the health board.

Founder members Mitchell Jones, Emma Walters and Matthew Haynes went on to win the Going the Extra mile category at ABMU's 2016 Chairman's Awards.

Emma and Mitchell said:

"We are so pleased that the health board has appreciated the importance of the network which is aimed at encouraging and supporting every staff member to bring their whole self to work.

"We at Calon are very proud to be part of an organisation that promotes equality and celebrates diversity in such a positive way, be it by marching at Pride, embracing the No Bystanders campaign, or joining Stonewall's Diversity Champion programme.

"When looking back on the 70th anniversary of the NHS, we realise how far we have come not just as an organisation, but as a society.

"ABMU is now a more inclusive organisation than it ever has been before, and it is comforting to know that with its commitment to living the values, it will continue to diversify, develop and become an even more inclusive organisation over the next 70 years."

ARCH — a unique collaboration

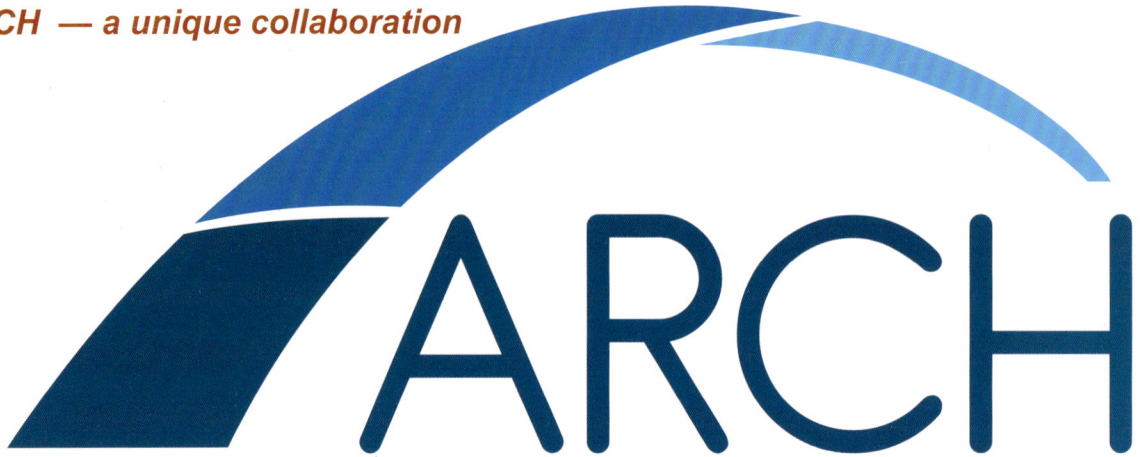

ARCH (A Regional Collaboration for Health) is a unique collaboration project between the three partners of ABMU Health Board, Hywel Dda University Health Board and Swansea University.

It spans six local authority areas of Ceredigion, Pembrokeshire, Carmarthenshire, Bridgend, Neath Port Talbot and Swansea and has three key aims:

- **To create a healthcare system fit for the 21st century;**

- **To drive investment and create jobs to boost economy of South West Wales; and**

- **To skill up the next generation of clinicians, researchers, academics, innovators and leaders.**

The partnership has already started to develop leading healthcare innovation which will benefit the entire population of the South West Wales region.

It focuses on keeping people healthy and better managing disease when they are ill. ARCH is bringing together industry, innovation, academic research and all health sectors to not only improve health and healthcare in South West Wales, but to drive inward investment and in turn boost the local economy.

ARCH Chairman Andrew Davies, who is also Chairman of ABMU, said:

"Nothing of this scale or complexity has been attempted in Wales before. Given the size of the ARCH ambition, the progress we are making is testament to the relationships built up between the three partners.

"I look forward to our continued work within ARCH which will establish this region as a world-leader in innovation, research, skills and healthcare."